Endobronchial Ultrasonography

Endobronchial Ultrasonography

Second Edition

Noriaki Kurimoto, MD, PhD
Department of Internal Medicine
Division of Medical Oncology and Respiratory Medicine
Shimane University Faculty of Medicine
Izumo, Japan

David I.K. Fielding, MD
Royal Brisbane and Women's Hospital
Herston, Queensland, Australia

Ali I. Musani, MD, FCCP
Division of Pulmonary Sciences & Critical Care Medicine
University of Colorado School of Medicine
Denver, CO, USA

Christopher Kniese, MD
Indiana University School of Medicine
Indianapolis, IN, USA

Katsuhiko Morita, MD, PhD
Department of Thoracic Surgery
Japan Community Health Care Organization (JCHO)
Shimonoseki Medical Center
Shimonoseki City, Yamaguchi Prefecture, Japan

Shimane University
Izumo City, Shimane Prefecture, Japan

WILEY Blackwell

This edition first published 2020

Registered Office(s)
John Wiley & Sons, Inc., 111 River Street, Hoboken, NJ 07030, USA
John Wiley & Sons Ltd, The Atrium, Southern Gate, Chichester, West Sussex, PO19 8SQ, UK

Editorial Office
9600 Garsington Road, Oxford, OX4 2DQ, UK

For details of our global editorial offices, customer services, and more information about Wiley products visit us at www.wiley.com.

Wiley also publishes its books in a variety of electronic formats and by print-on-demand. Some content that appears in standard print versions of this book may not be available in other formats.

Library of Congress Cataloging-in-Publication Data

Names: Kurimoto, Noriaki, editor. | I.K. Fielding, David, editor. | Musani, Ali I. editor | Kniese, Christopher, editor. | Morita, Katsuhiko, editor.
Title: Endobronchial ultrasonography / edited by Noriaki Kurimoto, St. Marianna University, School of Medicine, Division of Chest Surgery, Kawasaki City, Japan [and four others].
Description: Second edition. | Hoboken, NJ : Wiley-Blackwell, 2020. | Revision of: Endobronchial ultrasonography / Noriaki Kurimoto, David I.K. Fielding, Ali I. Musani, Christopher Kniese, Katsuhiko Morita | Includes bibliographical references and index.
Identifiers: LCCN 2019053505 (print) | LCCN 2019053506 (ebook) | ISBN 9781119233947 (cloth) | ISBN 9781119233930 (adobe pdf) | ISBN 9781119233954 (epub)
Subjects: LCSH: Bronchi–Cancer–Ultrasonic imaging. | Endoscopic ultrasonography. | Bronchi–Ultrasonic imaging.
Classification: LCC RC280.B9 K87 2020 (print) | LCC RC280.B9 (ebook) | DDC 616.99/423–dc23
LC record available at https://lccn.loc.gov/2019053505
LC ebook record available at https://lccn.loc.gov/2019053506

Cover Design: Wiley
Cover Image: © Life science/Shutterstock

Set in 9.5/12.5pt STIXTwoText by SPi Global, Pondicherry, India

10 9 8 7 6 5 4 3 2 1

Contents

Foreword

Seven years have passed since the first edition of *Endobronchial Ultrasonography* was published in 2011. During those seven years, endobronchial ultrasound-guided transbronchial needle aspiration (EBUS-TBNA) has become widespread throughout the world, and radial EBUS for peripheral pulmonary lesions has also shown signs of spreading.

Among a range of subjects, this second edition describes in detail the progress of EBUS-TBNA, outlines a method for determining the route of the bronchus reaching the peripheral pulmonary lesion, and explains the procedure for using EBUS with a guide sheath for peripheral pulmonary lesions. In addition, videos are available to help readers learn the practical aspects of EBUS techniques. Our authors, who are all highly experienced in using EBUS, provide detailed tips on the procedures they perform. I hope you will find the useful tips on EBUS procedures in each chapter.

There have also been remarkable advances in EBUS equipment and new functions. This book evaluates these advances as they are at present and considers how they will develop with diffusion and interpretation in the future. The general advantages of using EBUS for ultrasonic examination of the bronchial lumen have increased. An important issue is how to maximize the benefits of EBUS as it develops.

Finally, we would like to thank Yogalakshmi Mohanakrishnan and Kimiyoshi Ishibashi of Wiley-Blackwell, who put in a great deal of effort during the publication process.

Noriaki Kurimoto, MD, PhD

About the Companion Website

Endobronchial Ultrasonography, 2nd edition is accompanied by a companion website:

www.wiley.com/go/kurimoto2e

The videos are available to help readers learn the practical aspects of EBUS techniques.

1

Endobronchial Ultrasonography: An Overview

Noriaki Kurimoto

Department of Internal Medicine, Division of Medical Oncology and Respiratory Medicine, Shimane University Faculty of Medicine, Izumo, Japan

Introduction

Endobronchial ultrasonography (EBUS) is a diagnostic modality whereby a miniature ultrasonic probe is introduced into the bronchial (tracheal) lumen, providing tomographic images of the peribronchial (peritracheal) tissue. Endoscopic ultrasonography (EUS) is an established, indispensable technique for examining the gastrointestinal tract, particularly the stomach and large intestine. The applications of EUS include assessment of the depth of tumor invasion, detection of lymph node metastases, tumor staging, and fine-needle aspiration (FNA) under EUS guidance.

In 1988, Pandian et al. [1] were the first to report the clinical use of a narrow-gauge ultrasonic probe for intravascular ultrasonography. In 1990, EBUS was first mentioned in the study by Hürter et al. on EBUS of the lung and mediastinum. Since then, research and development in this field have been primarily conducted by Becker (Germany) and us (Japan).

Typically, radial EBUS probes are of the 20 MHz radial type. Therefore, tissue penetration of the ultrasound waves is of the order of approximately 2–3 cm; in other words, EBUS provides a tissue cross-section image with a radius of approximately 2–3 cm centered on the trachea or bronchus.

Some important EBUS studies are:

- Hürter and Hanarath [2]. Endobronchial sonography in the diagnosis of pulmonary and mediastinal tumors (in German).
- Iizuka et al. [3]: Evaluation of airway smooth muscle contractions in vitro by high-frequency ultrasonic imaging.
- Ono et al. [4]: Bronchoscopic ultrasonography in the diagnosis of lung cancer.
- Goldberg et al. [5]: US-assisted bronchoscopy with use of miniature transducer-containing catheters (delineation of central and peripheral pulmonary lesions).
- Becker [6]: EBUS – a new perspective in bronchology (tracheobronchial wall seven-layer structure).
- Kurimoto et al. [7]: Assessment of usefulness of EBUS in determination of depth of tracheobronchial tumor invasion (tracheobronchial wall five-layer structure).

Based on these studies, the current applications of EBUS are as follows:

- Determination of the depth of tumor invasion of the tracheal/bronchial wall (allocation of patients to localized endobronchial treatments such as photodynamic therapy).

Endobronchial Ultrasonography, Second Edition. Noriaki Kurimoto, David I.K. Fielding, Ali I. Musani, Christopher Kniese, and Katsuhiko Morita.

Companion website: www.wiley.com/go/kurimoto2e

- Identification of the location of a peripheral lung lesion during bronchoscopic examination (more accurate than fluoroscopy in determining contact between lesion and bronchus, thereby reducing abrasions, the time to determine biopsy sites, and duration of fluoroscopy).
- Qualitative diagnosis of peripheral lung lesions and differentiation between benign and malignant lesions.
- Determination of position and shape of peribronchial structures, particularly lymph nodes (at the time of transbronchial needle aspiration).
- Determination of the spatial relationship between bronchus and lesion in the short-axial image of the bronchus (if the bronchus is situated near the center of the lesion, the lesion might have arisen from the bronchus).

Issues arising from the application of EBUS to date and the results of studies include the following:

- Standardization of how the layers in the tracheobronchial wall structure are interpreted (how many layers are seen).
- Changes in the layer structure of the tracheobronchial wall with the use of higher frequencies (e.g. 30 MHz).
- Evaluation of the qualitative diagnosis accuracy and differentiation between benign and malignant lesions from EBUS images of peripheral lung lesions.
- Evaluation of peribronchial lymph node metastases.
- Complications of EBUS-guided transbronchial needle aspiration (TBNA).
- Technique of needle aspiration from the esophagus using the convex bronchoscope.

EBUS facilitates examining the state of the bronchial wall and extramural tissue that cannot be visualized with bronchoscopy alone. This book will present an overview of EBUS with reference to actual clinical cases.

Principles of Ultrasonography

What Is a Sound Wave?

Definition of Ultrasound

Typically, ultrasound refers to sound wavelengths >20 MHz that cannot be heard by the human ear. Because considerable variations exist in the range of frequencies audible to humans, we often define sounds in terms of their purpose. In this case, ultrasound is "sound not intended for humans to hear."

Frequency and Wavelength

The frequency of a sound tells us whether it is high or low in pitch. The unit of frequency is hertz (Hz), defined as the number of oscillations per second. For example, a sound with a frequency of 20 MHz has 20×10^6 oscillations per second. Medical ultrasonography equipment produces sounds with a frequency range of 2–50 MHz. Wavelength is the length of a soundwave, and it varies inversely with frequency; thus, the higher the frequency, the shorter is the wavelength (Figure 1.1).

Speed of Sound

Sound travels through various materials, such as air and water (hereafter media), and the speed at which it travels through each medium is the speed of sound for that medium. The speed of sound through the human body is generally considered to be 1530 m/s, although the actual speed of passage varies for different organs and tissues.

Production of Ultrasound Images

Transmitting and Receiving Ultrasound Waves

Ultrasonic probes used in medical ultrasonography comprise a sensor that transforms electrical signals into ultrasound and vice versa. When an electrical signal is applied to an electrode of an ultrasonic transducer (also known

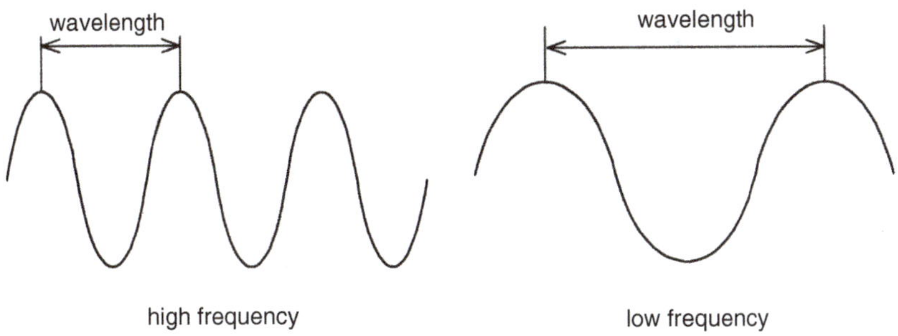

Figure 1.1 Correlation between frequency and wavelength.

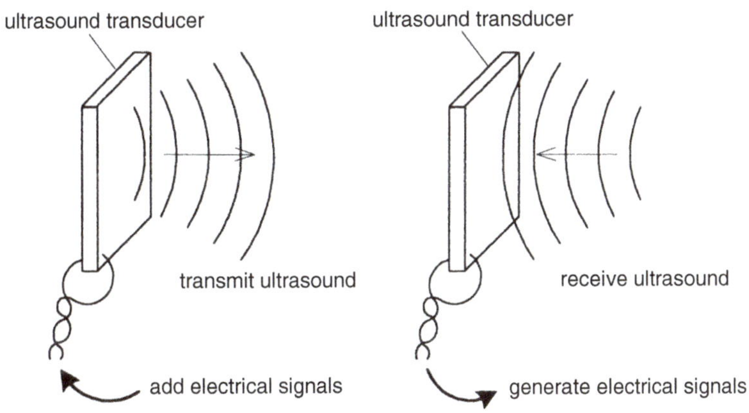

Figure 1.2 Transmitting and receiving ultrasound waves.

as an oscillator/transformer), ultrasound waves are transmitted from the device surface; when ultrasound waves are received by the device surface, an electrical signal is generated (Figure 1.2).

Propagation and Attenuation of Ultrasound Waves

Ultrasound waves produced by an ultrasonic transducer travel through a medium – called propagation. As the soundwave is propagated, the energy of its oscillations is absorbed and scattered, thereby weakening steadily; this phenomenon is called attenuation. Typically, the higher the frequency, the higher is the attenuation rate. Medical ultrasonography equipment uses high frequencies that do not propagate well through the air owing to the high attenuation ratio. Hence, a medium such as water is required between the ultrasonic transducer and the study object to allow the efficient propagation of ultrasound waves.

Reflection and Penetration

As with light, a proportion of ultrasound waves is reflected at the boundary between different media, and a proportion penetrates the boundary; the ultrasonic processor uses these reflections to construct images.

The ultrasonic transducer emits ultrasound pulses and receives ultrasound pulses reflected from the boundaries between media (Figure 1.3). In addition, the ultrasonic processor evaluates the positions (distance from the probe) of boundaries between media based on the time between transmitting and receiving ultrasound pulses and converts the strength of returning pulses into the brightness of the image.

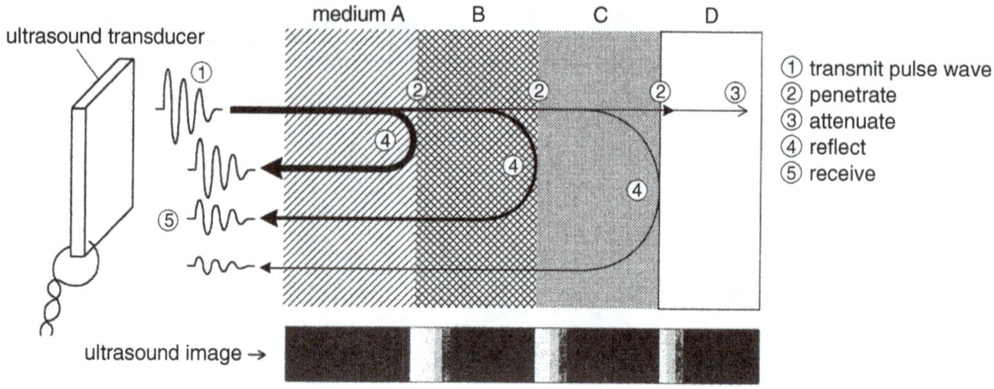

Figure 1.3 How an ultrasound image is made.

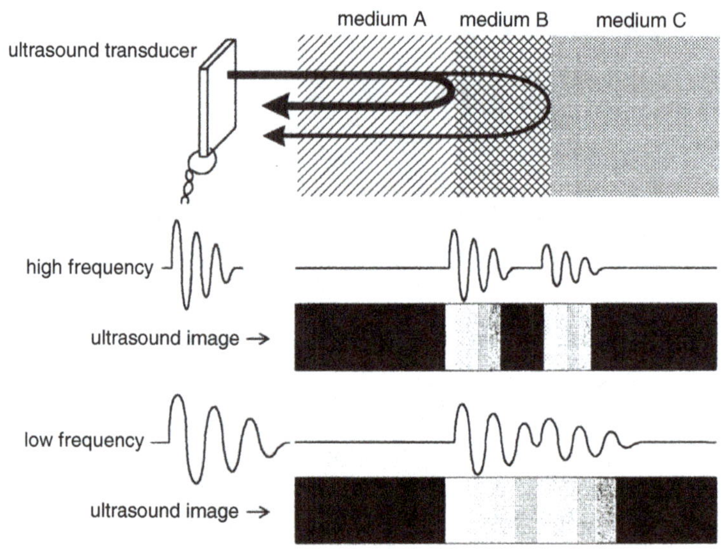

Figure 1.4 Difference in axial resolution between different frequencies.

Following these steps alone offers information about a body along a single line; thus, we obtain a two-dimensional image by moving the ultrasonic transducer (mechanical scanning) or using a linear array of multiple ultrasonic transducers that sequentially emit and receive ultrasound pulses (electronic scanning). This method of ultrasound imaging is called B-mode (B stands for brightness).

Resolution

Axial Resolution

Because an ultrasound pulse wave has a definite length, the boundary between media has a definite width on an ultrasound image. If the distance between the two boundaries of a medium is decreased, the pulse waves from the two boundaries will overlap, making it difficult to distinguish the two boundaries on the ultrasound image. The ability to distinguish objects on an ultrasound image is called resolution, and the resolution in the direction traveled by the ultrasound pulse is the axial resolution. Typically, higher the frequency, shorter is the ultrasound pulse; thus, distance resolution improves with higher frequencies (Figure 1.4).

Lateral Resolution

Resolution in the direction perpendicular to the direction traveled by the ultrasound pulse, in other words in the direction the probe moves

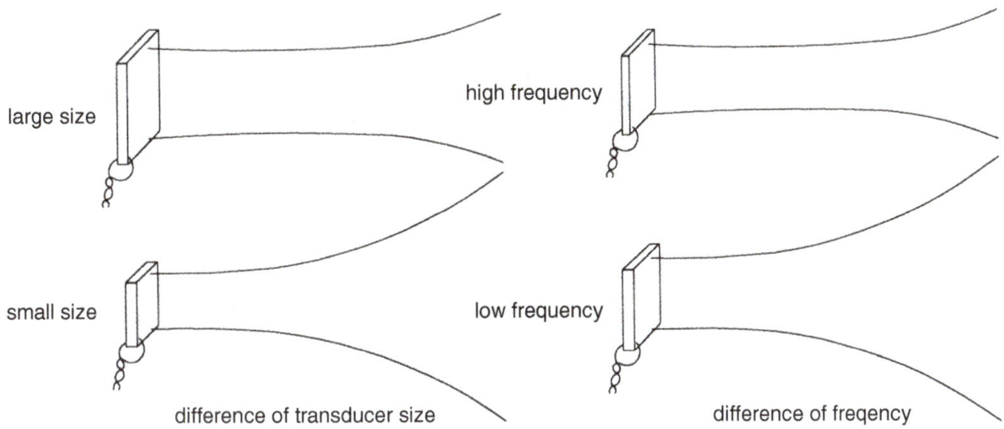

Figure 1.5 Pulse wave spreading.

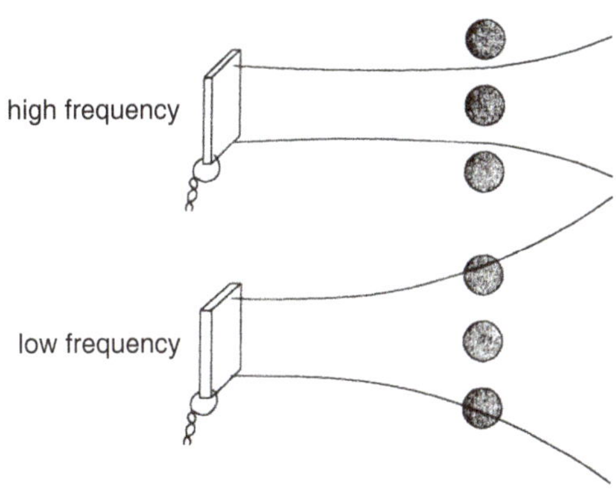

Figure 1.6 Lateral resolution.

or the direction of the array of transducers, is called lateral resolution. The ultrasound pulse wave emitted by a transducer gradually spreads out as it propagates through a medium. The degree of spreading depends on the transducer size (aperture area) and frequency. As the transducer size or frequency increases, the degree of spreading decreases (Figure 1.5). Lateral resolution improves with decreased spread (Figure 1.6).

Depth Penetration

Because ultrasound waves attenuate as they propagate through a medium, they can only reach a certain distance. Hence, ultrasound images can only be attained for a certain distance from the ultrasonic probe; this distance is called the depth penetration (or penetration). In addition, the depth penetration depends on the frequency and transducer size (aperture area). Because the attenuation rate of an ultrasound wave increases as its frequency increases, the depth penetration improves as the frequency decreases (Figure 1.7). As the aperture area of the ultrasonic transducer increases, it can emit a stronger pulse and can also convert weaker received pulses into electrical signals. Hence, the depth penetration increases as the transducer size increases.

Image Quality Adjustment

Despite using an ultrasonic probe appropriate to the task, its abilities cannot be completely harnessed unless appropriate image quality adjustment is performed. The fundamentals of image quality adjustment are gain, contrast, and sensitivity time control (STC).

Gain

Gain, also called brightness, is the mechanism for adjusting the overall brightness of an ultrasound image. Adjustment of the gain evenly increases or decreases the entire ultrasound signal (the signal from the ultrasonic transducer converted for display on the monitor). Changes in the gain make the entire image brighter or darker, but do not alter the differences in brightness between light and dark sections of the image (Figure 1.8).

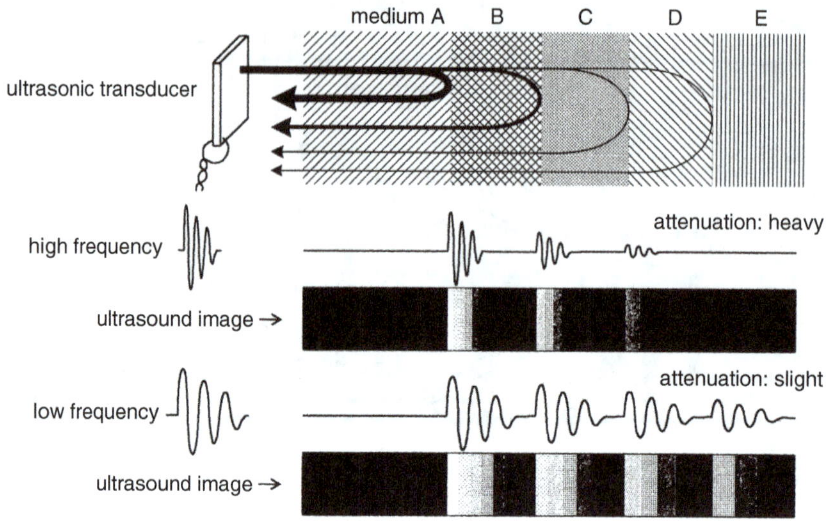

Figure 1.7 Differences in depth penetration at different frequencies.

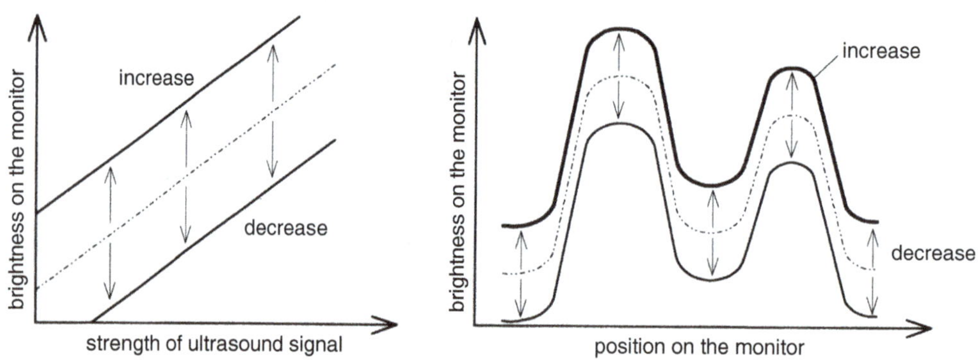

Figure 1.8 Adjustment of gain (brightness).

Contrast

Contrast is the mechanism for adjusting the difference in brightness between light and dark sections of an image. Adjustment of the contrast makes the most significant changes in the sections of an image with the strongest ultrasound signal; in other words, changing the contrast primarily alters the brightness of the lighter sections of an image, and the darker sections are changed only relatively little. Increasing the contrast of an ultrasound image yields an image with enhanced differences between light and dark areas, whereas decreasing the contrast yields an image with minimal differences between light and dark areas (Figure 1.9).

Sensitivity Time Control

STC, also known as time gain compensation, is the mechanism for adjusting the gain according to the distance (depth) from the ultrasonic probe. As shown in Figure 1.7, attenuation of the ultrasound wave increases with the distance from the probe; thus, ultrasound signals from distant (deep) regions are weaker than those from near (shallow) regions. To correct this and make the overall image as even as possible, the ultrasonic processor amplifies the

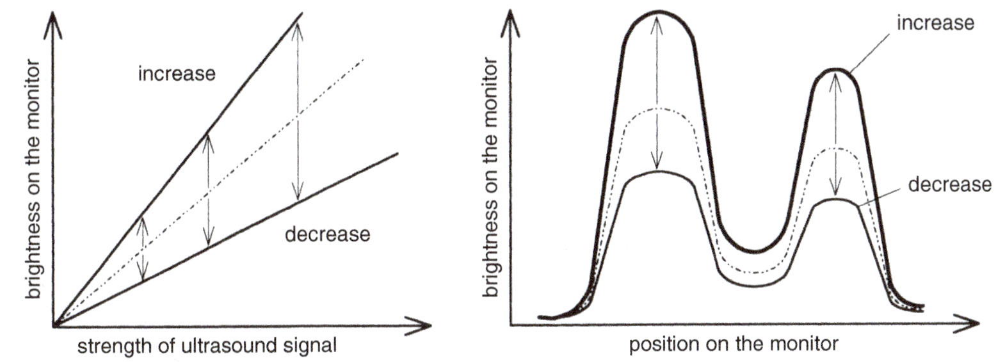

Figure 1.9 Adjustment of contrast.

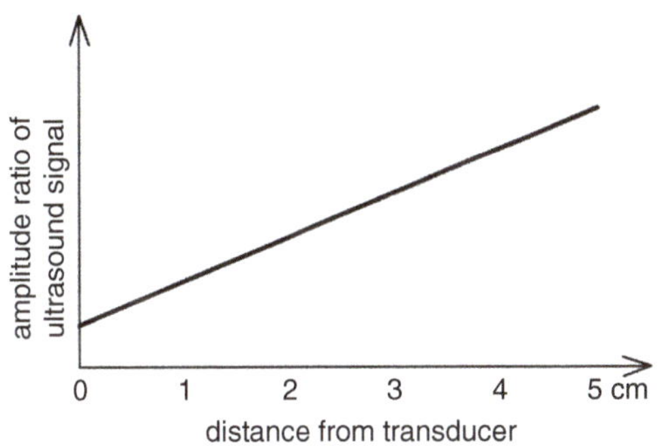

Figure 1.10 Sensitivity time control default settings.

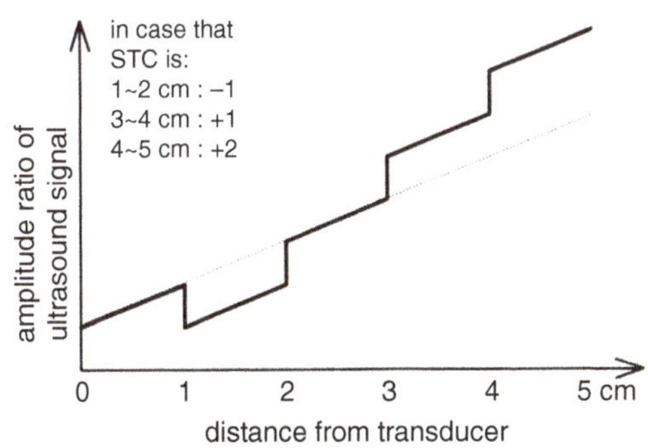

Figure 1.11 Adjustment of sensitivity time control (STC).

ultrasound signal based on the current distance from the probe (the time for the ultrasound pulse to return to the transducer; Figure 1.10). By altering the degree of amplification, adjustment of STC can make the ultrasound image lighter or darker based on the distance from the probe (Figure 1.11).

Equipment

Endoscopic Ultrasonic Probe

This section introduces the equipment (manufactured by Olympus Corporation, Tokyo, Japan) used by the author.

Table 1.1 shows the frequencies and outer diameters of the endoscopic ultrasonic probes used. Because the resolution and depth penetration of an ultrasonic probe depend on the frequency and size of the transducer (as the outer diameter of the probe increases, the size of the ultrasonic transducer increases), the probe needs to be selected to suit the aim of the procedure.

Ultrasound examinations can be performed using either the balloon (the probe contacts the study object through a balloon filled with a medium) or the direct contact method (the probe makes direct contact with the study object). The method is usually selected according to whether the study object is centrally or peripherally situated, and probe selection is also made according to the region being examined.

With the balloon method, the UM-BS20-26R ultrasonic probe (which can be inserted in a bronchoscope instrument channel with a diameter of at least 2.8 mm) is generally used (Figure 1.12). Other probes can also be used in the balloon method in combination with the

Table 1.1 Ultrasonic probes.

Model name	Maximum outer diameter	Frequency	Compatible biopsy channel
UM-2R	2.5 mm	12 MHz	2.8 mm or more
UM-3R	2.5 mm	20 MHz	2.8 mm or more
UM-4R	2.4 mm (2.0 mm at proximal side)	20 MHz	2.6 mm or more
UM-S20-20R	1.7 mm (2.0 mm at proximal side)	20 MHz	2.2 mm or more
	2.55 mm (incl. guide sheath SG-201C)		2.6 mm or more
UM-S30-20R	1.7 mm (2.0 mm at proximal side)	30 MHz	2.2 mm or more
	2.55 mm (incl. guide sheath SG-201C)		2.6 mm or more
UM-S30-25R	2.5 mm	30 MHz	2.8 mm or more
UM-BS20-26R	2.6 mm (incl. balloon sheath MAJ-643R)	20 MHz	2.8 mm or more
UM-S20-17S	1.4 mm (1.7 mm at proximal side)	20 MHz	2.0 mm or more
	1.95 mm (incl. guide sheath SG-200C)		2.0 mm or more

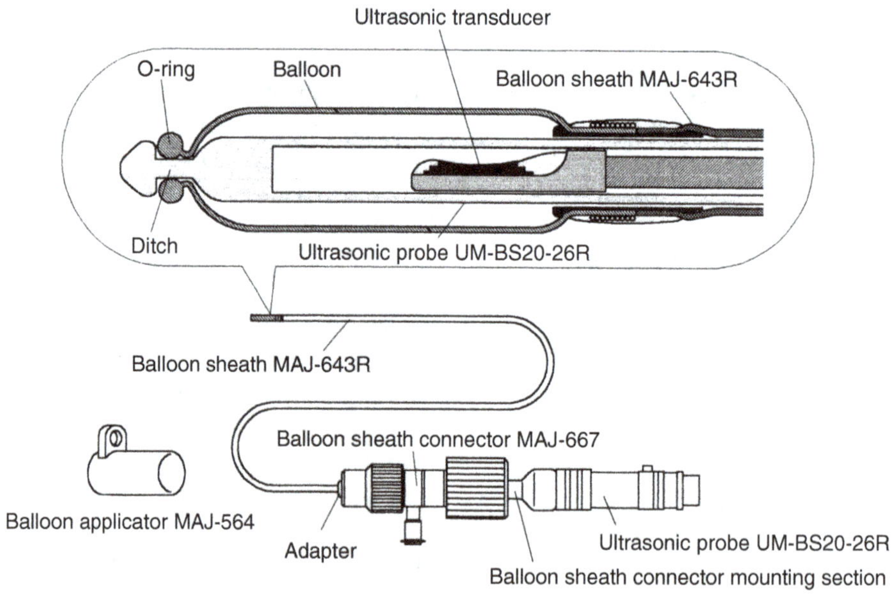

Figure 1.12 Structure of UM-BS20-26R.

balloon sheath MH-246R (outer diameter 3.6 mm); this will need a special bronchoscope, such as the BF-ST49, with an instrument channel and a diameter of at least 3.7 mm, or a rigid bronchoscope with an instrument channel of 11.5 Fr or more. Of note is that the direct contact method does not require a balloon; therefore, the probe is passed directly down the bronchoscope instrument channel.

Bronchoscope

Having selected an ultrasonic probe according to the aim of the investigation and the region being examined, it is then essential to select a bronchoscope suitable for use with that probe. In particular, when the balloon method is selected, care must be taken to prepare a bronchoscope with an instrument channel diameter of at least 2.8 mm.

Ultrasonic Processor and Probe Driving Unit

Ultrasound images are obtained by attaching the endoscopic ultrasonic probe to the Endoscopic Ultrasound Center EU-ME1 (Figure 1.13) and EU-ME2 (Figure 1.14) via the Probe Driving Unit MH-240; they are highly compact and fit in the standard endoscopic equipment trolley.

Preparations

Required Equipment

- Ultrasonic probe (sterilized)
- Balloon sheath
- Balloon sheath connector (for attachment of the balloon sheath to the probe)

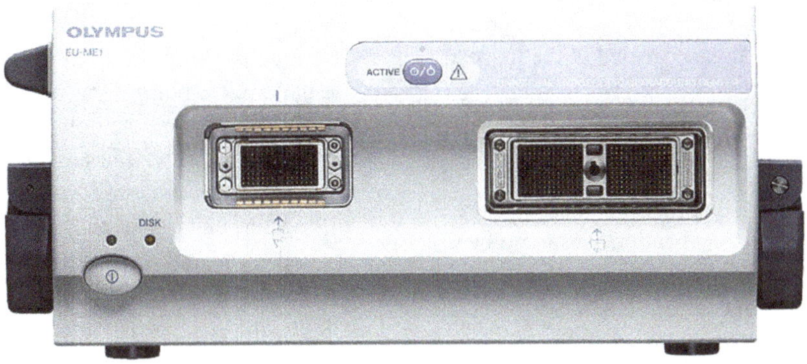

Figure 1.13 Endoscopic Ultrasound Center (EU-ME1). *Source:* Courtesy of Olympus.

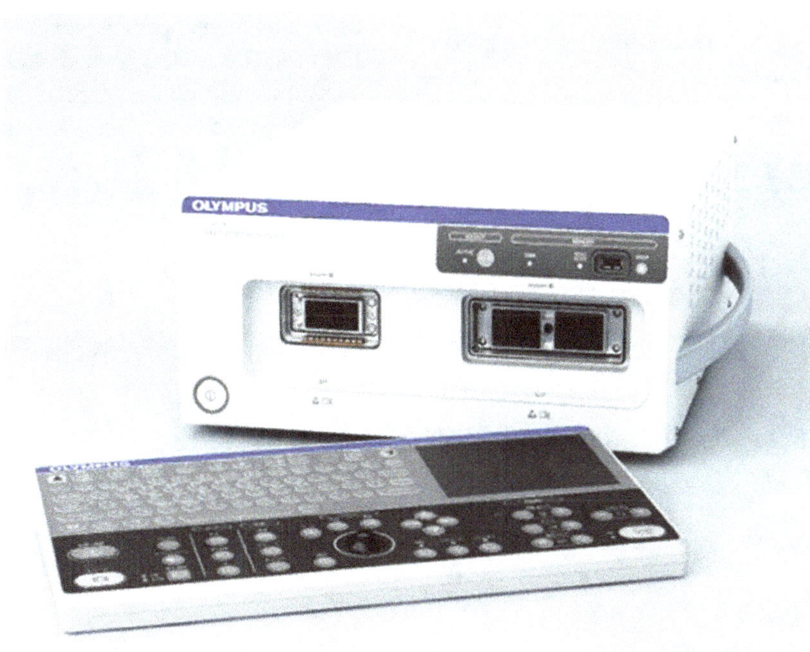

Figure 1.14 Endoscopic Ultrasound Center (EU-ME2). *Source:* Courtesy of Olympus.

- Three-way stopcock with an extension tube
- Physiological saline, 20 ml
- 20 ml syringe

Assembling the Balloon Probe

The advantage of the ultrasonic probe UM-BS20-26R is that it can be used with flexible bronchoscopes with a standard instrument channel with a diameter of at least 2.8 mm (BF-IT260, IT290, and IT240R).

Assemble the balloon probe in accordance with the instructions provided in the manual.

- Pass the balloon sheath connector from the probe tip down, and fix it to the balloon sheath connector attachment on the probe.
- Insert the balloon sheath from the probe tip, and press the balloon sheath clasp into the balloon sheath connector.
- The optimum position for the ultrasonic transducer is not in the center of the balloon, but the transducer should just protrude from the base of the balloon (Figure 1.15); this enables the transducer to rotate within the maximally expanded portion of the balloon when inflated.
- Draw up 15 ml of physiological saline into the syringe, fill the three-way stopcock extension tube with saline, and attach the extension tube to the balloon sheath connector inlet.
- Pull back on the syringe to create negative pressure, drawing out as much air as possible from between the balloon sheath and the probe. After repeating this step three times, slowly release the negative pressure and then slowly inject physiological saline into the balloon.
- Continue pushing the syringe plunger with the balloon tip pointing upward, filling the balloon with saline. Although a small bubble of air will enter the balloon, the tip of the balloon is separate, with a hole in it. Pulling the balloon in the direction of the tip, make a space between the probe tip and the balloon. The air in the tip of the balloon will go out.
- After eliminating all the air in the balloon, fix the probe by hand through the balloon, and push the O-ring on the balloon tip into the groove in the probe tip, either by hand or using a balloon applicator. Once the balloon has been filled with saline and checked for leaks and air bubbles, preparation is complete (Figure 1.16).

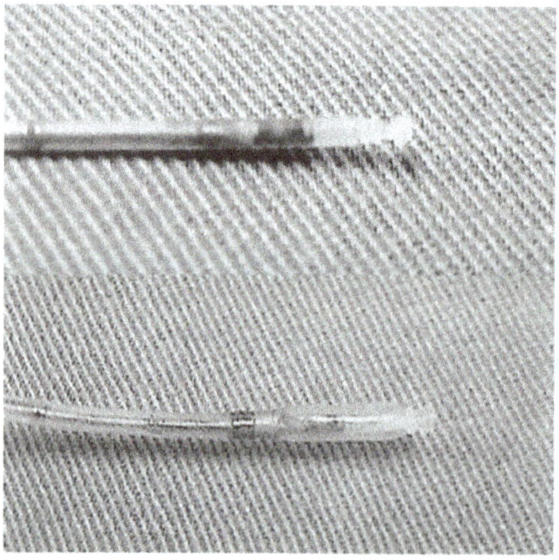

Figure 1.15 Probe (above) and probe inside balloon sheath (below).

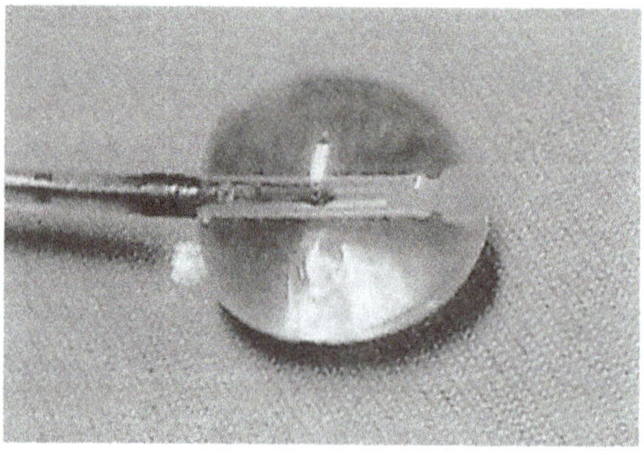

Figure 1.16 Balloon inflated with saline.

Connecting the Probe to the Driving Unit

Insert the connection of the ultrasonic probe into the connector on the driving unit, pointing the pin at the 12 o'clock position.

Connecting the Power and Data Entry

Only turn on the power to the Ultrasound Center after connecting the probe. The ultrasonic probe will be damaged if it is connected when the power is on. After the probe has been connected, switch the monitor to the ultrasound input, and enter the patient's identity number, age, and name.

Checking the Image

Unfreeze and rotate the ultrasonic probe. If it is working properly, multiple echoes with five to seven layers will be observed centered on the probe. If multiple echoes are not observed, the probe may be disconnected or there may be air bubbles in the medium in contact with the transducer of the probe.

Inverting the Image

Next, press the "Image Direction" switch to change the monitor image from Normal to Inverse; this inverts the ultrasound image, so that left and right are the same as the bronchoscopic image, to an image viewed from the proximal site (oral side). In gastrointestinal EUS, a normal ultrasound image is viewed from the caudal direction for easy comparison with computed tomography (CT) scans; however, in EBUS, it is desirable for the directions in the ultrasound image to coincide with those in the image from the bronchoscope. Of note is that the normal mode is only used in special situations, such as for comparison with CT images.

Operation

Anesthesia Application

In principle, anesthesia for EBUS is the same as that for regular bronchoscopic examinations. It should be kept in mind, however, that until the operator becomes more experienced, procedures will tend to be somewhat longer in duration. When EBUS is performed in conjunction with another procedure, such as laser-induced fluorescence bronchoscopy, intravenous anesthesia might be used, allowing spontaneous respiration. An important consideration for the anesthetist is to confirm, under direct observation using a laryngoscope, that local anesthetic spray is applied directly to the pharynx and larynx, particularly the vocal chords. After bronchoscopic examination of the trachea and bronchi, a local anesthetic is further applied to the bronchus (bronchi) into which the balloon probe will be introduced.

Inserting the Probe

Apply xylocaine jelly liberally to the distal end of the balloon probe, and slowly insert it into the instrument channel of the bronchoscope. During the insertion process, hold the probe at a point 2 or 3 cm away from the instrument port. Be aware that there are two places with high resistance in the instrument channel between the instrument port and the distal end of the bronchoscope. The first site is 4–5 cm from the instrument port, where the suction and instrument channels join, whereas the second is 2–3 cm from the bronchoscope tip, where the instrument bends. When resistance is high at either site and it is difficult to pass the probe, remove the probe and reapply jelly, and if that fails, remove the bronchoscope from the patient and reinsert the probe.

Operating the Probe

Advance the probe to a point slightly distal to the site of interest. Inject 1–3 ml of physiological saline, inflating the balloon while scanning so that it contacts the bronchial wall circumferentially. The optimum volume of saline is that which just enables circumferential contact of the balloon with the bronchial wall. Of note is that overinflation can cause bronchial wall structures to compress or the balloon to burst.

Then, while scanning and capturing images (always ensure video-recording), retract the probe from the distal to the proximal site. It is important to remember to retract the probe very slowly. If necessary, ask the patient to hold their breath while scanning. Advancing the probe from the proximal to the distal site can damage the probe and should be avoided.

Tips for Achieving Optimum Ultrasound Images

To obtain clear, easily understandable images, note the following:

- Rotate the ultrasound image so that it corresponds to the endoscopic images.
- To assess the depth of tumor invasion, the ultrasound pulse must penetrate the tracheal/bronchial wall perpendicularly.
- Rotate the ultrasound image so that it corresponds to the bronchoscopic images:
  - At a bifurcation (e.g. the opening of the right upper lobe bronchus), we can line up the direction that the balloon is not in contact with the bronchial lumen on the bronchoscopic image with the direction with no echo on the EBUS image. For example (Figure 1.17), in the left ultrasound image below, the direction with no echo, because the balloon is not in contact with the bronchial lumen, is from 4 to 6 o'clock. In the right bronchoscopic image, the direction that the balloon is not in contact with the bronchial lumen is from 2 to 4 o'clock. To match up the images, we need to rotate the EBUS image anticlockwise by about 45°.
  - Rotate the EBUS image according to the relative positions of the bronchial tree and the esophagus and great vessels. When scanning from the left main bronchus to the lower part of the trachea, the esophagus is located at the 6 o'clock direction (Figure 1.18, left). The right pulmonary artery runs anteriorly to the right intermediate trunk from 10 to 2 o'clock (Figure 1.18,

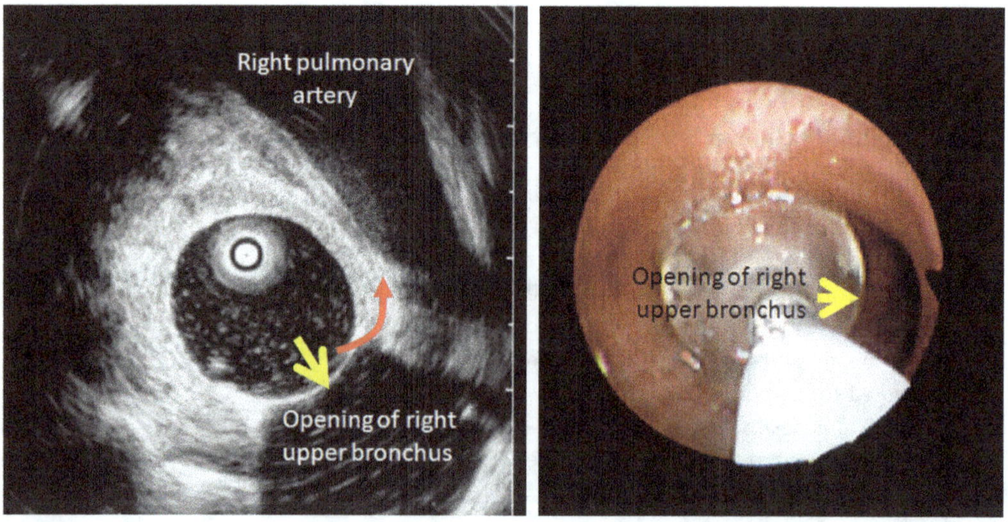

Figure 1.17 Tips for obtaining optimum ultrasound images: Rotation of the ultrasound image so that it corresponds to the bronchoscopic image. The arrows indicate a highly echoic first layer, with a clearly lineated layer structure in that region.

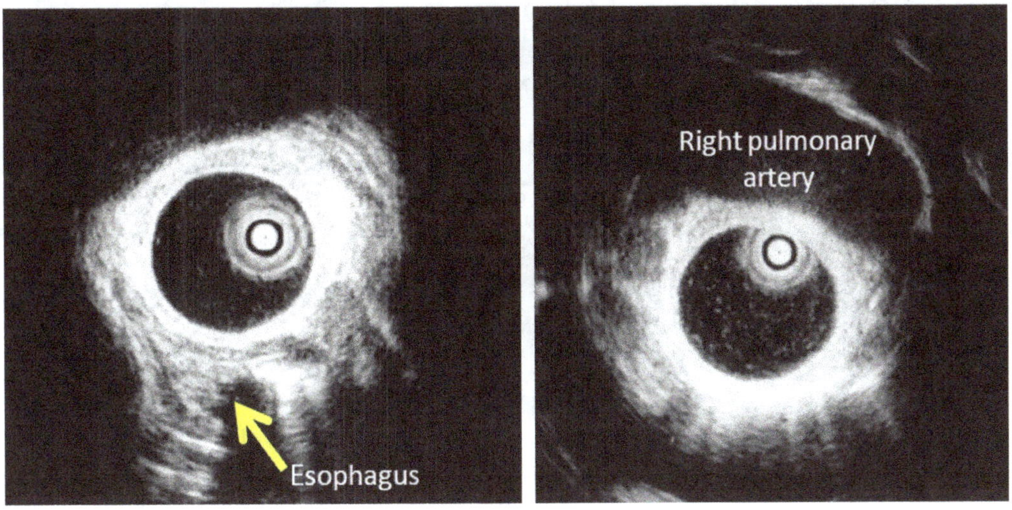

Figure 1.18 Tips for obtaining optimum ultrasound images: Rotation of the endobronchial ultrasonography image according to the relative positions of the bronchial tree and the esophagus and great vessels.

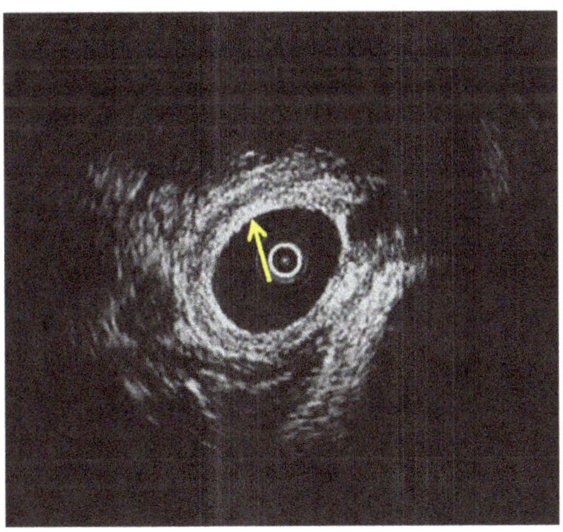

Figure 1.19 Tips for obtaining optimum ultrasound images: To assess the depth of tumor invasion, obtain images with the ultrasound pulse penetrating the tracheal/bronchial wall perpendicularly. The arrow indicates a highly echoic first layer, with a clearly lineated layer structure in that region.

right). Identify the position of these structures, and rotate the EBUS image accordingly.

- To assess the depth of tumor invasion, obtain images with the ultrasound pulse penetrating the tracheal/bronchial wall perpendicularly. If the first layer (marginal echo, reflected at the boundary between tissues) is highly echoic, the image can be said to be derived from an ultrasound pulse penetrating the tracheal/bronchial wall nearly perpendicularly (Figure 1.19).

Equipment for EBUS-Guided TBNA

A curved array transducer is combined at the tip of the bronchoscope for EBUS-TBNA (Figure 1.20; BF-UC290F, Olympus) [8–10]. This convex bronchoscope comprises an oblique forward viewing with a convex transducer mounted in front of the lens. This convex transducer is 5–12 MHz and covered with a balloon. In addition, this bronchoscope has a working channel with a diameter of 2.0 mm; we can insert the disposable biopsy instrument with a 22 G needle (Figure 1.21; Vizishot2, Olympus) through the working channel (Figure 1.22). After the convex-type probe is covered by the balloon, saline is

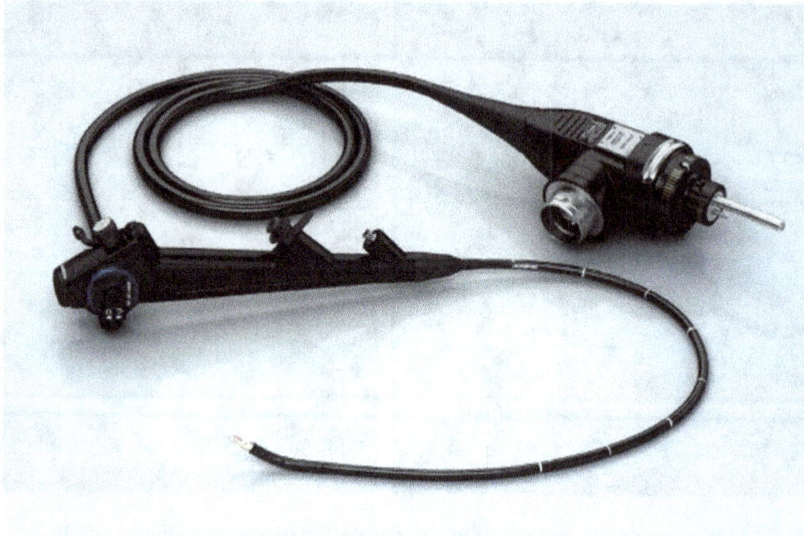

Figure 1.20 Ultrasonic bronchoscope (BF-UC290F). *Source:* Courtesy of Olympus.

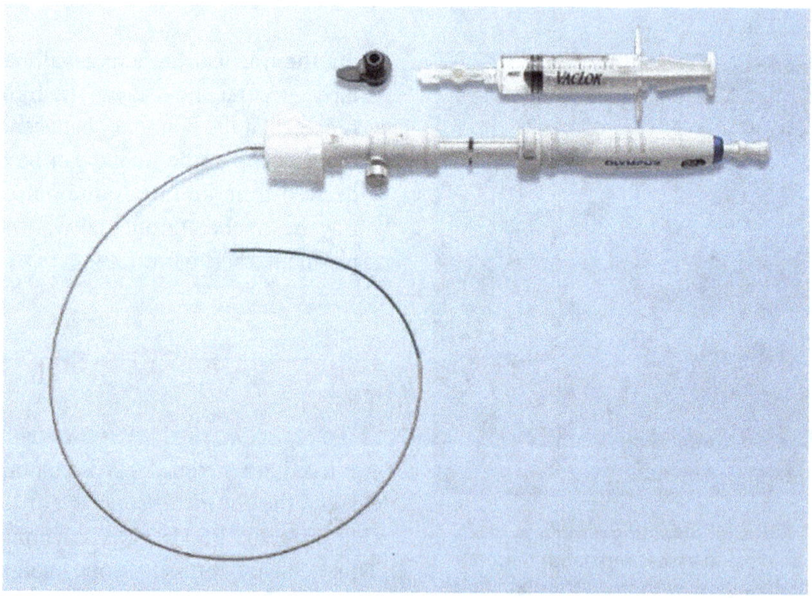

Figure 1.21 Aspiration needle (ViziShot 2). *Source:* Courtesy of Olympus.

injected into the balloon for filling its inner space. This bronchoscope is connected to the ultrasound unit, and the power switch should be turned on.

Because this convex bronchoscope has an oblique forward viewing, there is little difficulty in inserting this scope through the vocal cord. Watching the 12 o'clock direction of the vocal cord, the tip of this scope is straight, and it is easy to go into the trachea. The bronchoscope reveals the target lesion for TBNA beyond the bronchial wall; this transducer provides longitudinal planes of peribronchial areas, and the ultrasonographic image reveals the real-time movement of the TBNA needle.

Doppler Mode

The Doppler effect is that the frequency of sound increases while the source of sound moves to the ultrasound transducer, and the frequency of sound decreases while the source of sound removes from the ultrasound transducer. Using this effect, the Doppler mode of the Ultrasound Processor enables the visualization of vessels on EBUS images. The color Doppler mode reveals vessels based on the speed of the bloodstream, vessels coming up to the ultrasound probe as red and vessels removing from the ultrasound probe as blue (Figure 1.23). The power Doppler mode reveals vessels based on the amount of blood in the bloodstream.

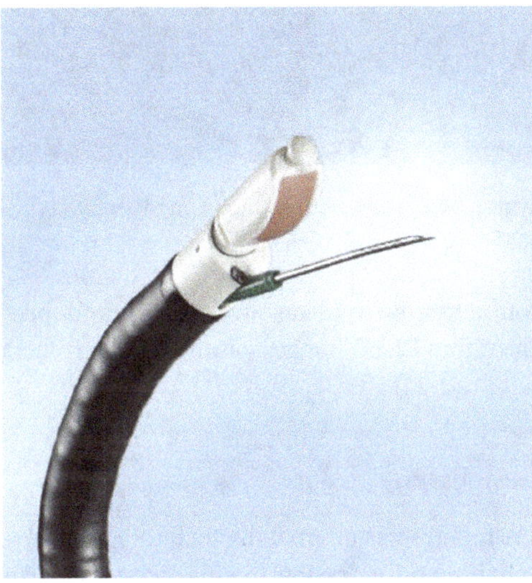

Figure 1.22 Ultrasonic bronchoscope with the needle. *Source:* Courtesy of Olympus.

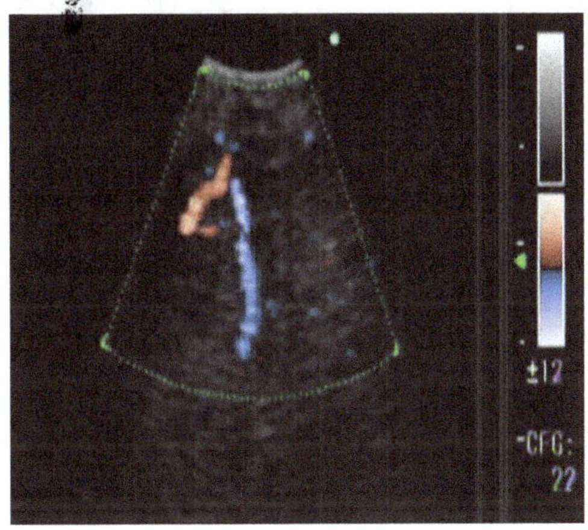

Figure 1.23 Doppler image of a representative case. The color Doppler mode shows vessels according to the speed of the bloodstream, vessels coming up to the ultrasound probe as red, and vessels removing from the ultrasound probe as blue.

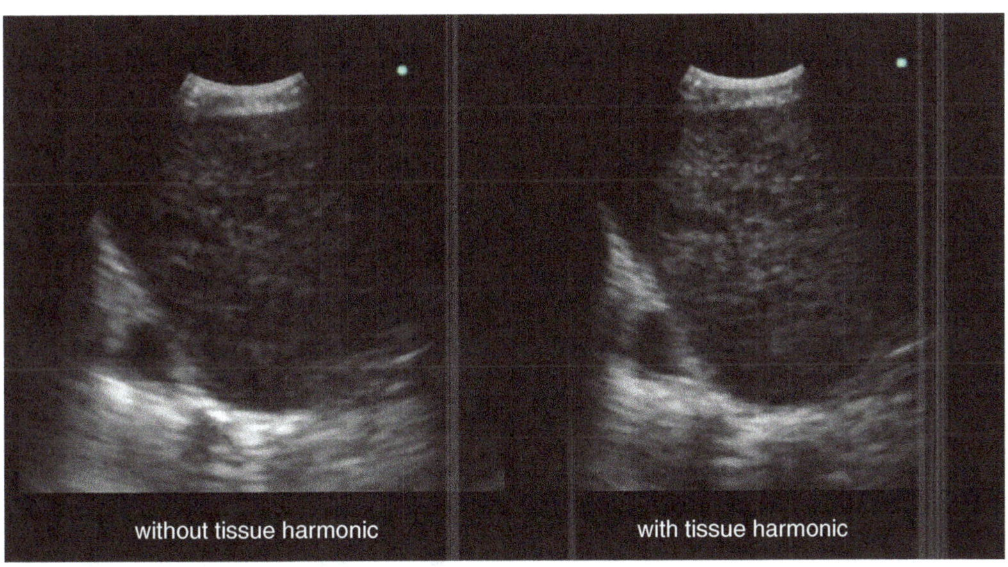

Figure 1.24 Tissue harmonic image of a representative case. The tissue harmonic image (right) is a fine image compared with the normal B-mode image.

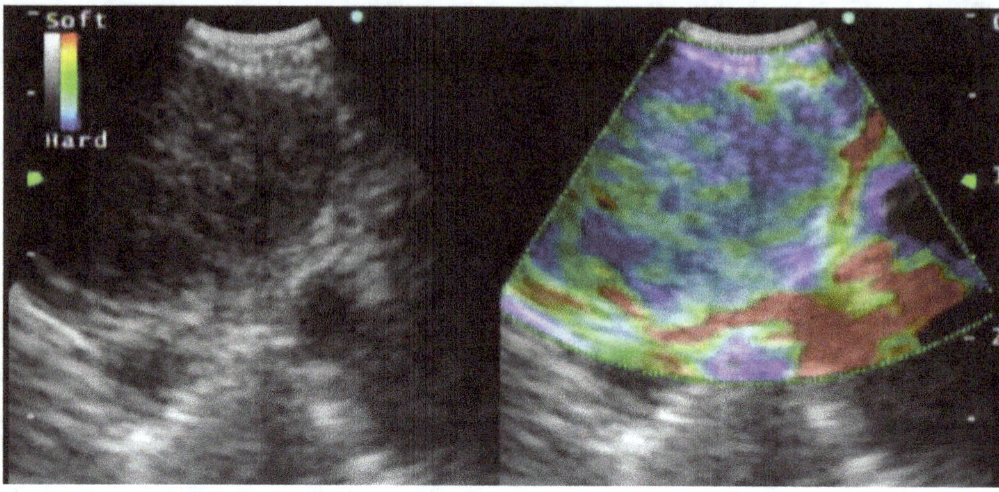

Figure 1.25 Elastography of a representative case. This lymph node shows mixed blue and green areas and is suspected of having heterogeneous internal structures.

New Functions of the Ultrasound Processor

The Ultrasound Processor (EU-ME2, premier; Olympus) provides some improvements.

Tissue Harmonic Echo

Some strains and harmonic components occur while the ultrasound wave is transmitting through organs. Harmonic components are produced from main lobes; then, harmonic components reduce artifacts from side lobes. Tissue harmonic echo visualizes these harmonic components of ultrasound waves and provides fine EBUS images with reduced artifacts (Figure 1.24).

Elastography

Elastography is an imaging technology for visualizing and assessing the elasticity when an external force compresses an elastic body. On the colored ultrasound strain image, which is superimposed on the B-mode image, each area is colored according to the amount of strain. While blue shows a relatively hard area, green and red show relatively soft areas (Figure 1.25).

References

1 Pandian, N.G., Kreis, A., Brockway, B. et al. (1988). Ultrasound angioscopy: real-time, two dimensional, intraluminal ultrasound imaging of blood vessels. *American Journal of Cardiology* 62: 493–494.

2 Hürter, T. and Hanarath, P. (1990). Endobronchiale Sonographie zur Diagnostik Pulmonaler und Medistinaler Tumoren. *Deutsche Medizinische Wochenschrift* 115 (50): 1899–1905.

3 Iizuka, K., Dobashi, K., Houjou, S. et al. (1992). Evaluation of airway smooth muscle contractions in vitro by high-frequency ultrasonic imaging. *Chest* 102: 1251–1257.

4 Ono, R., Suemasu, K., and Matsunaka, T. (1993). Bronchoscopic ultrasonography in the diagnosis of lung cancer. *Japanese Journal of Clinical Oncology* 23: 34–40.

5 Goldberg, B., Steiner, R., Liu, J. et al. (1994). US-assisted bronchoscopy with use of miniature transducer-containing catheters. *Radiology* 190 (1): 233–237.

6 Becker, H. (1996). Endobronchialer Ultraschall—Eine neue Perspektive in der Bronchologie. *Ultraschall in der Medizin* 17: 106–112.

7 Kurimoto, N., Murayama, M., Yoshioka, S. et al. (1999). Assessment of usefulness of endobronchial ultrasonography in determination of depth of tracheobronchial tumor invasion. *Chest* 115: 1500–1506.

8 Yasufuku, K., Chiyo, M., Koh, E. et al. (2005 Dec). Endobronchial ultrasound guided transbronchial needle aspiration for staging of lung cancer. *Lung Cancer* 50 (3): 347–354.

9 Yasufuku, K., Nakajima, T., Motoori, K. et al. (2006 Sep). Comparison of endobronchial ultrasound, positron emission tomography, and CT for lymph node staging of lung cancer. *Chest* 130 (3): 710–718.

10 Wahidi, M.M., Herth, F., Yasufuku, K. et al. (2016 Mar). Technical aspects of endobronchial ultrasound-guided transbronchial needle aspiration: CHEST Guideline and Expert Panel Report. *Chest* 149 (3): 816–835.

2

Identifying Peribronchial Organs during Endobronchial Ultrasonography

Noriaki Kurimoto

Department of Internal Medicine, Division of Medical Oncology and Respiratory Medicine, Shimane University Faculty of Medicine, Izumo, Japan

Overview of Ultrasound Imaging of the Bronchi as the Radial Probe Is Pulled in a Proximal Direction

Endobronchial ultrasonagraphy (EBUS) images are cross-sectional images of planes perpendicular to the long axis of the tracheobronchial tree. Because these images are used to assist endoscopic treatments, they are generally displayed as if looking from the rostral direction so that left and right match with the endoscopic images.

In EBUS images taken from the trachea, the positional relationship of the peribronchial organs corresponds to that in a reversed computed tomography (CT) image (CT scans are cross-sectional images seen from the caudal direction). However, EBUS images taken distal to the bifurcation of the left and right main bronchi are cross-sectional images of planes perpendicular to the long axis of the bronchus; therefore, the positional relationship of the peribronchial organs differs between EBUS images and CT images.

When EBUS is used to image centrally located lesions in clinical practice, the balloon is inflated distal to the lesion and the images are obtained while pulling the probe proximally. This is because it is difficult to push the probe distally with the balloon inflated, and pulling the probe proximally allows images to be obtained without bending the probe.

In this section we describe, using schematic diagrams and ultrasound images, the positional relationship of the peribronchial organs and the bronchial tree as seen while pulling the probe from the right or left lower lobe bronchus up to the right or left main bronchus, respectively. Understanding this positional relationship is essential for a full understanding of EBUS.

Right Bronchi

Right Lower Lobe Bronchus

When the balloon is inflated in the right basal bronchus, the inferior pulmonary vein (V^6) passes on the dorsal side of the bronchus (Figure 2.1 – 1), and the pulmonary artery, divided into the A^8, A^9, and A^{10} branches, is positioned between 9 and 2 o'clock anterior to the bronchus. As the probe is pulled back, A^8, A^9, and A^{10} meet in the 12 o'clock direction, and the pulmonary artery then moves gradually to the 3 o'clock direction (Figure 2.1 – 2, 3).

Endobronchial Ultrasonography, Second Edition. Noriaki Kurimoto, David I.K. Fielding, Ali I. Musani, Christopher Kniese, and Katsuhiko Morita.

Companion website: www.wiley.com/go/kurimoto2e

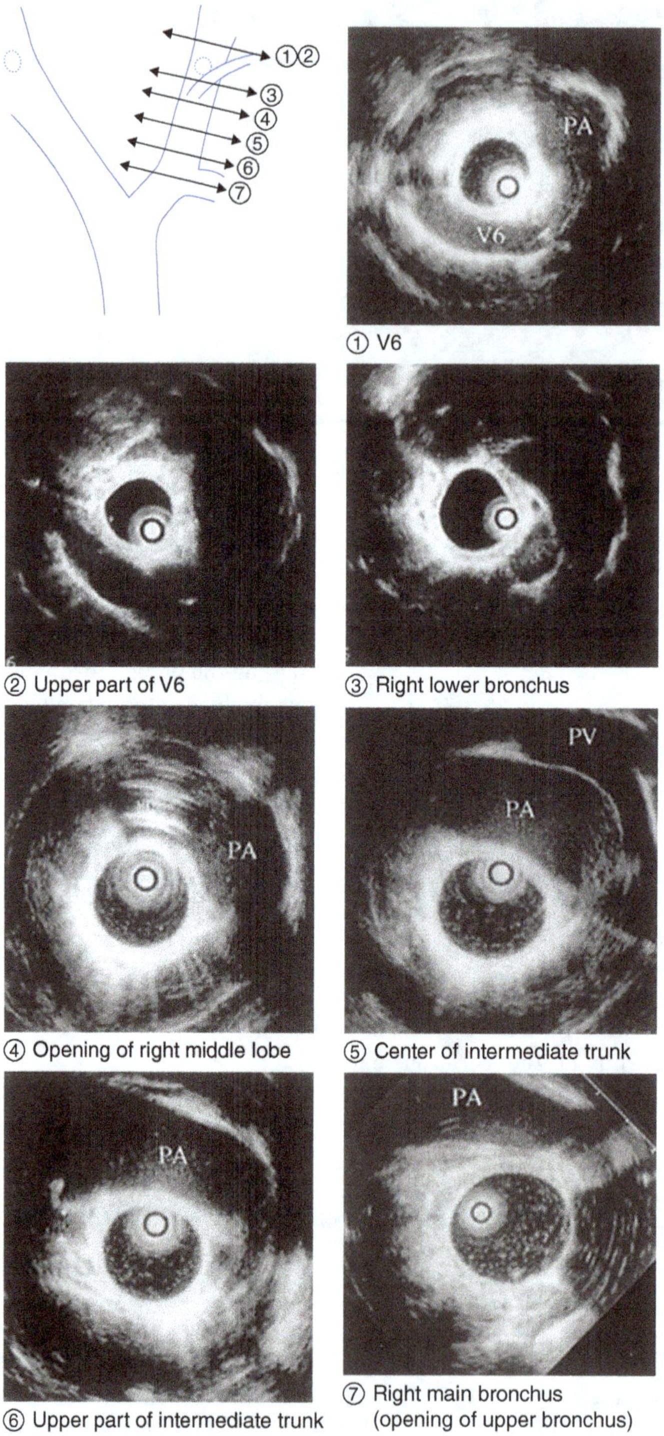

Figure 2.1 Positional relationship of the right peribronchial organs. PA, pulmonary artery; PV, pulmonary vein.

When the probe is pulled further back, it approaches the bifurcation of B^6, and part of the bronchial wall (in the 5 o'clock direction) loses contact with the balloon. This area therefore reflects back the ultrasound, resulting in the loss of the image of the layer that contains the bifurcation of B^6. As the probe is retracted further, the opening of the middle lobe bronchus appears at the 11 o'clock position, indicated by the reflection of the ultrasound pulse because of the loss of contact between the balloon and the bronchial wall at the bifurcation. By this point, the pulmonary artery has gradually moved round to the 2 o'clock position (Figure 2.1 – 4).

From the Right Intermediate Bronchus to the Right Main Bronchus

As the probe is pulled from the distal intermediate bronchus to a point immediately below the origin of the upper lobe bronchus, the pulmonary artery crosses the bronchus from the right to the left (Figure 2.1 – 5, 6, 7). The superior pulmonary vein can sometimes be seen in the central section of the intermediate bronchus, anterior to the pulmonary artery (Figure 2.1 – 5). As the probe reaches the bifurcation of the upper lobe bronchus, the balloon again loses contact with the bronchial wall; therefore, the upper lobe bronchus appears as a reflection of the ultrasound pulse in the 3 o'clock direction (Figure 2.1 – 7). Pulling the probe back further, A^{1+3}, which originate from the pulmonary trunk, can be seen crossing horizontally, anterior to the right main bronchus. Retracting the probe further, the origin of the left main bronchus at the carina is indicated by the reflection of the ultrasound pulse in the 9 o'clock direction.

The key to reading EBUS images of the right bronchi is to recognize the anatomy of the peribronchial organs as the probe is retracted from the lower lobe bronchus to the main bronchus.

Right Side

Right basal segment bronchus:	inferior pulmonary vein, V^6, at 6 o'clock
	PA^{7-10} at 2 o'clock
Right lower lobe bronchus:	PA^{6-10} between 2 and 3 o'clock
Right intermediate bronchus:	right pulmonary artery at 12 o'clock
Right main bronchus:	A^{1+3} at 12 o'clock
PA:	pulmonary artery

Left Bronchi

Left Lower Lobe Bronchus

With the balloon inflated in the left basal bronchus, the inferior pulmonary vein (V^6) passes on the dorsal side of the bronchus, and the A^8, A^9, and A^{10} branches of the pulmonary artery meet at the 10 o'clock position (Figure 2.2 – 1, 2). As the probe is pulled proximally toward the bifurcation of B^6, there is loss of contact between the balloon and part of the bronchial wall in the 7 o'clock direction. This reflects the ultrasound, resulting in the loss of the image of the layer containing the bifurcation of B^6. As the probe is retracted further, the opening of the upper lobe bronchus appears at the 11 o'clock position, indicated by the reflection of the ultrasound pulse because of the loss of contact between the balloon and bronchial wall at the bifurcation (Figure 2.2 – 3). Here, the pulmonary artery is located below the origin of the upper lobe bronchus.

Left Main Bronchus

The distal section of the left main bronchus is characterized by the left pulmonary artery in the 10 o'clock direction, the descending aorta in the 7 o'clock direction, and the left atrium between the 1 and 3 o'clock directions (Figure 2.2 – 4, 5). As the probe enters the central section of the left main bronchus, the left atrium disappears and the esophagus appears in the 6 o'clock direction. The subcarinal (#7)

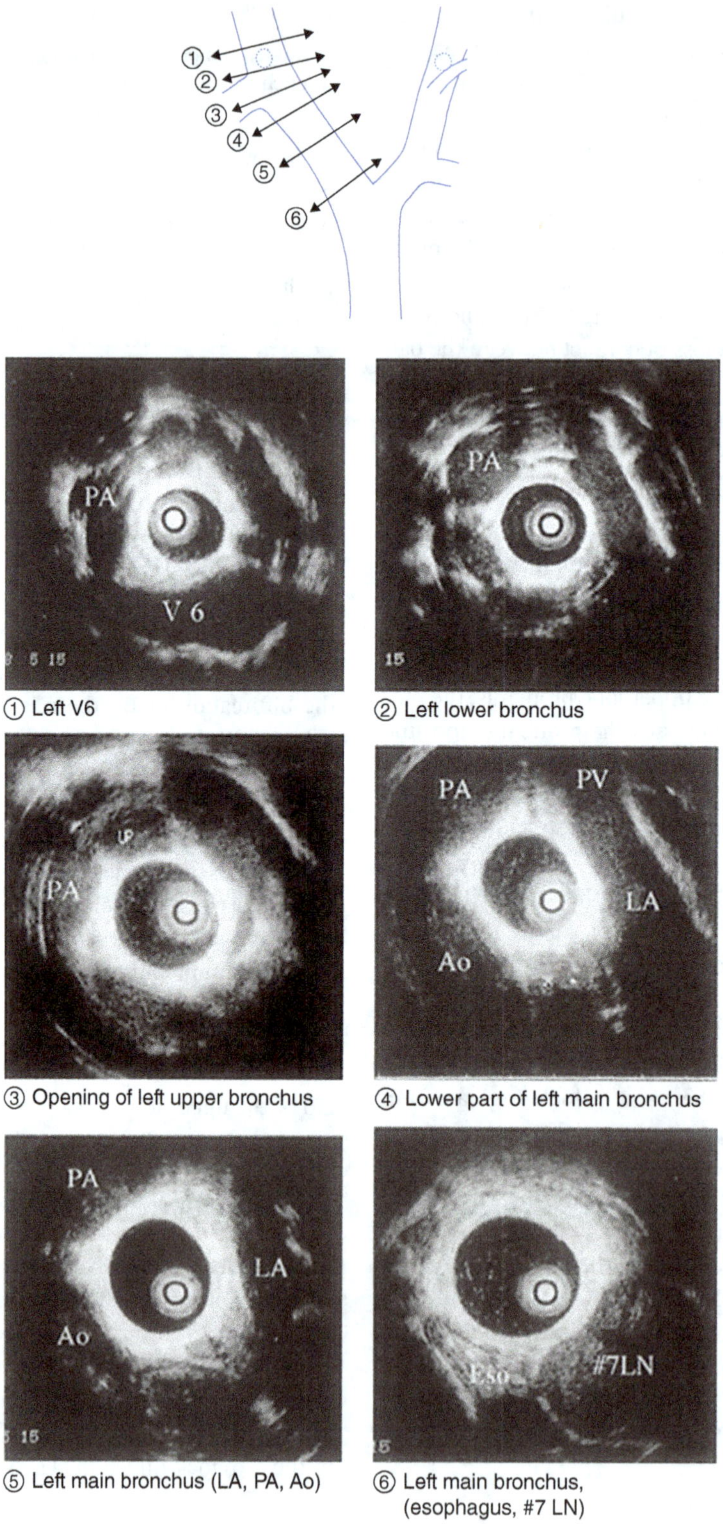

Figure 2.2 Positional relationship of the left peribronchial organs. Ao, aorta; Eso, esophagus; LA, left atrium; PA, pulmonary artery; PV, pulmonary vein.

lymph node (LN) is often visible medial to the esophagus (Figure 2.2 – 6). When the probe is pulled further back, the origin of the left main bronchus at the carina is indicated by the reflection of the ultrasound pulse at the 3 o'clock position because of the loss of contact between the balloon and the bronchial wall at the bifurcation.

The key to reading EBUS images of the left bronchi is to recognize the anatomy of the peribronchial organs as the probe is retracted from the lower lobe bronchus to the main bronchus.

Left Side

Left basal segment bronchus:	inferior pulmonary vein, V^6, at 6 o'clock
	PA^{8-10} at 9 o'clock
Left lower lobe bronchus:	PA^{6-10} at 10 o'clock
	superior pulmonary vein between 1 and 4 o'clock
Left main bronchus (distal):	left pulmonary artery at 10 o'clock
	aorta at 7 o'clock
	left atrium between 1 and 3 o'clock
Left main bronchus (proximal):	left pulmonary artery at 10 o'clock
	aorta at 7 o'clock
	left atrium between 1 and 3 o'clock
	esophagus at 6 o'clock
PA:	pulmonary artery

Ultrasound Imaging of Mediastinal and Hilar Lymph Nodes for EBUS-TBNA Using a Convex Bronchoscope

An understanding of ultrasonographic images of the peribronchial vessels and lymph nodes is necessary for performing EBUS-TBNA successfully.

#7 LN: Subcarinal Lymph Node

To approach this lymph node, the convex bronchoscope is inserted into the right main bronchus. Scanning in the 9 o'clock direction allows confirmation of the largest area of the lymph node. The right main pulmonary artery can then be viewed by rotating clockwise to scan in the 11 o'clock direction (Figure 2.3).

#11Ri LN: Right Interlobar Lymph Node between the Right Lower and Middle Lobe Bronchi

To approach this lymph node, the convex bronchoscope is inserted into the right basal bronchus. Scanning in the 11 o'clock direction allows confirmation of the largest area of the lymph node. The right pulmonary artery can then be viewed by rotating clockwise to scan in the 2 o'clock direction (Figure 2.4).

#11Rs LN: Right Interlobar Lymph Node between the Right Intermediate Trunk and Upper Lobe Bronchus

To approach this lymph node, the convex bronchoscope is inserted into the right intermediate trunk. Relative to the intermediate trunk, the right upper bronchus is located in the 11 o'clock direction. Scanning in the 11 o'clock direction allows confirmation of the largest area of the lymph node. The right main pulmonary artery can then be viewed by rotating anticlockwise to scan in the 9 o'clock direction (Figure 2.5).

#11L LN: Left Interlobar Lymph Node

To approach this lymph node, the convex bronchoscope is inserted into the left basal bronchus. On the bronchoscopic image, the left upper lobe bronchus is located in the 11 o'clock direction relative to the left lower lobe bronchus. Scanning in the 11 o'clock direction

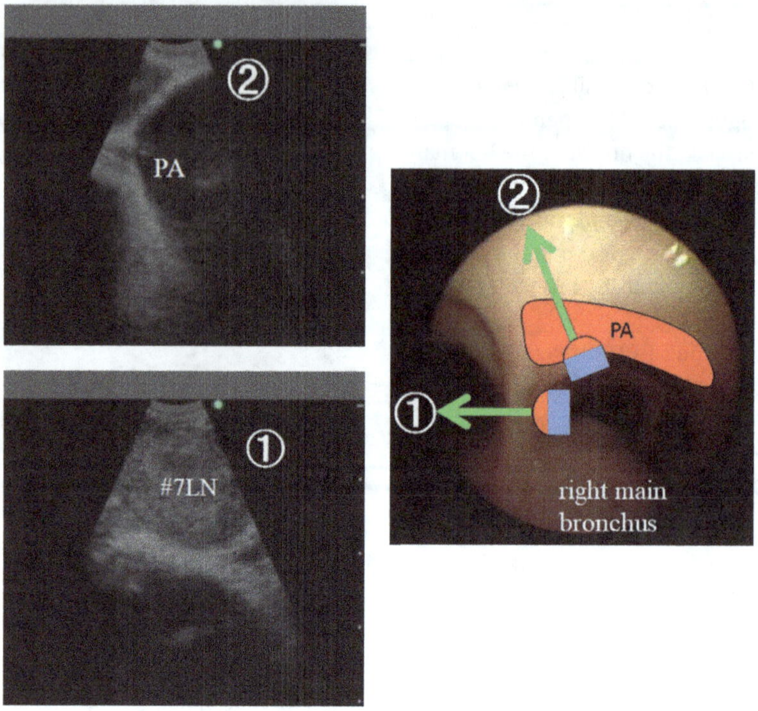

Figure 2.3 #7 LN: Subcarinal lymph node. The numbers indicate the distinction of scanning direction by ultrasound. PA, pulmonary artery.

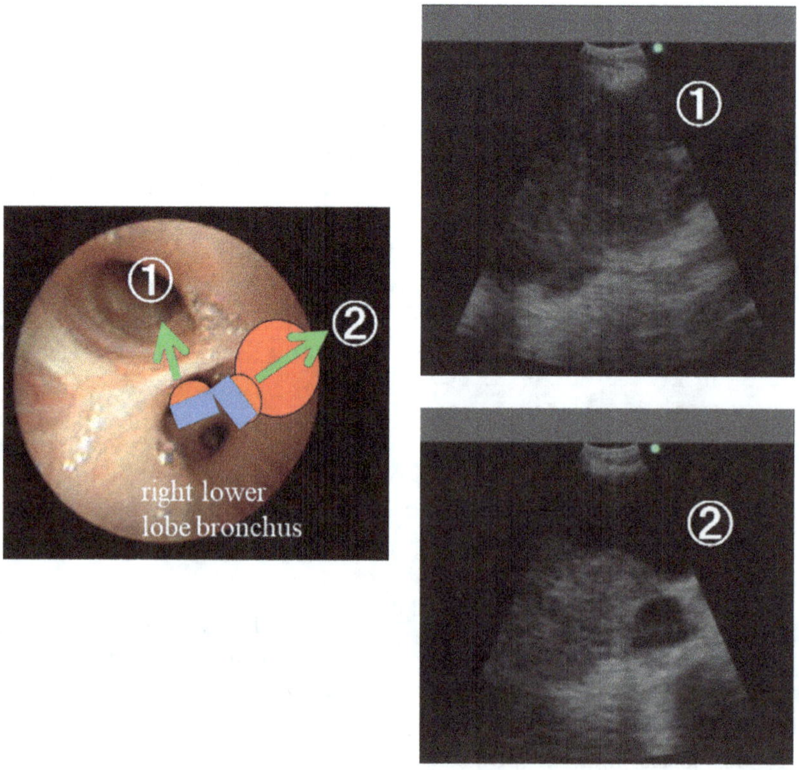

Figure 2.4 #11Ri LN: Right interlobar lymph node between the right lower and middle lobe bronchi. The numbers indicate the distinction of scanning direction by ultrasound.

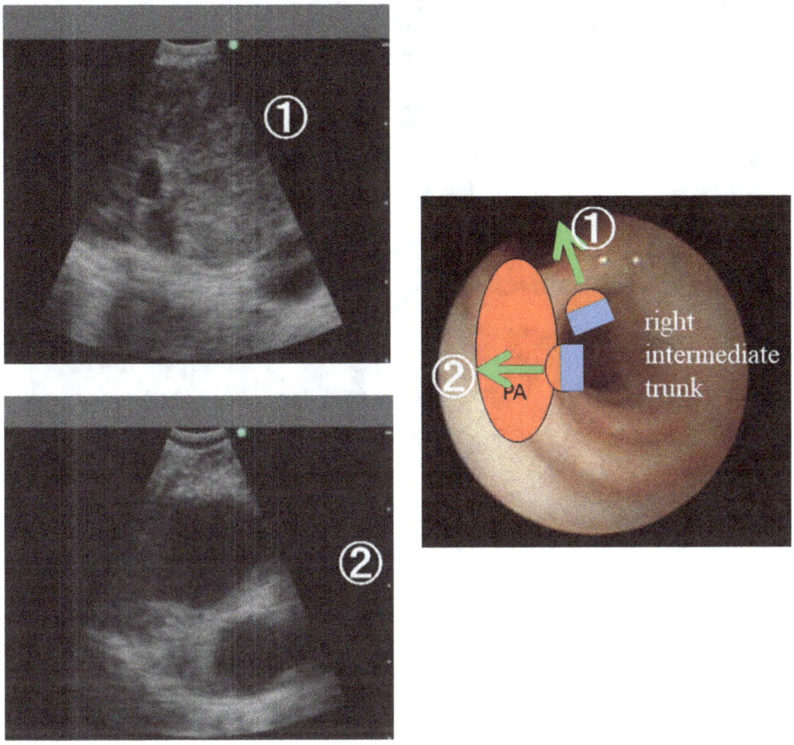

Figure 2.5 #11Rs LN: Right interlobar lymph node between the right intermediate trunk and upper lobe bronchus. The numbers indicate the distinction of scanning direction by ultrasound. PA, pulmonary artery.

allows confirmation of the largest area of the lymph node. The left pulmonary artery can then be viewed by rotating anticlockwise to scan in the 10 o'clock direction (Figure 2.6).

#4L LN: Left Lower Paratracheal Lymph Node

To approach this lymph node, the convex bronchoscope is inserted into the most distal site of the trachea. Scanning in the 11 o'clock direction allows confirmation of the largest area of the lymph node. The left main pulmonary artery can then be viewed by pushing the scope approximately 1–2 cm distally, whereas pulling the scope proximally by approximately 1–2 cm allows the aortic arch to be viewed (Figure 2.7).

#4R LN: Right Lower Paratracheal Lymph Node

To approach this lymph node, the convex bronchoscope is inserted into the distal site of the trachea. On the bronchoscopic image, the membranous portion of the trachea is located in the 6 o'clock direction. Scanning in the 2 o'clock direction allows confirmation of the largest area of the lymph node. The superior vena cava (SVC) can be seen just beside this (Figure 2.8).

Azygous Vein and Esophagus

The azygous vein runs beside the right side of the lowest part of the trachea. The azygous vein forms an important border between the #4R LN and #10 LN. By rotating the tip of the bronchoscope, the azygous vein can be followed from the posterior direction to the anterior direction, checking the connection to the SVC (Figure 2.9, red arrow).

The esophagus is located just to the left at the lower part of the trachea and posterior to the left main bronchus (Figure 2.10, yellow

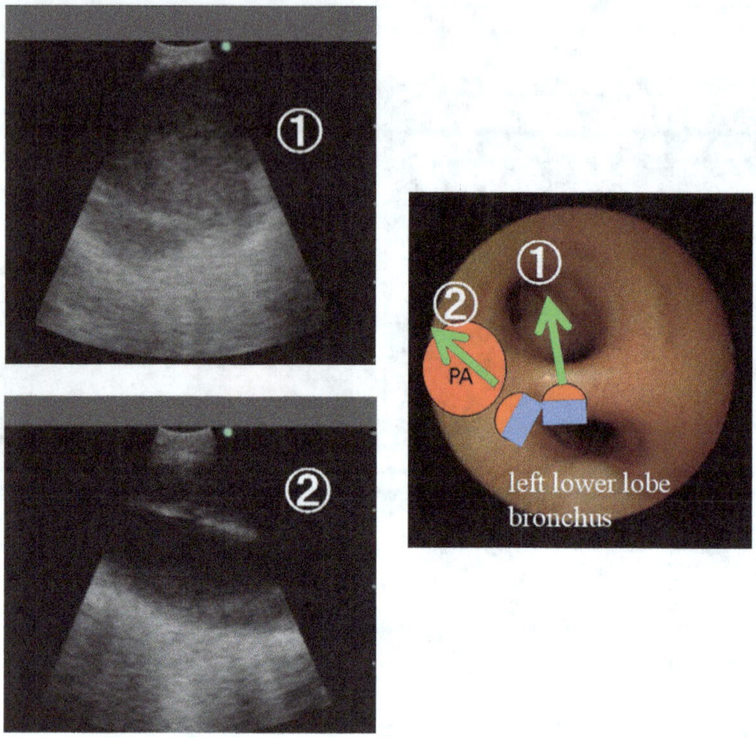

Figure 2.6 #11L LN: Left interlobar lymph node. The numbers indicate the distinction of scanning direction by ultrasound. PA, pulmonary artery.

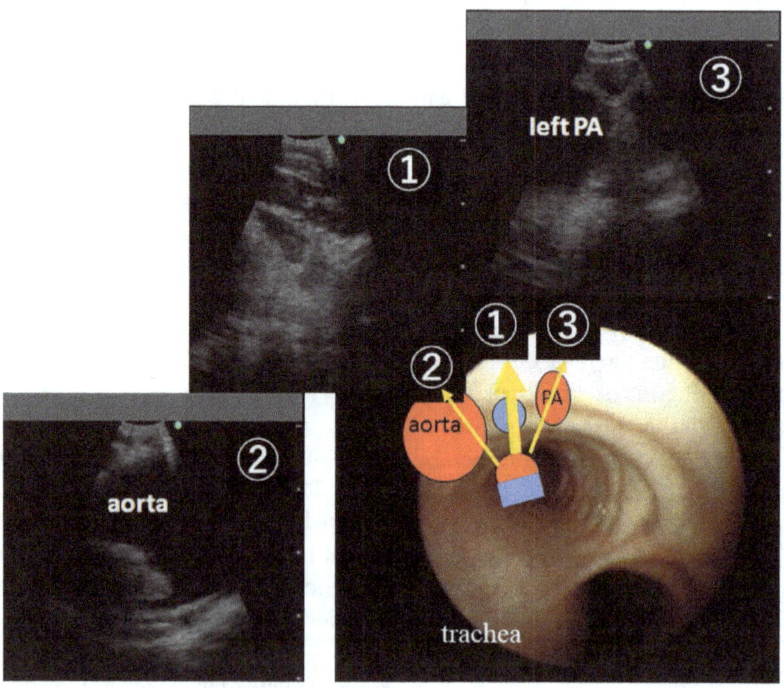

Figure 2.7 #4L LN: Left lower paratracheal lymph node. The numbers indicate the distinction of scanning direction by ultrasound. PA, pulmonary artery.

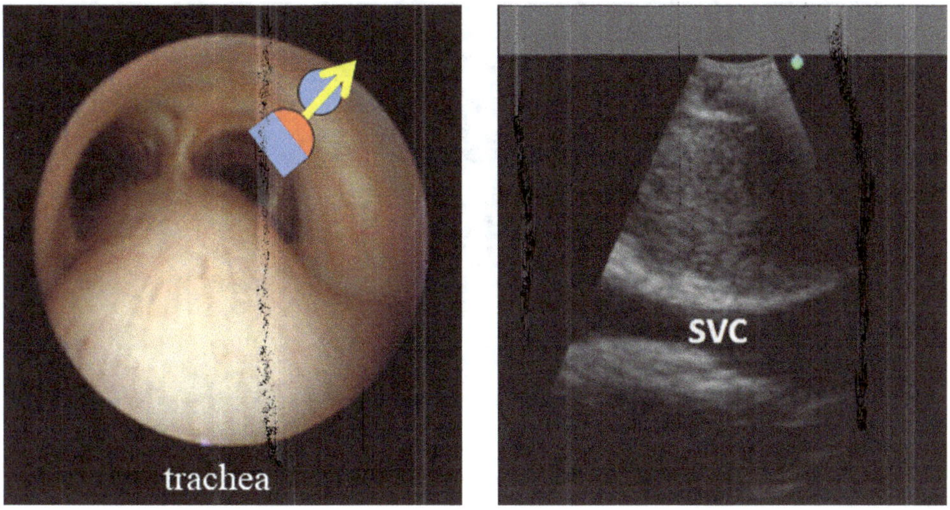

Figure 2.8 #4R LN: Right lower paratracheal lymph node. SVC, superior vena cava.

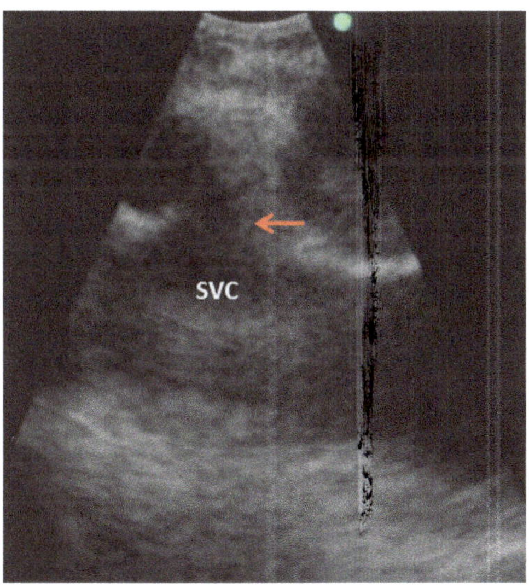

Figure 2.9 Azygous vein. SVC, superior vena cava.

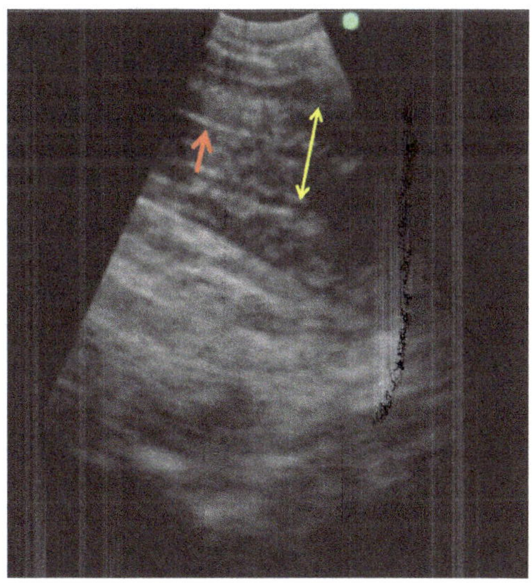

Figure 2.10 Esophagus.

arrow). EBUS confirms the presence of air in the lumen of the esophagus (Figure 2.10, red arrow) and that the esophagus follows its characteristic path in the longitudinal direction.

Bronchial Artery

The bronchial artery branches from the thoracic descending aorta and eventually arrives at the trachea and bronchi after distributing blood to the mediastinal and hilar lymph nodes (Figure 2.11). The bronchial artery is a high-pressure blood vessel, but it has thin walls. During EBUS-TBNA, there is a high risk of forming a hematoma by puncturing the bronchial artery between the lymph node and bronchial wall, so it should be confirmed that there is no bronchial artery on the

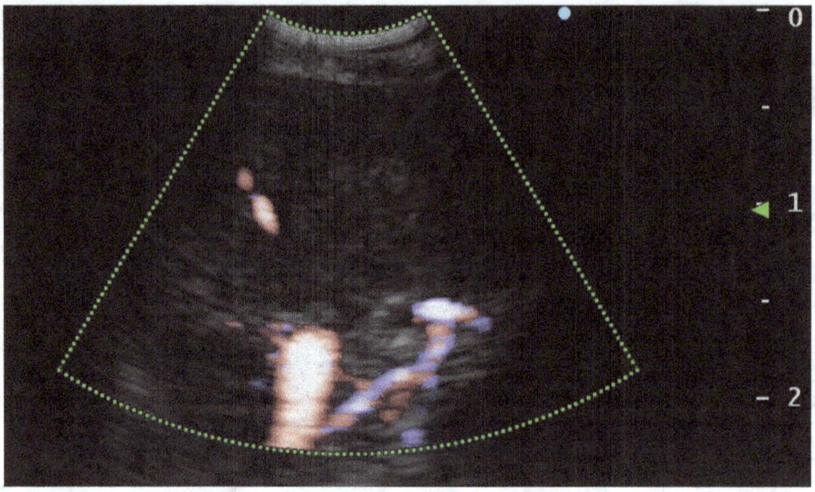

Figure 2.11 Bronchial artery.

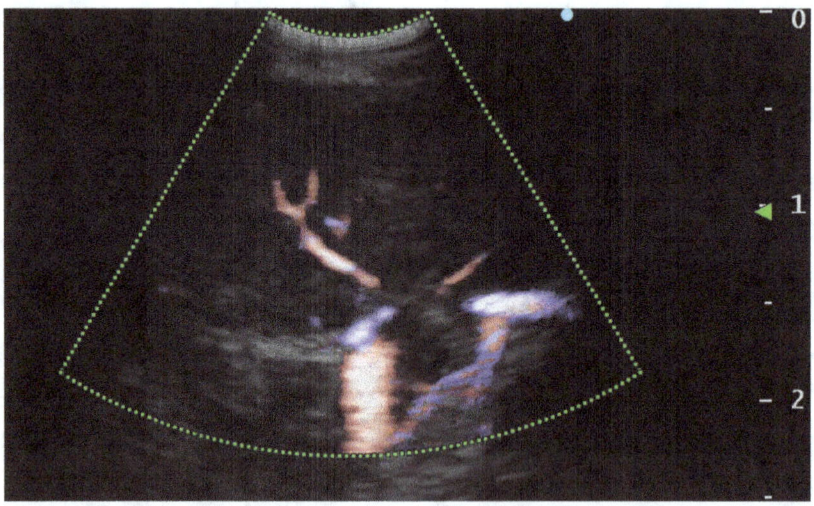

Figure 2.12 Bronchial artery in a benign lymph node.

puncturing line. The bronchial artery often passes the boundary of the proximal side of especially the #11L LN, and attention to this is required during puncturing. With benign diseases, the routes of the bronchial artery in the lymph nodes often appear dendritic (Figure 2.12), whereas they meander in the lymph nodes of patients with malignant diseases (Figure 2.13). It has been reported that EBUS using a convex bronchoscope is useful for differentiating between benign and malignant lymph nodes [1].

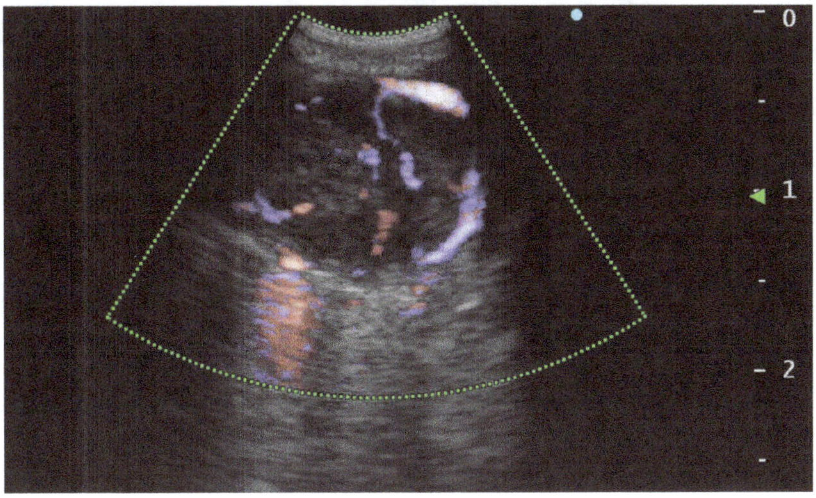

Figure 2.13 Bronchial artery in a malignant lymph node.

Reference

1 Nakajima, T., Anayama, T., Shingyoji, M. et al. (2012). Vascular image patterns of lymph nodes for the prediction of metastatic disease during EBUS-TBNA for mediastinal staging of lung cancer. *Journal of Thoracic Oncology* 7 (6): 1009–1014.

3

How to Perform Endobronchial Ultrasonography

Noriaki Kurimoto

Department of Internal Medicine, Division of Medical Oncology and Respiratory Medicine, Shimane University Faculty of Medicine, Izumo, Japan

Introduction

I first performed endobronchial ultrasonography (EBUS) in August 1994. Initially, I performed EBUS using a radial probe without a guide sheath for the diagnosis of peripheral pulmonary lesions. Guide sheaths became available in 1996 and helped with identifying the accurate location of the peripheral pulmonary lesions. Another early application of EBUS was the use of the radial probe with a balloon to visualize the layer structures of the tracheobronchial wall. In recent years, there has been a rapid increase in many countries in the use of convex probes with the bronchoscope for EBUS-guided transbronchial needle aspiration (EBUS-TBNA). In this chapter, I describe the equipment used for EBUS with a radial probe and EBUS-TBNA, along with tips for performing various procedures successfully. All equipment is from Olympus Corporation, Tokyo, Japan.

Balloon Probes for Central Lesions

Air inhibits the visualization of ultrasound images; therefore, the probe should be kept in direct contact with the bronchial wall wherever possible. Beyond the subsegmental bronchi, the outer surface of the probe fits snugly against the bronchial surface, but a balloon probe is needed to obtain EBUS images of central lesions located between the trachea and subsegmental bronchi.

Equipment

In the past, I used a 20 MHz mechanical radial ultrasonic probe (UM-3R) with a balloon-tip sheath (MH-246R). However, the diameter of the sheath was 3.6 mm, which required the use of a bronchoscope with a large-diameter channel (BF-ST40, with a working channel diameter of 3.7 mm). In recent years, I usually use a narrower 20 MHz mechanical radial ultrasonic probe (UM-BS-20-26R; see Figure 1.16) with a balloon-tip sheath (MH-676R) and a flexible bronchoscope (BF-1T260, with a working channel diameter of 2.8 mm). These probes can be connected to an endoscopic ultrasound system (EU-ME-1 and EU-ME-2).

Preparation of the Balloon Probe

To prepare the balloon probe, the ultrasonic probe is first inserted into the balloon sheath; then both are fixed in place by the connecting unit. A 25 ml syringe containing approximately

Endobronchial Ultrasonography, Second Edition. Noriaki Kurimoto, David I.K. Fielding, Ali I. Musani, Christopher Kniese, and Katsuhiko Morita.

Companion website: www.wiley.com/go/kurimoto2e

15 ml of saline is connected to the injection port in the connecting unit. Most of the air between the inner surface of the sheath and the outer surface of the probe is removed using the syringe in two or three aspirations. Saline is then injected from the syringe into the sheath and the balloon at its tip. The tip of the balloon is slightly compressed to collect the small amount of remaining air in the uppermost part of the balloon; this air is then withdrawn into the sheath. This completes the preparation of the balloon probe.

Performing EBUS Using a Balloon Probe

For all EBUS procedures using a balloon probe, we use a flexible bronchoscope (BF-1TQ290, BF-1T260) with a working channel diameter ≥2.8 mm. To avoid coughing by the patient during the procedure, we apply local anesthetic to the bronchi that the balloon probe will come into contact with. After inserting the balloon probe into the working channel of the bronchoscope, we advance it beyond the lesion and then inflate it with the minimum amount of saline required to obtain an EBUS image of the entire circumference of the bronchial wall (Figure 3.1). Scanning is performed while retracting the probe slowly in a proximal direction (i.e. toward the mouth). Advancing the probe in the other direction (distally) can damage it and should be avoided.

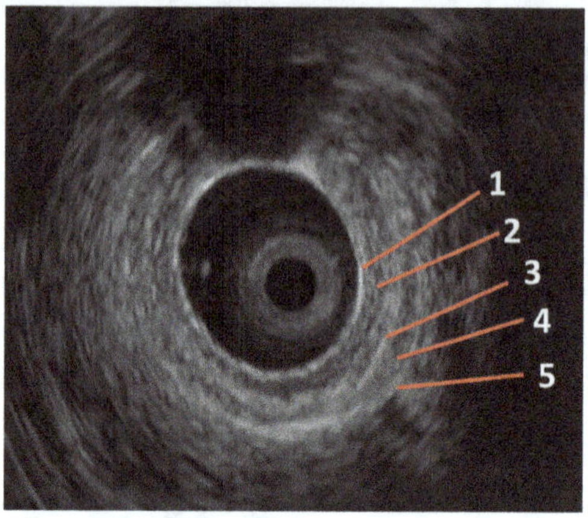

Figure 3.1 Endobronchial ultrasound (EBUS) image obtained using a balloon probe. The balloon probe is inserted into the bronchoscope working channel and inflated with the minimum volume of saline needed to obtain an EBUS image of the entire circumference of the bronchial wall. The bronchial wall is visualized as five layers.

Because the 12 o'clock direction for the EBUS image does not correspond to that of the bronchoscopic image, we routinely rotate the EBUS image to match the orientations. The correct angle to rotate the EBUS image can be judged from the peribronchial anatomy (Figure 3.2). The balloon probe is withdrawn gradually to enable the acquisition of EBUS images in the short axis of the lesion and tracheobronchial wall.

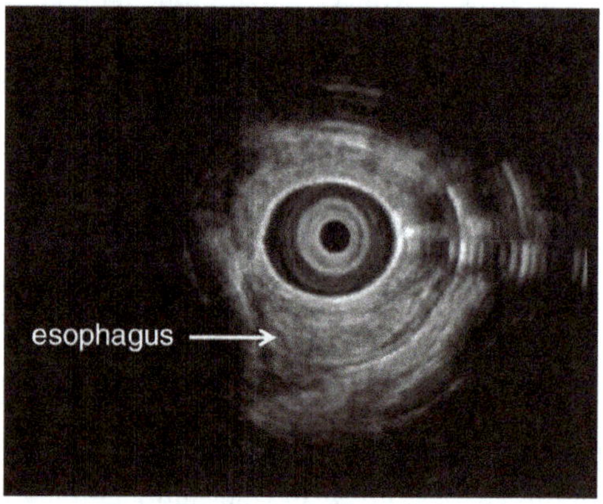

Figure 3.2 Orientation of the radial probe. The direction of the 12 o'clock position differs between the bronchoscopic and endobronchial ultrasound (EBUS) images. The peribronchial anatomy shows the correct angle to rotate the EBUS image. On this image of the left main bronchus, the location of the esophagus is posterior to the bronchus, providing the correct orientation for the radial probe.

Tips for successful EBUS using a balloon probe:

- Keep the probe at the center of the balloon. When the probe is at the center of the balloon, the ultrasound wave enters the bronchial wall perpendicularly.
- Assess the depth of the tumor at a site where the first layer is a thick hyperechoic layer. Here, the bronchial wall can be visualized clearly, with the ultrasound pulse penetrating the bronchial wall perpendicularly [1].

Bronchial lesions are often thin. This can make it difficult to ascertain whether the balloon is actually covering a lesion that has been seen bronchoscopically to allow successful ultrasound scanning. There are two ways to address this problem. The first is to confirm the presence of the lesion by placing the probe directly against it with the balloon deflated, and then to reinflate the balloon and scan the entire 360° circumference for an accurate identification of the position of the lesion. The other method is to make a 360° circumferential scan with the balloon inflated and then to retract the balloon a short way into the instrument channel, so that the bronchoscope tip indents the balloon; the positions of the probe transducer and lesion can then be directly observed through the saline-filled balloon and the lesion identified in the ultrasonic images.

Performing EBUS Using a Guide Sheath for Examining Peripheral Pulmonary Lesions

EBUS has some advantages over fluoroscopy when performing transbronchial biopsy (TBB). For example, it is not possible to use fluoroscopy to confirm whether a brush or forceps have reached the site for endobronchial brushing and TBB. Although EBUS cannot create images of normal air-filled lungs, it can delineate peripheral pulmonary lesions because only small amounts of air are in contact with the probe. Exploring bronchi with the miniature probe allows a more definitive determination of which bronchus should be selected for endobronchial brushing and TBB than is possible with fluoroscopy. EBUS is also useful for examining lesions that are difficult to visualize by fluoroscopy, such as lesions behind the mediastinum or diaphragm, ill-defined opacities, small lesions, and lesions behind other lesions. In addition, EBUS can be used to identify the bronchus most closely related to the lesion that should be subjected to biopsy. Using fluoroscopy, the probe appears to be at a slight distance from the lesion even when it is adjacent. This has been demonstrated by the definitive diagnosis of adenocarcinoma by endobronchial brushing at the site using EBUS, which suggested that the area at the margins of a lesion contained air; the margins may therefore appear normal on fluoroscopy, leading to an underestimation of the size of the lesion.

A technique we have been using since 1996 is to deploy the ultrasonic probe in a guide sheath with the active part of the probe protruding from the tip. We identify the location of the lesion ultrasonically and then pass instruments, such as brushes and biopsy forceps, down the guide sheath to collect cells or tissue specimens [2].

Equipment

For EBUS with a guide sheath (EBUS-GS), we use two miniature 20 MHz mechanical radial ultrasonic probes (UM-S20-17R and UM-S20-20R) with outer diameters (ODs) of 1.4 and 1.7 mm, respectively. The probes are connected to an endoscopic ultrasound system (EU-ME1, EU-ME2). The Guide Sheath Kit (K-201-202, K-203-204) contains a guide sheath (OD 1.95 and 2.55 mm, respectively), a disposable brush (BC-204D-2010, BC-202D-2010; OD 1.4 and 1.8 mm, respectively), and disposable biopsy forceps (FB-233D, FB-231D; OD 1.5 and 1.9 mm, respectively).

Preparation for EBUS-GS

- The bronchial brush (BC-202D-2010 or BC-204D-2010), or biopsy forceps for TBB (FB-231D or FB-233D), is introduced into the guide sheath such that the tip of the brush or forceps reaches the far end of the sheath to facilitate manipulation (Figure 3.3). The forceps are opened and closed, retrieving tissue of 4 mm from the sheath for TBB by the hinge of the forceps. During EBUS-GS, the stopper on the forceps is used to protrude the cups of the forceps out of the distal end of the sheath.

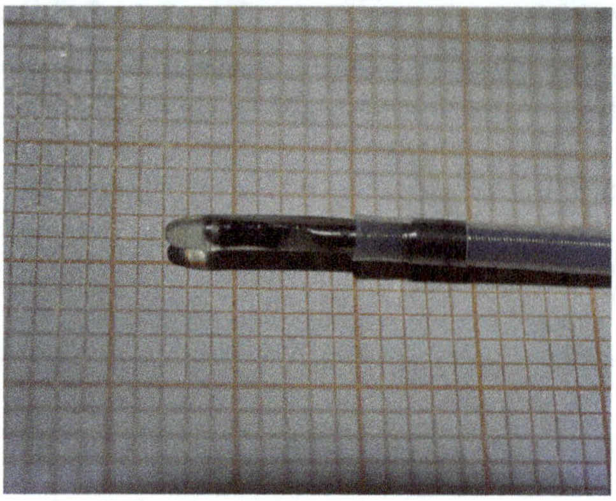

Figure 3.3 A probe and a guide sheath.

- A miniature probe is introduced into the guide sheath (SG-201C or SG-200C) until the center of the transducer at the tip of the probe protrudes at 4 mm away from the far end of the sheath. This ensures that the EBUS image will be at the same position as the biopsy site, 4 mm from the end of the sheath. The probe and sheath are then bound together at the proximal end of the sheath with the stopper, to ensure that the tip of the probe remains positioned at 4 mm far from the distal end of the sheath.

How to Perform EBUS-GS

We use a flexible bronchoscope for all procedures. When the bronchoscope is advanced beyond the vocal cords, all the segments of the bronchial tree can be visualized. The bronchus leading to the lesion is chosen by carefully studying the computed tomography (CT) image at the segment where the lesion lies, and the miniature probe with the guide sheath is negotiated into the bronchus of interest. When the lesion is small, choosing the correct bronchus can be difficult; in such cases, a list of possible fifth- or sixth-generation candidate bronchi can be made by the bronchoscopist before the procedure.

The probe is advanced until it reaches a point where the operator feels resistance, and it is then pulled back to perform the scanning. Once an EBUS image of the lesion has been obtained and the location of the lesion has been identified precisely, the probe is withdrawn, leaving the guide sheath in place.

Biopsy forceps or a bronchial brush is introduced into the sheath until the point marked by the stopper reaches the proximal end of the sheath. Under fluoroscopic guidance, the brush is moved vigorously backward and forward a few times to collect cells. After the brush is withdrawn, the biopsy forceps are once again introduced into the sheath until the stopper on the surface of the forceps reaches the proximal end of the sheath. The forceps cups are opened, the forceps advanced about 3 or 4 mm into the lesion, and the cups closed under imaging guidance. Once an adequate biopsy specimen is obtained, it is placed in formalin.

The guide sheath is left in place for approximately two minutes to exert pressure on the biopsy site to control bleeding. The procedure is concluded after confirmation that hemostasis has been achieved (Figure 3.4).

Evaluation of Diagnostic Yield Using EBUS-GS for Peripheral Pulmonary Lesions

We conducted a study to assess the ability of EBUS-GS to diagnose peripheral pulmonary lesions [2]. The overall diagnostic yield for EBUS-GS using a thick guide sheath (OD 2.5 mm) was 77% (116/150 patients), with diagnostic yields of 81% (82/101) for malignant lesions and 73% (35/45) for benign lesions. In addition, we found diagnostic yields of 60% (90/150) for brushing cytology and 70% (89/128) for TBB. The diagnostic yield when the probe was within the lesion on the ultrasound image was 87% (105/121), which was considerably better than the diagnostic yield of 42% (8/19) when the probe was adjacent to the lesion (Figure 3.5). The results showed that EBUS-GS can diagnose large and small lesions with equal accuracy, with no statistically significant difference in diagnostic yield according to lesion size; the diagnostic yields were

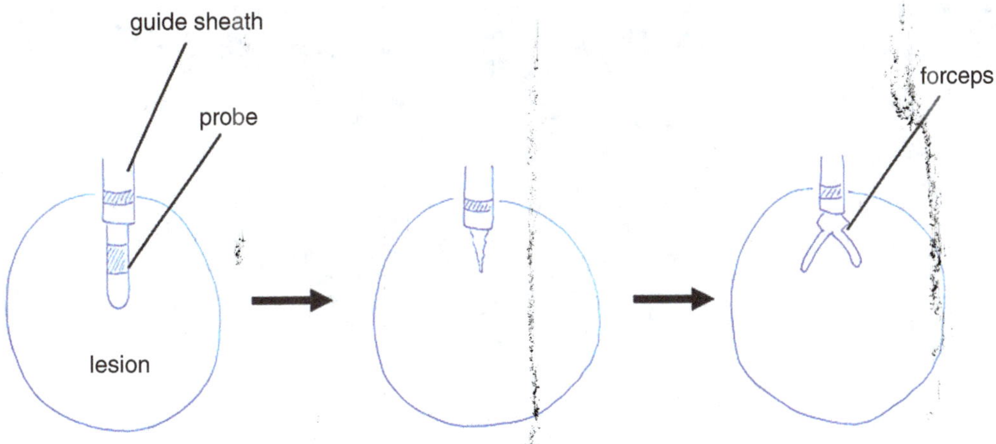

Figure 3.4 Procedure for endobronchial ultrasound with a guide sheath (EBUS-GS). Once an EBUS image of the lesion has been obtained, the probe is withdrawn, leaving the guide sheath in place. A bronchial brush or biopsy forceps is advanced into the sheath to collect cells and tissues.

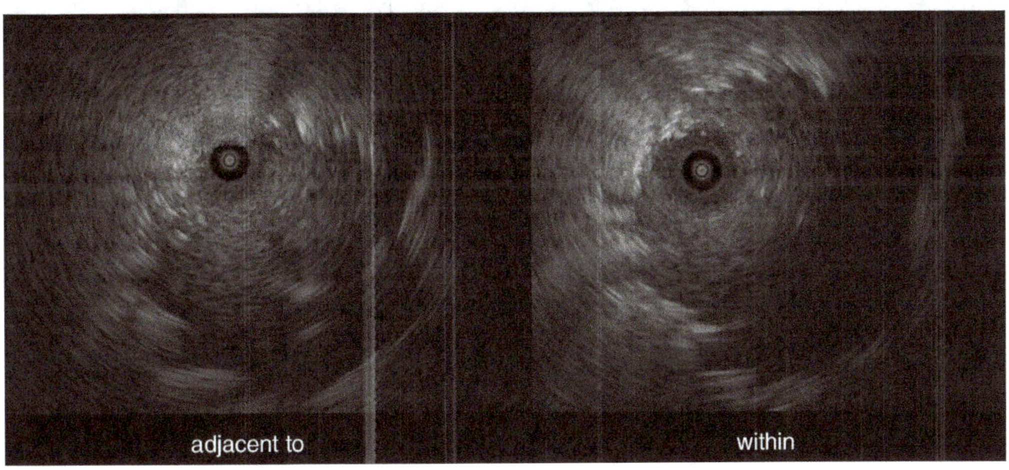

Figure 3.5 Location (adjacent to, within) of the probe in endobronchial ultrasound with a guide sheath for peripheral pulmonary lesions.

76% (16/21) for lesions ≤10 mm, 76% (19/25) for lesions >10 mm and ≤15 mm, 69% (24/35) for lesions >15 mm and ≤20 mm, and 77% (33/43) for lesions >20 mm and ≤30 mm. Notably, a high diagnostic yield of 74% (40/54) was achieved with lesions ≤20 mm, which cannot be detected using fluoroscopy.

We now achieve favorable diagnostic results using ultrasonic probes in smaller-gauge guide sheaths with smaller-diameter bronchoscopes. The route to the lesion is determined by virtual bronchoscopy using a CT-based navigation system.

Tips for Successful EBUS-GS

We suggest the following tips for using a guide sheath and for introducing the probe into the lesion.

- Use the signal attenuation caused by the guide sheath to place it accurately (Figure 3.6). This offers a method for accurately placing the guide sheath within a peripheral pulmonary lesion. The lesion should first be delineated using EBUS. Then, keeping the guide sheath stationary at the point where the lesion appears at its largest and clearest, the

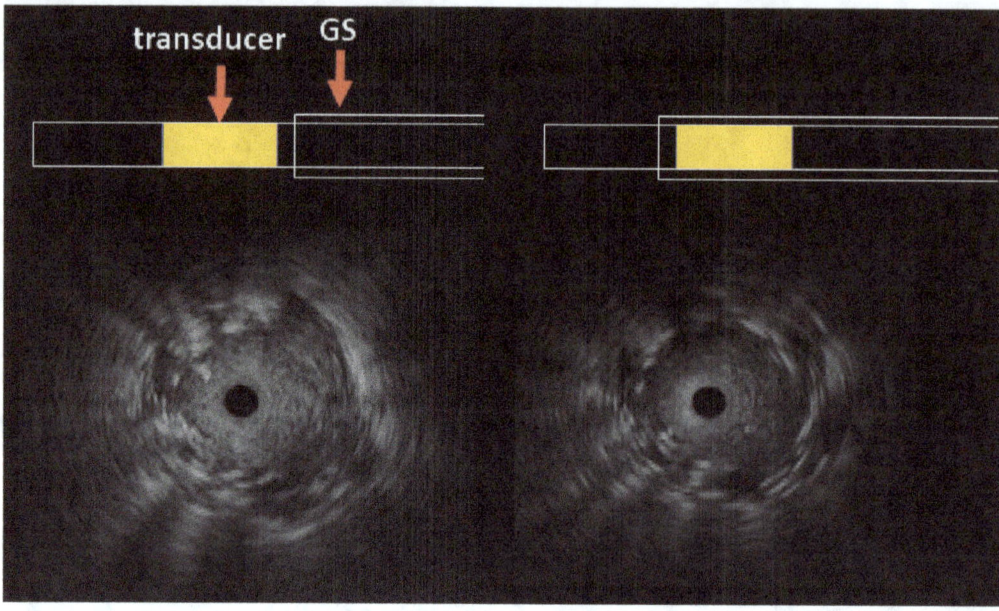

Figure 3.6 Confirmation of the location of the guide sheath (GS) within the lesion. Once a peripheral lesion has been delineated using endobronchial ultrasound, the guide sheath should be kept stationary at the point where the lesion appears at its largest and clearest, and the assistant should then withdraw the ultrasonic probe approximately 2–3 mm at a time until the probe transducer enters the guide sheath. When the transducer has completely entered the sheath, the ultrasonic pulse will be reflected by the sheath, and the ultrasound image will suddenly become darker.

assistant should undo the connection of the ultrasound probe to the guide sheath and slowly withdraw the probe 2–3 mm at a time until the probe transducer enters the guide sheath. When the transducer has completely entered the sheath, the sheath will block the ultrasonic pulse and the ultrasound image will suddenly become darker. If the site where this happens is within the peripheral pulmonary lesion, the guide sheath will have been placed precisely within the lesion.

- Move the probe and the guide sheath from adjacent to the lesion to within the lesion. In the study described earlier, we found that the diagnostic yield was superior when the probe was within the lesion than when it was adjacent to the lesion [2]. With the 4 mm diameter bronchoscopes commonly used today, when the probe is introduced into the selected sub-subsegmental bronchus to delineate a lesion using EBUS, it sometimes ends up next to the lesion rather than within it. In that case, the probe should be introduced into another sub-subsegmental bronchus in an attempt to place it within the lesion.
- When a lesion cannot be visualized with EBUS, use the lever that controls the up-down angle of the bronchoscope to bring the probe and guide sheath in the working channel closer to the lesion while looking at the monitor of fluoroscopy. Again using the up-down lever, pull back the probe and guide sheath and insert it toward the lesion; the probe and guide sheath then sometimes reaches the lesion (see Figure 9.2).
- If the probe and guide sheath end up at a position adjacent to the peripheral pulmonary lesion, try to move them to a location within the lesion. Using the bronchoscope's up-down lever, move the probe and guide sheath through the working channel to a position closer to the lesion on the EBUS

image. When the probe and guide sheath are close to the lesion, pull them from the lesion and insert them in the back; then, try to reach within the lesion.

- When using the bronchoscope's up–down lever, the probe and guide sheath may move in a direction tangential to the boundary of the lesion on the EBUS image. If this happens, it is sometimes possible, when rotating the bronchoscope and applying the up–down lever to move the probe and guide sheath closer to the lesion, to insert them within the lesion by withdrawing them proximally and then advancing them distally to reach the lesion.

Main benefits of EBUS-GS

- It can accurately determine the position of lesions.
- Forceps can be introduced any number of times to the same site.
- It allows analysis of the internal structure of the lesion.
- There is very little post-TBB bleeding.

EBUS-TBNA

Equipment

For EBUS-TBNA, we use a convex bronchoscope (see Figure 1.22) connected to an endoscopic ultrasound system (EU-ME1, EU-ME2).

How to Perform EBUS-TBNA

We usually perform EBUS-TBNA with a topical pharyngeal anesthesia and sedation (e.g. midazolam). The assistant elevates the patient's jaw to maximize the pharyngeal space, and the convex bronchoscope is inserted into the pharynx, keeping the 12 o'clock position of the vocal cord under close observation to ensure that the larynx is passed smoothly because this scope has an oblique forward view.

Another way of introducing the bronchoscope into the trachea is to insert an endotracheal tube, leaving this in place for the duration of the procedure. An 8.0–8.5 Fr endotracheal tube is placed over the commonly used bronchoscope, and the tip of the bronchoscope is introduced into the trachea. With the end of the patient's jaw elevated, the endotracheal tube is introduced into the trachea using the bronchoscope as a guide. The advantage of this method of intubation is that emergency treatment for hemorrhages can be administered even if the visual field is obscured by blood on the bronchoscope lens.

While the location of the lesion is assessed on chest CT, the inflated balloon containing the probe should be in contact with the bronchial wall adjacent to the lesion. The target lesion is clearly outlined by EBUS. By rotating the bronchoscope on its axis slightly in each direction, the transducer at its tip will scan and delineate the entire target lesion, allowing the size of the lesion to be measured (Figure 3.7).

First, B-mode scanning is used to determine whether the internal echoes of the lesion to be punctured are homogeneous or heterogeneous. Power Doppler mode should then be used to scan the target lesion and the path that the needle is expected to traverse. This additional information should help to avoid the unintended puncture of any small vessels and bronchial arteries interposed between the bronchial wall and target lesion. Sometimes, the target lesion is a lymph node with necrotic areas. In this case, optional power Doppler mode scanning will show the necrotic areas with reduced blood flow, which are to be avoided, and identify regions with tortuous blood flow (in 1 mm vessels) within the target lesion that is to be punctured.

The Doppler effect describes the phenomenon where the frequency of sound increases when the source of the sound moves toward the observer and decreases when the source moves away. Because of the movement of blood, the Doppler mode of an ultrasound processor enables the visualization of blood vessels on the EBUS images. The color Doppler mode shows vessels according to the speed and

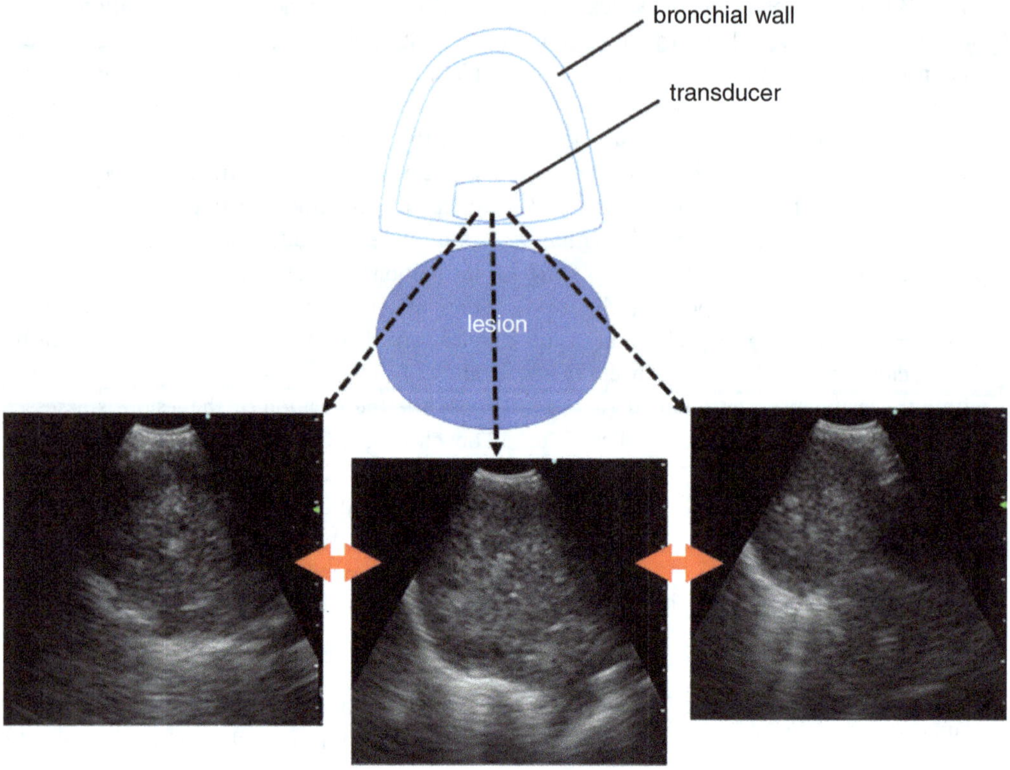

Figure 3.7 Rotating the convex bronchoscope to delineate the target lesion. The target lesion is clearly outlined by endobronchial ultrasound. By rotating the bronchoscope on its axis a little in each direction, the transducer at its tip will scan and delineate the entire target lesion.

direction of the bloodstream, with vessels approaching the ultrasound probe appearing in red and those moving away from the ultrasound probe appearing in blue.

Doppler mode is prepared by selecting the best Doppler gain. To do this, the assistant should increase the Doppler gain to show noise on the Doppler image (Figure 3.8 – 1, 2) and then reduce the Doppler gain until the noise fades away, at which point the Doppler gain should be stopped immediately on the Doppler image (Figure 3.8 – 3).

During puncture, the transducer must constantly be held in firm contact with the tracheobronchial wall. The needle should be prepared immediately before performing the puncture and then inserted into the working channel of the bronchoscope, watching until the edge of the outer sheath just protrudes from the bronchoscope. The stylet is then withdrawn a few centimeters to expose the sharp needle. With the needle we used to use (Vizishot), the outer sheath often protruded too far when the needle was advanced. To overcome this problem, we pushed the needle anteriorly within the bronchus so that when it neared the tip of the outer sheath, the sheath approached the transducer; through the bronchoscope, we could see the tip of the outer sheath suddenly drop down a millimeter or so. The needle was stopped at this point, and the outer sheath was withdrawn once again until the tip of the sheath could just be seen through the bronchoscope. Now, when the needle was advanced, the puncture could be performed with almost no movement of the outer sheath. When using the currently

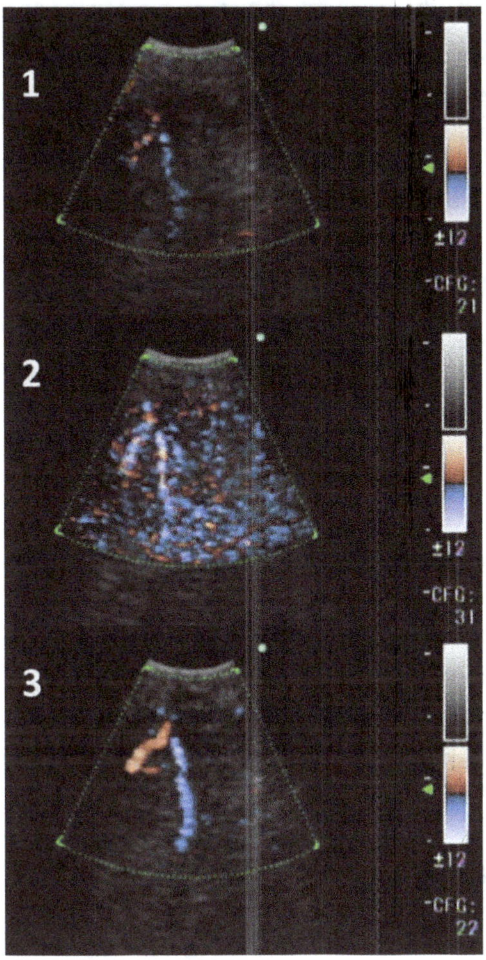

Figure 3.8 Preparation of Doppler mode. The Doppler gain should be increased until noise appears on the Doppler image (1, 2) and then reduced until the noise fades, at which point the Doppler gain should be stopped immediately on the Doppler image (3).

available aspiration needle (Vizishot2), the outer sheath does not protrude when the needle is advanced. This means that the needle no longer needs to be prepared as just described.

The tip of the outer sheath is then advanced toward the bronchial wall, aiming for the membranous part between cartilages. A tip for locating the tip of the outer sheath of the needle between cartilages is first to push the outer sheath of the needle against the bronchial wall, and then to push and pull the scope to select the position between the cartilages with the tip of the outer sheath [3]. This step is of great importance for a successful puncture. The needle is placed against the tracheobronchial wall and target lesion. The needle, with the partially withdrawn stylet, is then advanced into the lesion under real-time ultrasound guidance. Before the stylet is withdrawn, the stylet is repositioned to remove the primary tissue plug containing superficial layers and bronchial cartilage from the needle. Suction is then applied through the needle using a 10 or 20 ml syringe. The needle is advanced further into the lesion and moved back and forth under ultrasound control; usually, 5–10 strokes within the lesion is sufficient. With the tip of the needle still within the lesion, suction is equilibrated. The needle is then withdrawn and removed with the outer sheath.

To retrieve the tissue sample from the needle, the stylet is inserted into the needle and the sample emerges from the needle tip. This is deposited on a piece of filter paper to facilitate the histopathological examination. Any cellular material remaining inside the needle is then flushed out using air from the syringe and sent off for cytological examination.

New Functions of Ultrasound Processors

There have been some developments to ultrasound processors.

Tissue Harmonic Echo

Some strains and harmonic components occur while the ultrasound wave transmits through organs. Harmonic components are produced from main lobes; then, harmonic components reduce artifacts from side lobes. Tissue harmonic echo visualizes these harmonic components of ultrasound waves and provides fine EBUS images with reduced artifacts (see Figure 1.24).

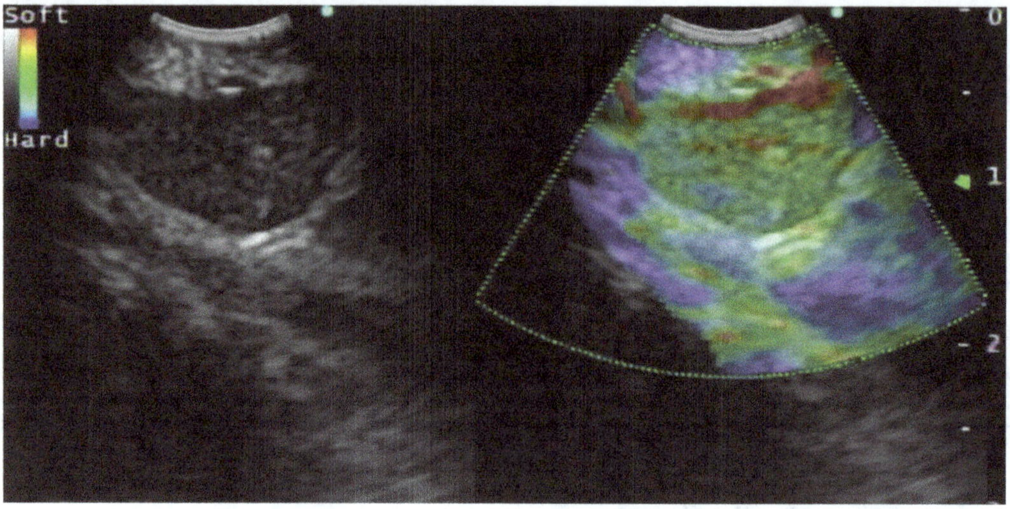

Figure 3.9 Elastography of a subcarinal lymph node with sarcoidosis. The lymph node is shown as homogeneous green, suggesting it to be a soft lymph node.

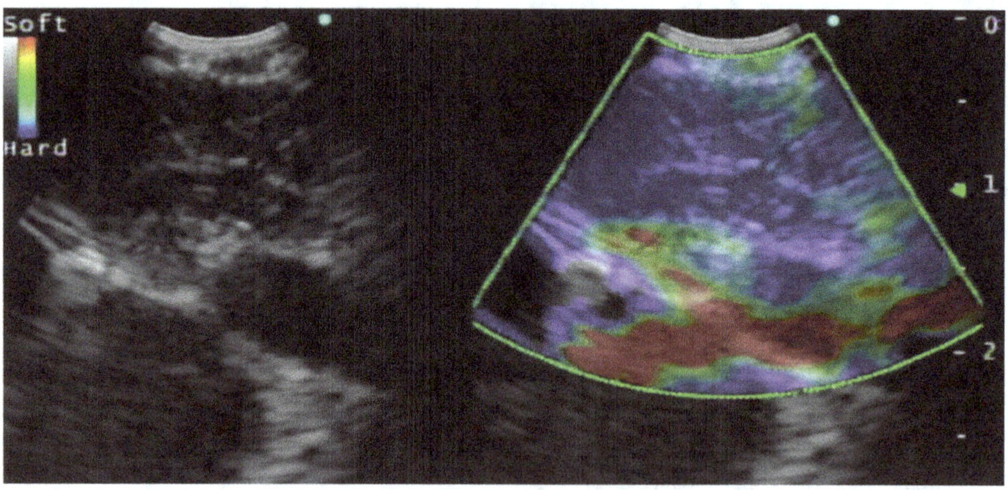

Figure 3.10 Elastography of a subcarinal lymph node with metastasis. The lymph node is shown as homogeneous blue, suggesting it to be a hard lymph node.

Elastography

Elasticity refers to the recovery of the shape of a substance when it has been deformed by an external force and then the force is removed. Tissue elasticity is an important characteristic for evaluating tissue and an important diagnostic factor closely related to pathological findings. Most cancerous lesions are harder and less elastic than normal tissue.

Elastography is an imaging technology for visualizing and assessing elasticity. On the colored ultrasound strain image, which is superimposed on the B-mode image, each area is colored according to the amount of strain. Blue indicates areas that are relatively hard (inelastic), whereas green and red show relatively soft (i.e. elastic) areas. Figures 3.9 and 3.10 show examples of strain images for sarcoidosis and metastasis, respectively.

References

1 Kurimoto, N., Murayama, M., Yoshioka, S. et al. (1999). Assessment of the usefulness of endobronchial ultrasonography in tracheobronchial depth diagnosis. *Chest* 115: 1500–1506.

2 Kurimoto, N., Miyazawa, T., Okimasa, S. et al. (2004). Endobronchial ultrasonography using a guide sheath increases the ability to diagnose peripheral pulmonary lesions endoscopically. *Chest* 126: 959–965.

3 Inoue, T., Kurimoto, N., Furuya, N. et al. (2013). New technique for endobronchial ultrasound-guided transbronchial needle aspiration to improve diagnostic yield. *Journal of Bronchology and Interventional Pulmonology* 20 (1): 28–32.

4

Endobronchial Ultrasound-Guided Transbronchial Needle Aspiration

Christopher Kniese[1] *and Ali I. Musani*[2]

[1] *Indiana University School of Medicine, Indianapolis, IN, USA*
[2] *Division of Pulmonary Sciences & Critical Care Medicine, University of Colorado School of Medicine, Denver, CO, USA*

Anatomy

The nomenclature for mediastinal lymph nodes involves both anatomic descriptions and a numeric system, with the letters "R" and "L" signifying right and left, respectively. In 2009, the International Association for the Study of Lung Cancer (IASLC) released a proposal to establish this system in order to standardize the way lymph nodes are described, released concurrent with the seventh edition of the tumor, node, metastasis (TNM) staging system [1]. While the TNM system has been recently updated to the eighth edition, this naming system remains in place [2]. Despite this, there are still discrepancies in the way these lymph nodes are described, particularly within different geographic realms. In the United States there is still a tendency to use anatomic location to describe the nodes, whereas in Europe and Asia they generally use the international nomenclature. Figure 4.1 shows the tracheobronchial tree with associated mediastinal and hilar lymph node structures using both the anatomic locations and numeric stations. It is important that providers are comfortable with both of these naming systems to ensure clear communication with other colleagues in the field.

The lymph node stations accessible using endobronchial ultrasound-guided transbronchial needle aspiration (EBUS-TBNA) include the following: highest mediastinal (station 1), upper paratracheal (stations 2R and 2L), lower paratracheal (stations 4R and 4L), subcarinal (station 7), hilar (stations 10R and 10L), interlobar (stations 11R and 11L), and lobar (stations 12R and 12L). Refer to Figure 4.1 for further reference.

There are some important discrepancies between the US and international nomenclatures. For example, station 4L (left lower paratracheal) is often incorrectly referred to as the aortopulmonary (AP) window node, given its position between the aorta and pulmonary artery on ultrasound. However, the true AP window node is station 5, which sits a few centimeters from the trachea, and is thus not accessible via EBUS-TBNA. In addition, station 11 nodes are often referred to as hilar nodes in the United States, whereas the international nomenclature labels these nodes interlobar, given their location adjacent to the takeoff of the upper lobes bilaterally. Station 10

Endobronchial Ultrasonography, Second Edition. Noriaki Kurimoto, David I.K. Fielding, Ali I. Musani, Christopher Kniese, and Katsuhiko Morita.

Companion website: www.wiley.com/go/kurimoto2e

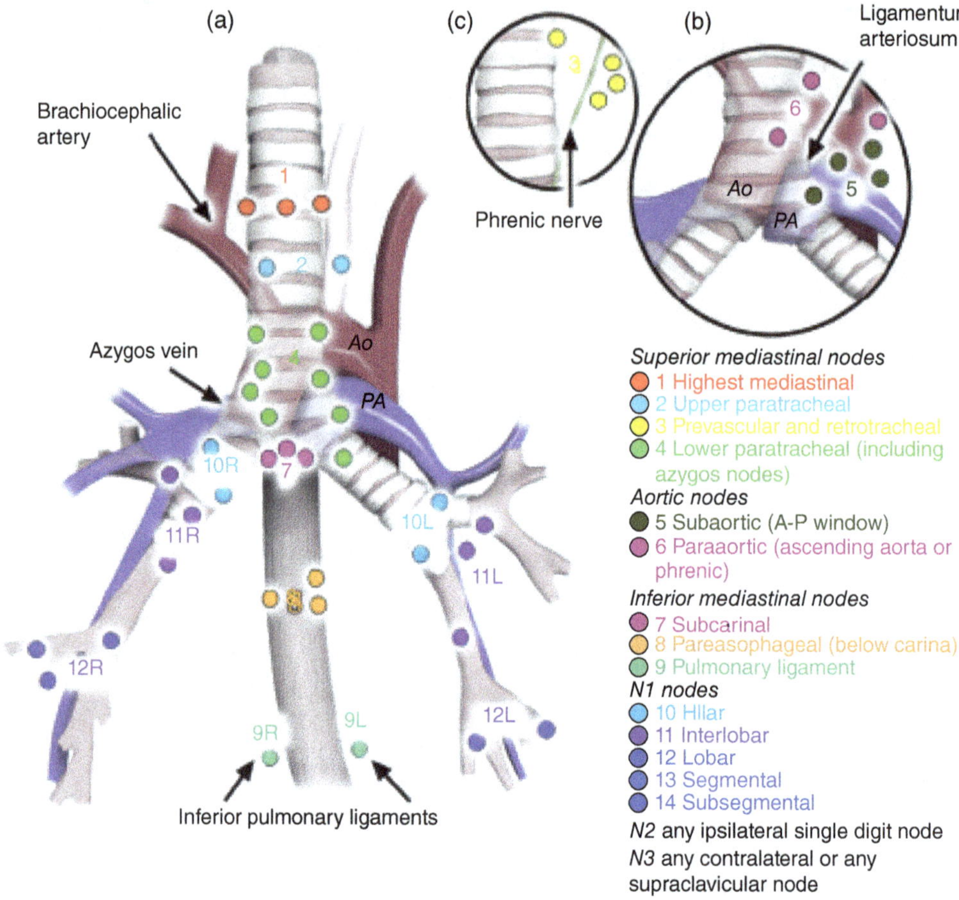

Figure 4.1 (a) Anterior view of mediastinal lymph node stations in relation to major airways and vascular structure. (b) Lateral view of stations 5 and 6 in relation to aorta and main pulmonary artery. (c) Station 3 node along trachea with close proximity to phrenic nerve.

lymph nodes, on the other hand, represent true hilar nodes.

Lymph node stations are not the only important anatomic structures adjacent to the airways. There are several vital vascular structures, and their location relative to the airways and lymph node stations should be committed to memory. Figures 4.2–4.6 demonstrate various portions of the tracheobronchial tree with the adjacent vascular structures. The ascending aorta lies anterior and subsequently runs along the left side of the distal trachea, then curves around the left hilum and begins descending in posterior fashion (Figures 4.2 and 4.3). The main pulmonary artery also lies anterior to the left side of the distal trachea, then bifurcates near the carina, with the right and left main branches running along the right and left mainstem bronchi, respectively (Figures 4.3 and 4.4). The pulmonary arteries then divide into smaller branches mimicking the branches of the distal airways (Figure 4.4). Station 7, which can be accessed via either mainstem bronchus, lies just below the carina (Figures 4.5 and 4.6), with the left atrium often visible behind the lymph node structures. It is vital to understand this anatomy so that TBNA can safely be performed at the various lymph node stations, with care taken to avoid injury to these vascular structures.

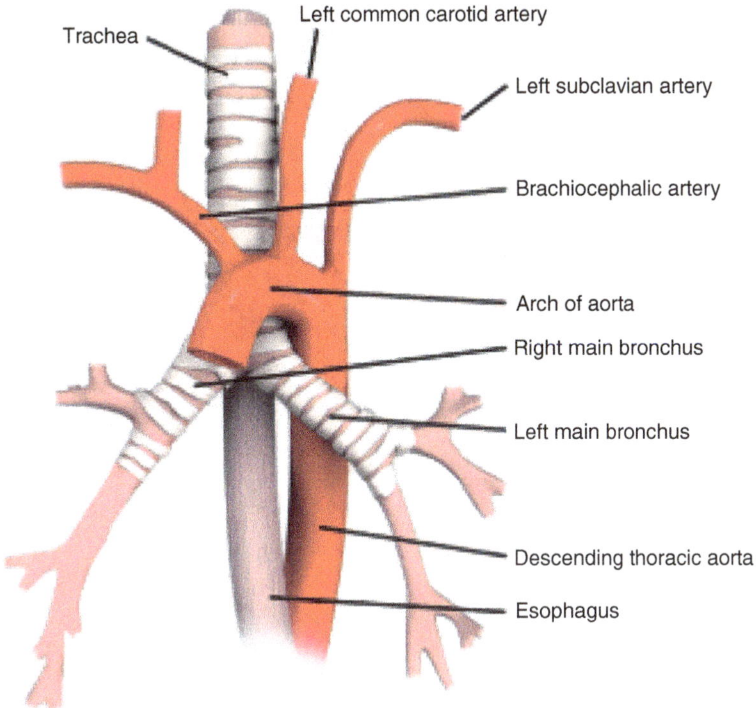

Figure 4.2 Anatomy of trachea and major airways in relation to the arch of aorta and its main branches, anterior view.

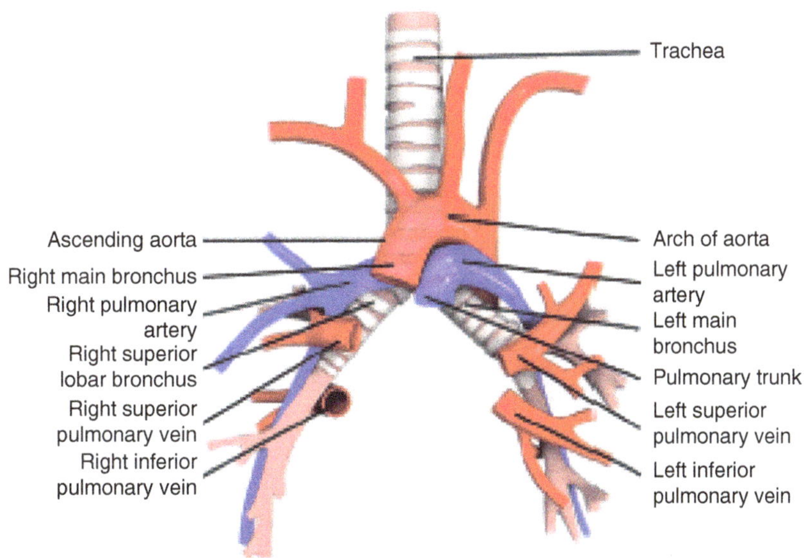

Figure 4.3 Anatomy of major airways in relation to aorta, pulmonary artery, pulmonary vein, and their branches.

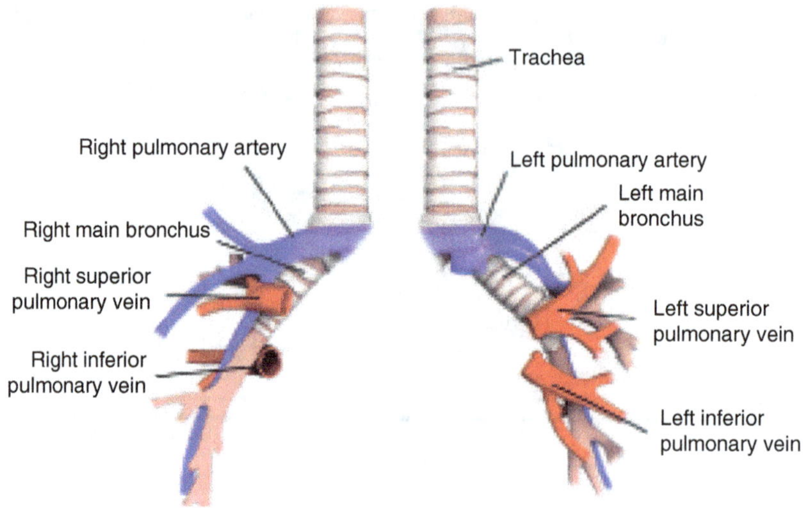

Figure 4.4 Anatomy of trachea and bilateral main stem bronchi with major vessels.

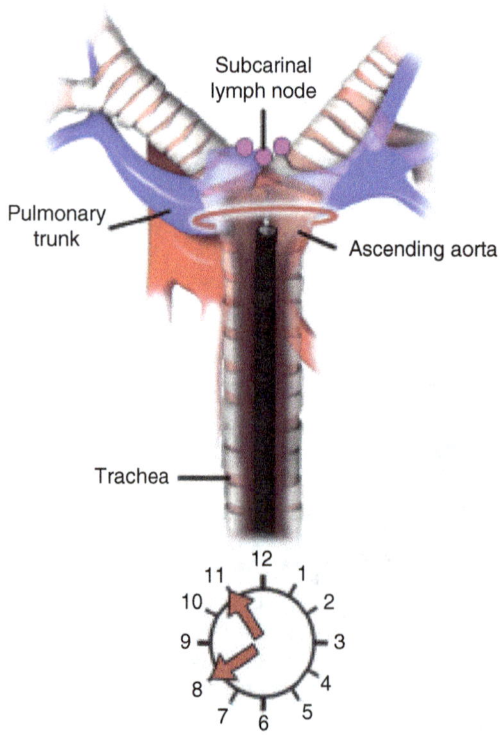

Figure 4.5 Locations of subcarinal (station 7) lymph nodes in relation to trachea, main stem bronchi, aorta, and pulmonary artery. The anatomic clock at the bottom shows unsafe areas for needle insertion by red arrows pointing in that direction.

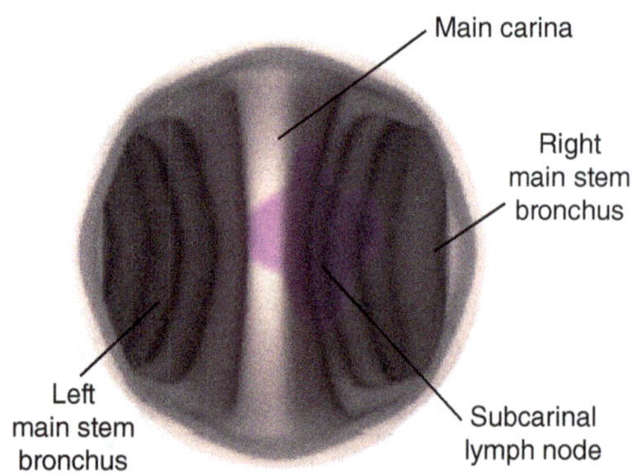

Figure 4.6 Endotracheal and endobronchial area is highlighted to show the proper site for needle insertion for subcarinal node transbronchial needle aspiration.

Transbronchial Needle Aspiration (TBNA)

TBNA was traditionally performed without imaging guidance, termed conventional transbronchial needle aspiration (c-TBNA; see Figure 4.7). However, the diagnostic yield of this procedure was widely variable across different studies and was historically dependent on the skill level of the bronchoscopist. TBNA

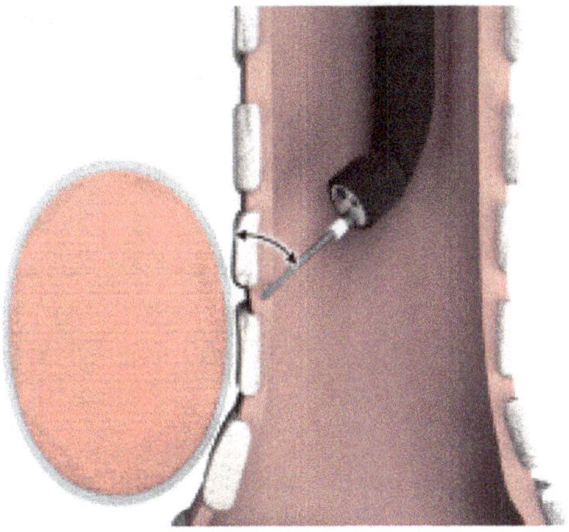

Figure 4.7 Transbronchial needle aspiration: the needle is passed through the airway wall in between the cartilage, with an angle as perpendicular as possible. The lymph node or mass lying outside of the airways is traversed blindly or under ultrasound guidance.

without EBUS required knowledge of the mediastinal anatomy, including location of lymphatic structures, and willingness to biopsy these structures without real-time imaging guidance. Recent studies have shown some significant improvement in the diagnostic yield of TBNA when performed with ultrasound guidance, termed EBUS-TBNA. The AQuIRE study, published in 2011, demonstrated that the diagnostic yield of EBUS-TBNA is heterogeneous across different institutions, with higher-volume centers reporting higher yield [3]. EBUS-TBNA, like other forms of bronchoscopy, can be performed through either the nasal or oral routes, although given the larger size of the scope, the oral route is more routinely used [3, 4]. In addition, a recent study has shown similar diagnostic yield and risk of major complications with EBUS-TBNA performed with either general anesthesia or moderate sedation, thus choice of sedation technique often depends on individual patient factors and local practice [5].

As previously mentioned, the success of EBUS-TBNA depends heavily on operator experience. A recent study evaluating trainees in interventional pulmonology demonstrated that "expert level skill" was obtained by trainees for efficiency and correct lymph node identification after a median of 212 and 164 procedures, respectively [6]. This study was performed at large academic centers and may not represent experience at non-academic centers; regardless, this suggests a substantial learning curve with EBUS-TBNA.

Several recent studies have assessed EBUS-TBNA with c-TBNA. One such study, published in 2017, suggested that the overall yield of EBUS-TBNA was similar to that of c-TBNA, while a staged approach (using c-TBNA and if initial on-site examination was negative, then EBUS-TBNA) may be better than either approach alone [7]. A separate study showed that in patients with initial non-diagnostic c-TBNA examinations, follow-up EBUS-TBNA significantly increased yield, in both benign and malignant disease [8].

Mediastinoscopy has long been held as the gold standard for staging of non-small cell lung cancer (NSCLC). However, a recent study from Korea (single-center, prospective trial) showed EBUS-TBNA had superior sensitivity, accuracy, and negative predictive value compared to mediastinoscopy [9]. Given the less invasive nature of EBUS-TBNA, the authors recommended it as the first-line procedure for mediastinal staging. However, this was a single-center trial. A prospective, multicenter randomized control trial comparing the two strategies is currently ongoing [10]. A separate recent trial demonstrated similar survival and improved cost-effectiveness of an endosonographic approach as compared to a surgical staging approach in patients with NSCLC [11]. Likewise, EBUS-TBNA can be used to provide tissue sampling for molecular markers, which is an integral part of modern lung cancer treatment [12].

EBUS-TBNA can play a role in mediastinal adenopathy outside of lung cancer as well. EBUS-TBNA is a useful tool in the diagnosis and subtyping of mediastinal lymphoma [13, 14]. As in previous instances, the minimally invasive nature of EBUS compared to surgical lymph node biopsy makes it an attractive option in this case. Likewise, the role of EBUS in sarcoidosis has recently been studied. EBUS-TBNA appears to be superior to c-TBNA in sarcoidosis, with a demonstrated yield of 75–80% [15, 16]. It remains to be seen whether combining EBUS-TBNA with rapid on-site cytologic evaluation (ROSE) will improve yield further [17].

In order to use EBUS-TBNA to its maximum potential, the bronchoscopist must first hone his or her standard TBNA skills. EBUS merely provides real-time images to prevent non-nodal needle insertion. Good samples ultimately depend on good TBNA technique, and the feeling of EBUS-TBNA is very similar to standard TBNA, albeit with the added benefit of visualization. Comfort with standard TBNA removes much of the "mystery" about EBUS-TBNA and makes clear the intuitive aspects of the design of the EBUS-TBNA needle. In the following section, the knowledge and instruments necessary for successful TBNA are briefly reviewed.

Needles

TBNA needles generally range in size from 19 to 22 gauge (G), although 25 G needles have been trialed in certain settings. Needle length usually varies from 13 to 15 mm, and needle stiffness varies depending on the manufacturer (see Figure 4.8).

There are few evidence-based guidelines governing choice of needle size, but a common convention is to start with a smaller-gauge needle (21 or 22 G) for the initial puncture, then progress to larger sizes if initial samples are deemed inadequate. This helps to confirm the safety of the biopsy site. If desired, larger-bore needles (19 G) or histology needles can then be employed.

Certain conditions may dictate the use of a larger needle. For example, lymphoma and sarcoid are two conditions in which tissue architecture plays an integral role in making the diagnosis. As such, many providers opt for larger needles (such as 19 G) when these are suspected. Interestingly, a large retrospective study from the AQuIRE registry compared sample adequacy between specimens obtained with 21 and 22 G needles, and found no significant difference, although the combination of 21 G needle and ROSE led to fewer needle passes [18]. Many new needle products are in development, and the use of needle forceps for mediastinal lymph node sampling has been preliminarily studied [19].

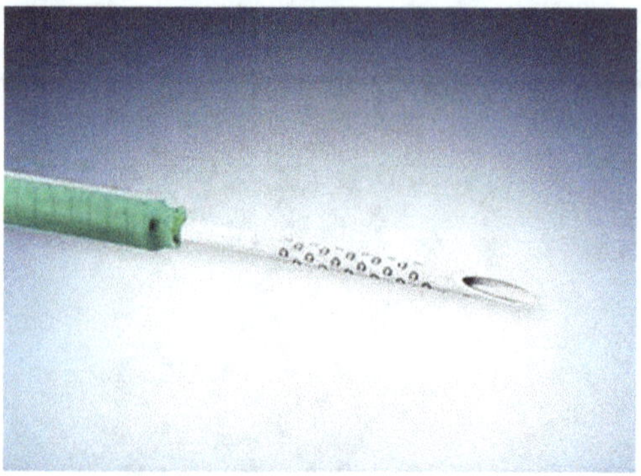

Figure 4.8 An example of an endobronchial ultrasound-guided transbronchial needle aspiration (EBUS-TBNA) needle with associated catheter, the ViziShot 2 Needle (Olympus America). Source: Image obtained with permission from http://medical.olympusamerica.com/products/vizishot2-ebus-tbna-needles.

Planning the Procedure

The chest computed tomography (CT) scan, ideally with intravenous contrast, should be thoroughly reviewed prior to the planned procedure. Some prefer to reverse the CT image so that anatomic structures will be viewed in the same orientation they will appear during bronchoscopy. Contrast-enhanced CT should allow for detailed evaluation of lymph nodes, and their relationship to nearby airways and vascular structures. All of the nodal stations should be assessed, and a strategic plan to approach different stations in order of preference should be made.

When lung malignancy is suspected, one should always attempt to sample the node that would provide the highest stage first, as this can potentially limit the number of sites that need to be sampled, thus exposing the patient to less cumulative risk. This requires knowledge of the nodal stations and their respective designations per the TNM staging system (N1, N2, and N3 nodes). For example, in a patient with a 1 cm left upper lobe nodule (T1 disease) and adenopathy at left lower paratracheal (4L), subcarinal (7), and right lower paratracheal (4R), the station 4R node should be sampled first, as this would represent N3 disease, whereas stations 7 and 4L would both be N2 disease. This is significant, given that the presence of N3 disease, regardless of tumor status, would upstage the patient to IIIB. Figure 4.9 shows a representative CT from a patient with a large right upper lobe mass and associated mediastinal adenopathy.

This approach allows one to diagnose and stage the patient appropriately in a single, minimally invasive, outpatient procedure and precludes unnecessary surgical staging. If the highest station lymph nodes cannot successfully be sampled, then one should proceed to the next highest station, and so on. It is generally accepted that one can continue using the same needle if prior sites were negative. However, if another site, such as the primary tumor, has already been sampled, then a separate needle should be employed to reduce the risk of tumor contamination of the needle and false-positive staging [20].

Insertion Technique

The four most common techniques for needle insertion during TBNA described in the literature are the so-called hub, jab, piggy-back, and cough techniques. The technique used is purely a matter of personal preference. I prefer the hub technique, mainly because it is safer and easier to teach. The "hub" technique (Figure 4.10) involves placing the hub of the needle and catheter at the desired insertion site, watching for needle movement during a few respiratory cycles, and pushing the needle out while holding the scope and hub in place. The "jab" technique (Figure 4.11) involves first advancing the needle out of the catheter and then entering the target area by pushing the catheter down while holding the scope in place. The "piggy-back" technique (Figure 4.12) entails having the needle out of the catheter while the catheter is outside of the working channel of the scope, at a fixed distance from the site in the airway lumen. The entire scope is then advanced to the target in one motion.

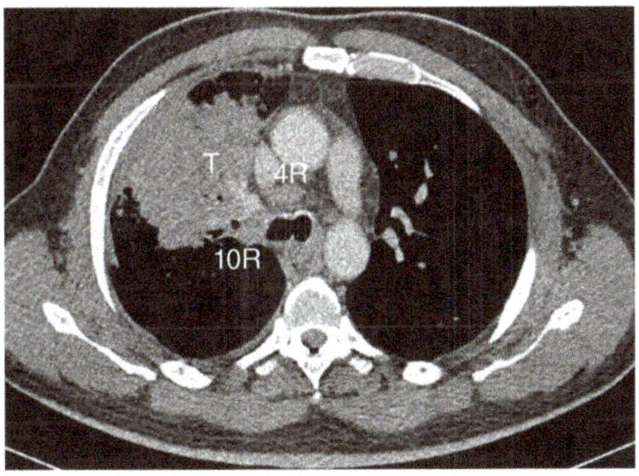

Figure 4.9 Axial cut of computed tomography (CT) chest demonstrating a large right upper lobe mass (T), with mediastinal adenopathy at stations 10R (N1 disease) and 4R (N2 disease).

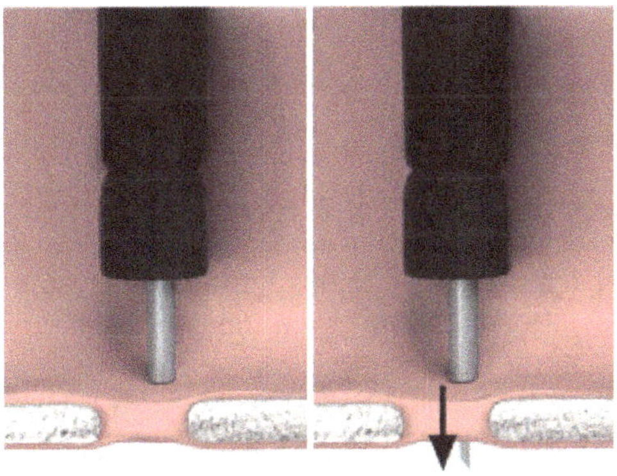

Figure 4.10 Hub technique – by placing the hub of the needle at the desired site of insertion, the needle is pushed out while holding the scope and the catheter in place.

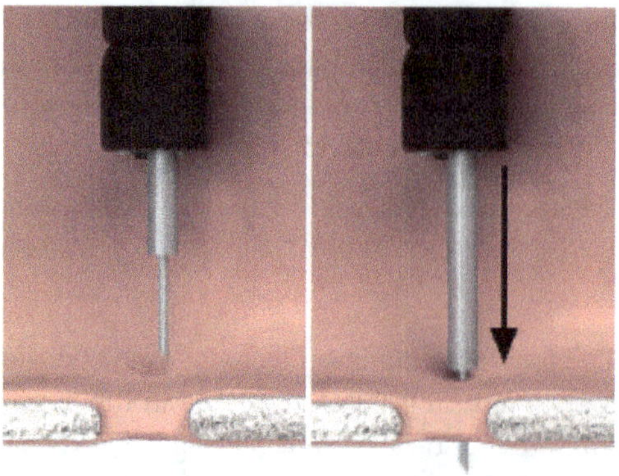

Figure 4.11 Jab technique – having the needle out of the catheter and then entering the target area by pushing the catheter down while holding the scope in place.

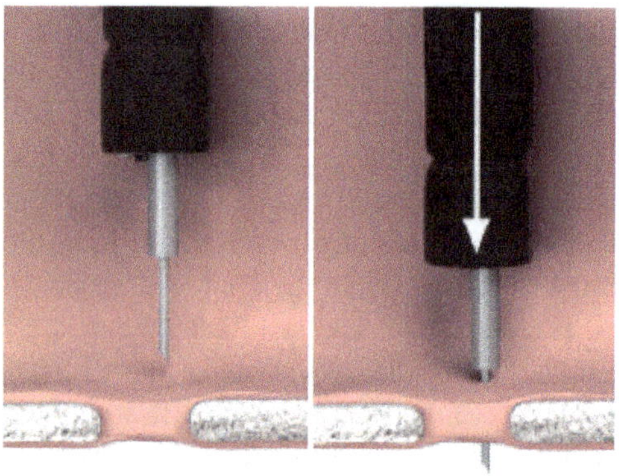

Figure 4.12 Piggy-back technique – having the needle out of the catheter while holding the catheter out of the working channel at a fixed distance in the lumen of the airway. The scope is then driven down into the target by the operator as one unit.

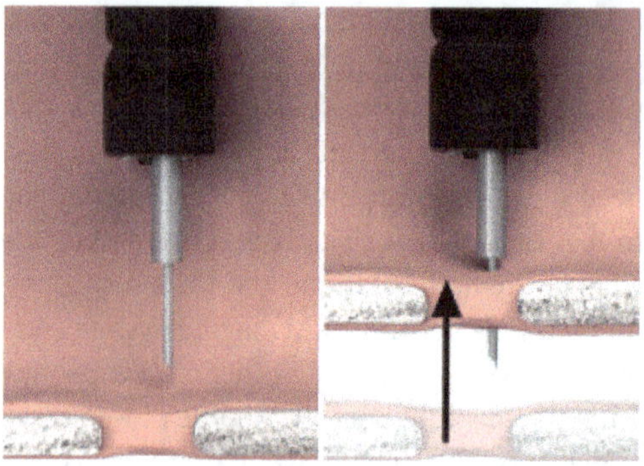

Figure 4.13 Cough technique – the patient is asked to cough while the needle is held in a steady position on the airway wall. The cough brings the airway wall onto the needle, allowing it to penetrate the tissue.

Lastly, the "cough" technique (Figure 4.13) requires a relatively awake and cooperative patient. In this technique the patient is asked to cough while the needle (outside of the catheter) is held in a steady position on the airway wall. The cough brings the airway wall onto the needle, allowing it to penetrate into the tissue.

Regardless of technique, the needle is generally inserted with the stylet in place. However, a recent study has shown that the presence or absence of the stylet may not have a significant impact on diagnostic yield [21]. Once the needle is firmly in place, the stylet is typically "jostled" to remove bronchial epithelial tissue from the needle that could contaminate the specimen, and then removed. It is generally recommended that one only jostle the stylet once or twice, as research has suggested that metal contamination is possible in needle specimens and may become more likely with increase repeated stylet manipulation [22]. Once the stylet is removed, many bronchoscopists opt to apply suction to the needle. While studies have shed doubt on the notion that this increases diagnostic yield, it does help to confirm the avascular nature of the insertion site [23]. If bloody return is seen, then suction should be removed immediately, and the needle should be retracted and removed from the working channel in order to allow suction in case bleeding from the site is encountered. A common practice is to apply suction on the first pass, and if a bloody specimen is obtained, then perform subsequent passes without suction. In general, bleeding in these situations is minor and resolves spontaneously. Once bleeding stops, another attempt can be made, albeit in a different location.

Once the needle is in the desired tissue, and the site is confirmed to be avascular, a rapid and shallow in-and-out motion is used to obtain the sample. Throughout this motion, the scope should remain fixed at the patient's nose or mouth. It may help to have an assistant hold the scope for this purpose. Motion should be deliberate and swift. The scope should be kept straight between the patient and the operator's hand, as slack or curvature in the scope will cause much of the jabbing motion to be lost before it reaches the needle. I commonly jab between five and ten times during each TBNA pass. Suction should be released before pulling the needle back into the catheter to prevent aspirating bronchial cells on the way out. Once the needle is fully inside the catheter, it can then be removed from the working channel of the scope. Care must be taken to ensure that the needle is fully inside the catheter when going in and out of the working channel, otherwise the scope can be lacerated. Once the needle assembly is removed, the bronchoscopist should deliberately pause to clear any secretions from the tip of the scope, to allow as clear a view as possible for subsequent TBNA attempts. It is now widely accepted that when evaluating lymph nodes, particularly during mediastinal staging for suspected or confirmed malignancy, each lymph node should be sampled three times to ensure adequate sensitivity [24].

Sample Handling

Cytopathology in the setting of EBUS will be discussed elsewhere in this text. If available, ROSE may allow for deferring additional biopsy passes without sacrificing diagnostic yield, ultimately lowering procedural risk. In addition, it appears to be cost-effective [25]. If ROSE is available, the needle sample should be transferred directly to slides. If possible, two slides from each pass can be made; the first for Diff-Quik, the second for hematoxylin and eosin (H&E) stain. The air-drying method is employed to prepare the slides. The remaining sample is then expressed from the needle and into a saline container for cell block. First saline, then air is used to purge the needle of all specimen. This prevents clotting and maximizes the tissue sample available for evaluation. This process is generally repeated for every needle specimen, although in the event of a positive specimen, one may skip the step of making slides and place all samples into cell block on subsequent passes.

Endobronchial Ultrasound

Endobronchial ultrasound was developed by modifying and miniaturizing the endoscopic ultrasound used by gastroenterologists. Refer to Chapter 1 of this text for a review of the physical principles of ultrasound. The initial design was a radial ultrasound probe (termed a radial probe; see Figure 4.14). The probe was designed such that it could be passed through the working channel of the bronchoscope and into the airway, where it could rotate to provide a 360° image. A balloon sheath over the probe would inflate with saline to fill the airway lumen and provide contact with the wall, thus providing a medium for sonic coupling between the probe and the target tissue. Once the lesion was located, and images were captured and recorded, the probe was removed, and TBNA needles were passed through the working channel to perform biopsy. As a result, the operator needed to make a mental picture of the potential needle insertion site in reference to the airway and vascular structures. Hence, this was a "blind" technique, which limited its utility and popularity. It did allow for more confidence in less commonly needled sites such as hilar or left paratracheal. For more applications of this technology, see Chapter 11 in this book.

In early 2000, a real-time EBUS device was introduced. The major difference between the EBUS scope (linear or convex probe scope) and the radial probe is its capacity to provide real-time images during TBNA. The EBUS scope (BF-UC260F-OL8, Olympus Corporation, Tokyo, Japan; Figure 4.15) has a convex/linear transducer (7.5 MHz) extending ahead of the

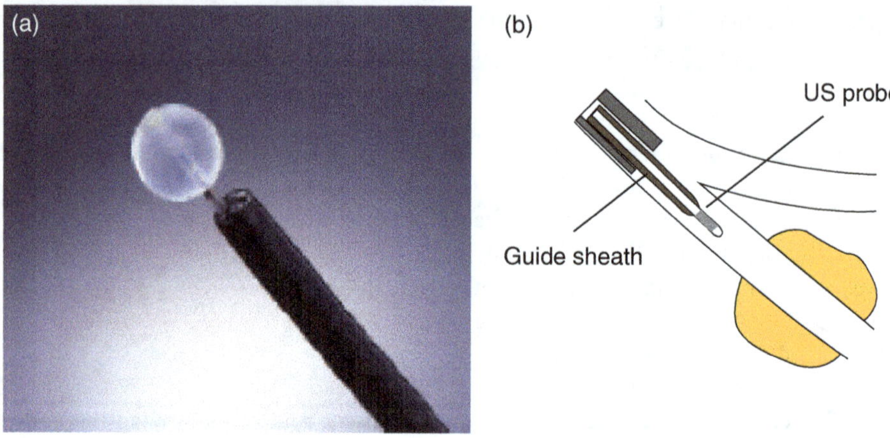

Figure 4.14 (a) Endobronchial ultrasound balloon probe (UM-BS20-26R) extending out of the working channel of a flexible bronchoscope. The balloon over the probe is inflated with normal saline. (b) Endobronchial ultrasound probe is extended in the lumen of the airway through the working channel of a flexible bronchoscope. Once the balloon is inflated, the probe can pick up the sonographic features of a mass around the airways.

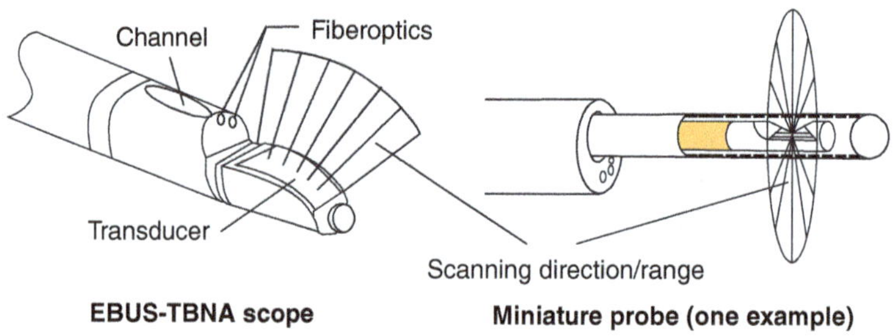

Figure 4.15 Comparative structures of endobronchial ultrasound (EBUS) scope and radial probe. The EBUS scope (XBF-UC260F-OL8, Olympus, Tokyo, Japan) has a convex/linear transducer (7.5 MHz) extending ahead of the light source and camera. The outer diameter of the scope itself is 6.7 mm, whereas that of a tip is 6.9 mm. The angle of the view is 90° and the direction of the view is 30° forward oblique. The radial probe can pass through the working channel of the bronchoscope into the lumen of the airway. It rotates 360° and gives a circular image of objects all around it.

light source and camera. The outer diameter of the scope is 6.7 mm, whereas the tip is 6.9 mm (Figure 4.16). The angle of view is 90°, and the direction of view is 30° forward oblique. The convex surface of the probe needs to be in good contact with the airway wall, or the space between them should be filled with a good sound-conducting medium, such as saline. This is accomplished with a balloon sheath that covers the convex probe. The ultrasound image is processed in the ultrasound scanner (EU-C2000, Olympus, Tokyo, Japan). The small balloon (Figure 4.17) is mounted over the convex probe, and once the probe is in the airway lumen, the balloon is again filled with saline. The scope has a specially designed channel to allow inflation and deflation of the balloon by the scope operator (Figure 4.18). Because the camera faces 30° forward and upward, maneuvering the scope can be somewhat more challenging compared to a traditional flexible bronchoscope. An appropriate analogy would be lying on one's back in a tunnel looking up and ahead while moving forward. Despite this challenge, the value of the real-time imaging provided by convex probe

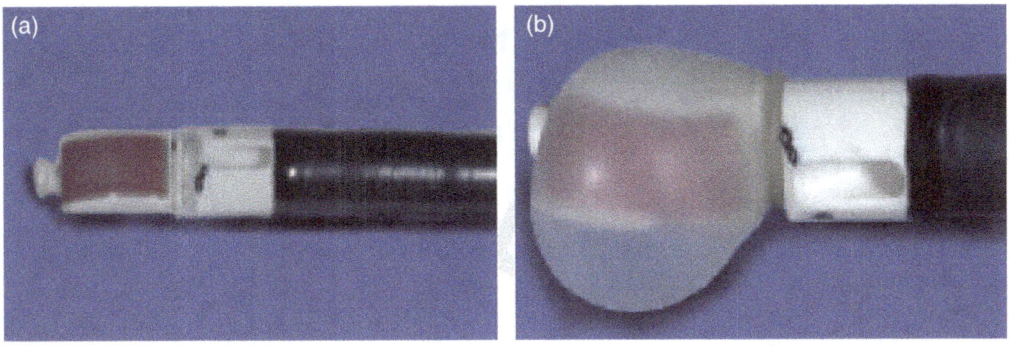

Figure 4.16 (a) Endobronchial ultrasound (EBUS) scope (XBF-UC260F-OL8, Olympus, Tokyo, Japan). (b) The balloon over the transducer is inflated with saline.

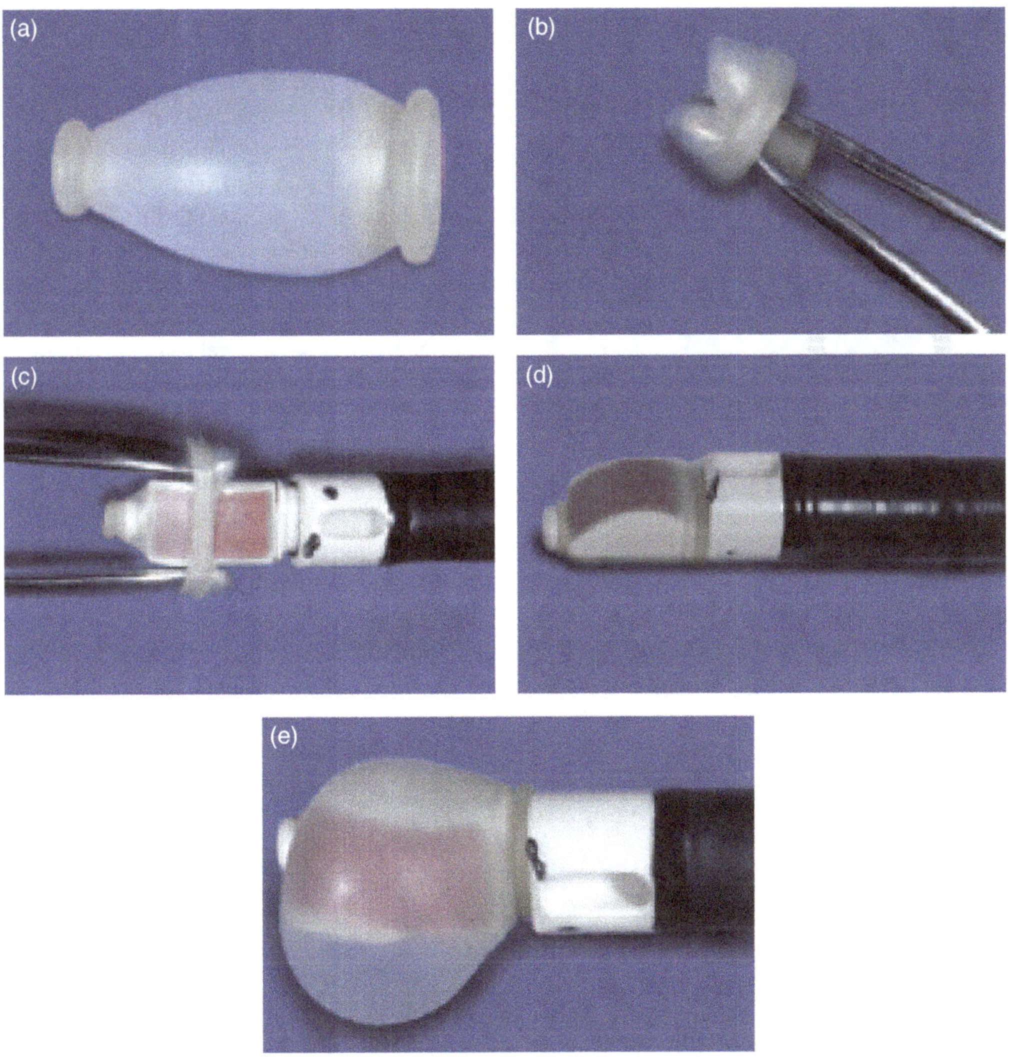

Figure 4.17 (a) Balloon to go over the convex probe. (b) The balloon is held between the two arms of the application forceps at half length and reversed over it. (c) The balloon is applied over the convex probe, with the wider opening of the balloon sitting in the crease on the distal aspect of the convex probe. (d) The smaller opening of the balloon is pushed down with the pad of the index finger over the tiny knob at the distal-most aspect of the convex probe. All the bubbles should be released from the tip of the balloon after the first inflation with saline before pushing the tip of the balloon onto the tip of the convex probe. (e) Inflated balloon on the convex probe without any air bubbles.

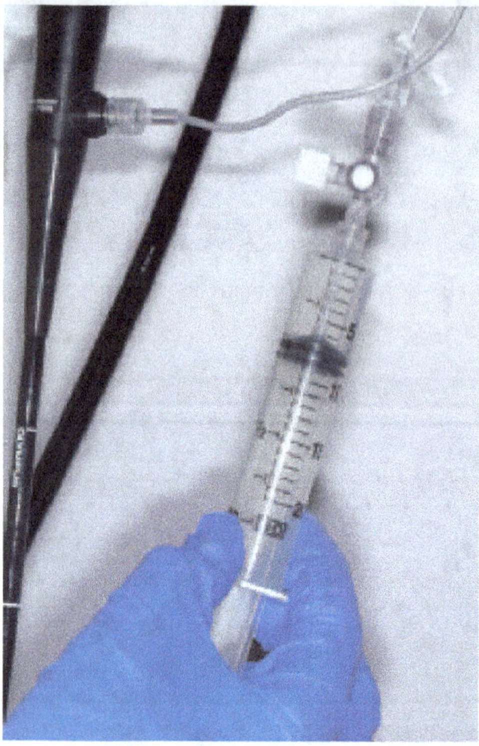

Figure 4.18 An extra opening under the working channel port of the scope allows for inflation of the balloon over the transducer with saline. This opening is connected with the 20 cc syringe filled with saline via intravenous tubing and a stopcock.

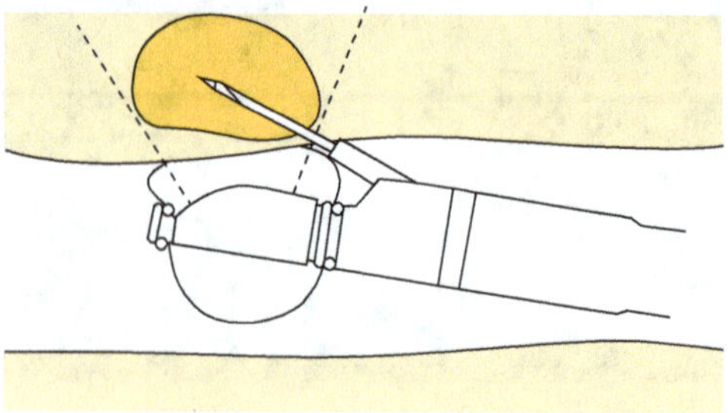

Figure 4.19 The relationship between the convex probe, the balloon covering the convex probe, and the needle extending from the working channel and penetrating the lymph node behind the airway wall.

EBUS cannot be overstated. With experience, clear imaging of lymph nodes and surrounding vascular structures can be obtained, to allow for assessment of the proper depth of needle insertion. In addition, studies have begun assessing whether ultrasound characteristics of lymph node tissue can be used to predict benign or malignant potential [26].

The needle assembly of the EBUS scope can appear complex at first and requires a good understanding of its operation prior to use during TBNA. The needle exits the working channel of the scope at a 45° angle, passing above and away from the balloon sheath (Figure 4.19). Nowadays needles range in size from 19 to 22 G. The most proximal portion of the needle assembly is the stylet, which sits within the needle during insertion (Figure 4.20). Just under the handle portion of the needle device is a needle lock that controls the length of the needle outside of the sheath, thus controlling the depth of needle penetration during insertion. Most needle assemblies include a locking device (stop bar) that limits the depth of needle insertion. When set at level three, as an example, the stop bar limits the functional length of the needle to 20 mm. Under the stop bar, there is a separate sheath locking device. This device allows the sheath covering the needle to be moved forward or backward (Figures 4.21 and 4.22). Most operators prefer the sheath to be advanced out until the tip is just visible in the right upper portion of the monitor screen. This prevents the scope from being pushed away from the tissue when trying to introduce the needle into the tissue. Under the sheath lock, there is a safety adaptor to lock the needle assembly to the working channel of the scope, thus preventing movement of the needle assembly during TBNA.

To properly set up the EBUS scope, one must also know how to plug the scope into the control tower, including connecting the scope via cable to the control panel (see Figure 4.23). Once connected properly, monitor settings should be chosen for optimal picture quality. Our usual settings are depth 4 cm, penetration mode, and GI2 (contrast 2). The gain is certain at every start- up of the ultrasound machine (Figure 4.24).

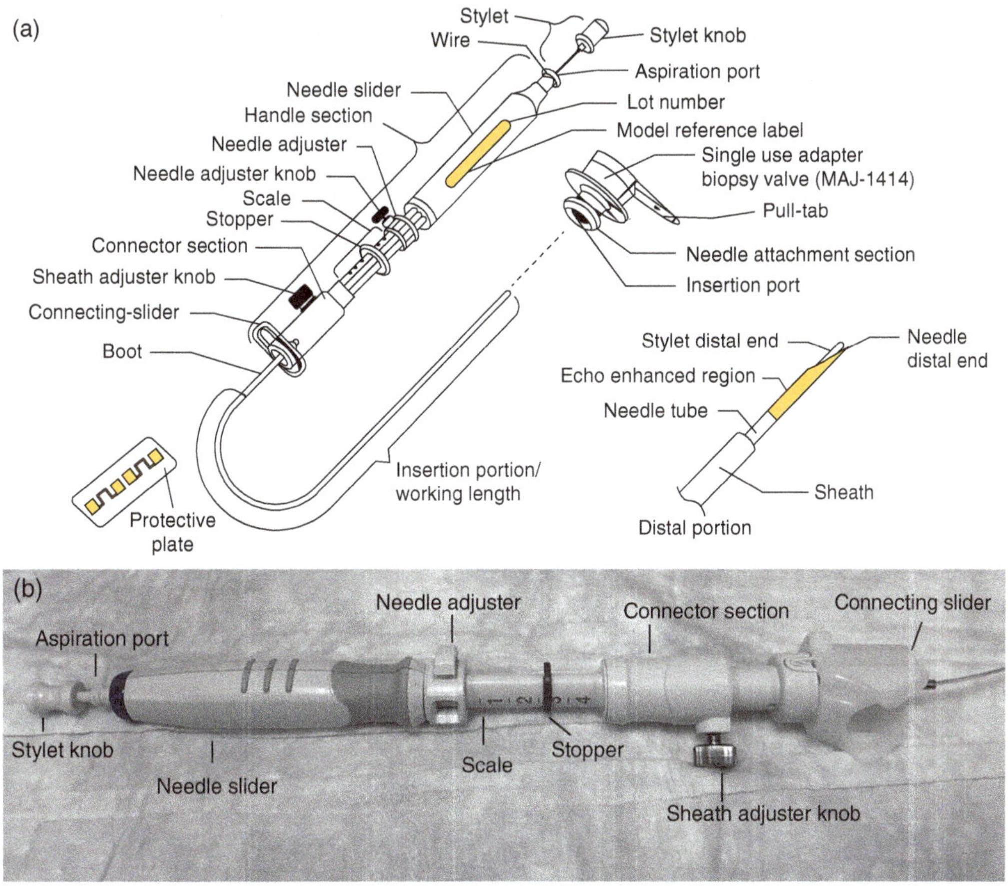

Figure 4.20 (a) A complete needle assembly system for endobronchial ultrasound-guided transbronchial needle aspiration (EBUS-TBNA). (b) Proximal portion of the needle assembly focusing on the needle and sheath adjuster knobs and the needle stopper to determine the functional length of the needle.

Step-by-Step EBUS-TBNA

A thorough examination of the airway is performed with a conventional (non-EBUS) bronchoscope prior to EBUS-TBNA. Endobronchial lesions should be excluded which may obviate the need for EBUS-TBNA. Once the inspection is done, the conventional bronchoscope is removed and the EBUS scope is deployed, through either the oral or nasal route. Some experts direct the scope directly to the first planned TBNA site, while others perform a thorough ultrasound examination of the mediastinum prior proceeding to the pre-selected site (see Section 4.4, Planning the Procedure). I prefer the latter approach, because the ultrasound survey often provides more practical information about the location and accessibility of nodes, compared to a CT scan. However, it is important to abide by the predetermined plan, even if alternative nodes appear easier to biopsy, in order to sample the lymph nodes that would, if positive, stage the disease to the highest level in the smallest number of attempts.

After ultrasound-guided mediastinal survey is performed, and the target node is identified, the scope should be retracted into the neutral (non-flexed) position. We will now outline the steps for performing EBUS-TBNA. First, the needle is inserted through the working channel of the EBUS scope, until the needle

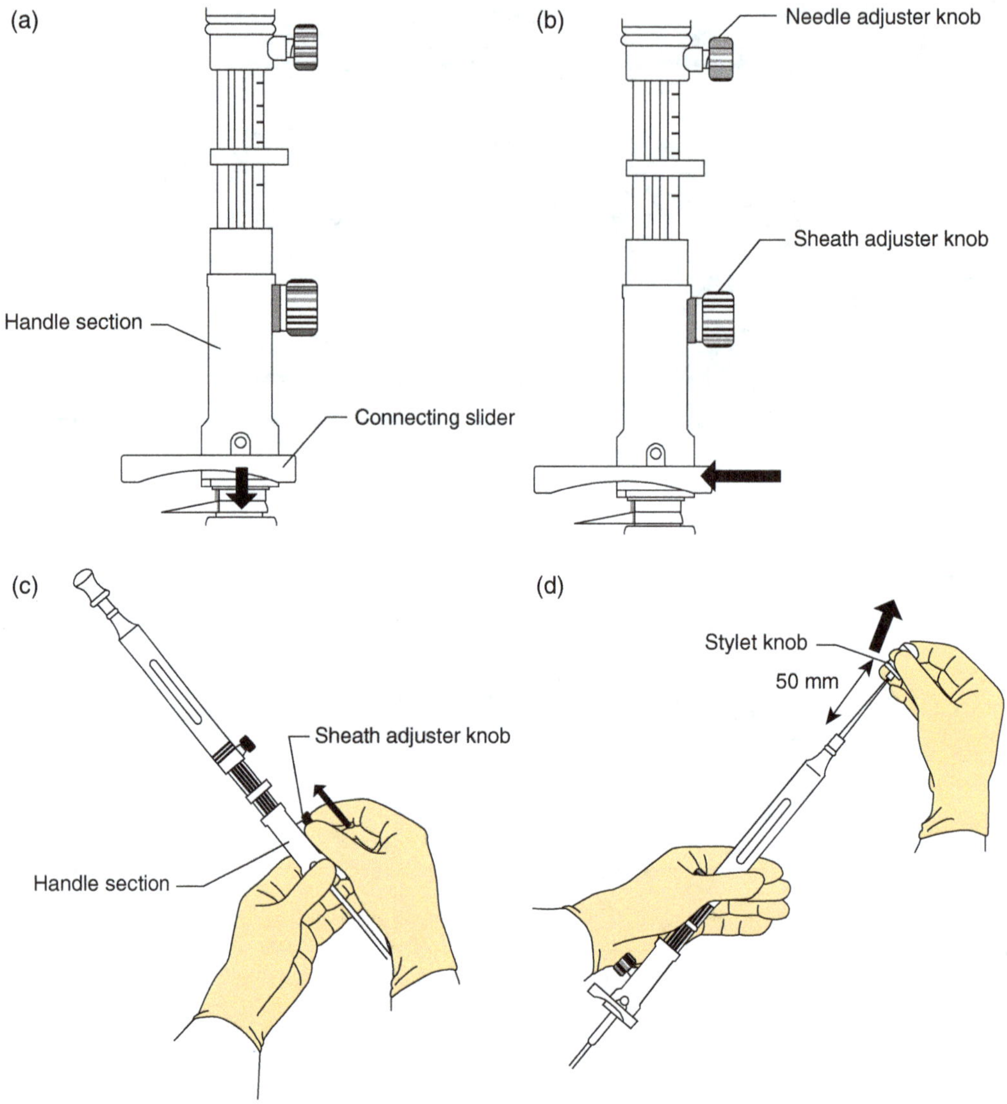

Figure 4.21 Different parts of a needle assembly system used with an endobronchial ultrasound- guided transbronchial needle aspiration (EBUS-TBNA) scope. (a) The needle assembly's handle section showing how the connecting slider fits on the adaptor attached to the working channel port of the scope. (b) The connector slider is pushed backward. The needle adjustor knob is located above the sheath adjuster knob. (c) The sheath adjuster knob is loosened by rotating it counterclockwise. (d) The stylet is pulled back by holding the stylet knob.

assembly is connected with the working channel of the scope. The needle assembly is then locked, keeping it fixed to the scope. This step must be performed with the EBUS scope in a neutral position in order to avoid damage to the working channel of the scope. Next, the needle sheath is advanced out of the working channel, by manipulation of the needle assembly, until the tip of the sheath is just visible in the right upper quadrant of the bronchoscope screen (see Figure 4.25). The sheath is then locked using the screw locking device on the needle assembly. This will fix the sheath in the appropriate position for the duration of the

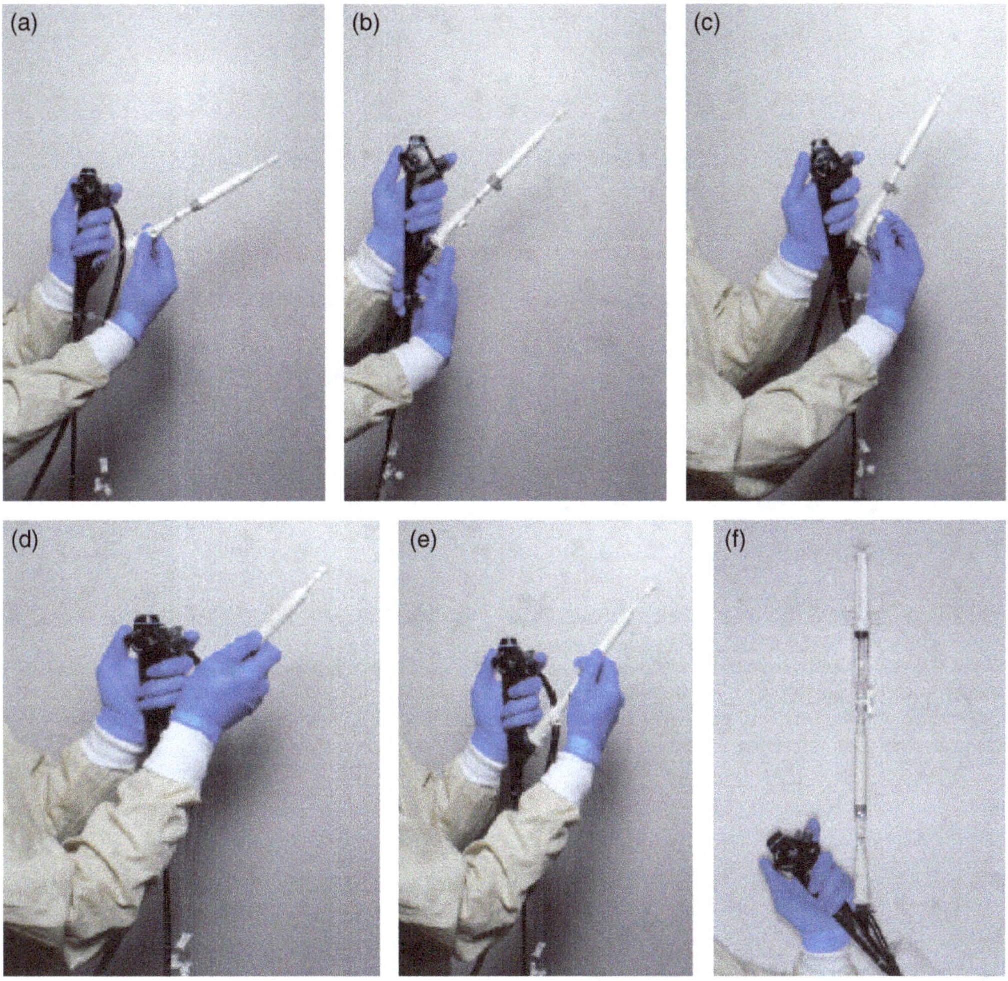

Figure 4.22 Proper technique for loading the needle assembly on the scope, step by step. (a) The needle is passed through the working channel and the entire needle assembly is loaded in the special working channel cap provided with the needle kit. The tightening knobs should face forward. The sheath and the needle should be completely retraced by pulling their sliders all the way up. (b) Once the needle assembly is tightly fitted in the working channel, the lock should be applied by sliding it backward. (c) In preparation for needle insertion, the sheath is pushed out by loosening the sheath lock (lower knob on the assembly). (d) Before lowering the needle, the position of the needle length slide lock should be confirmed at 3, allowing only about 20 mm of needle to come out of the scope. (e) The stylet is pulled back a couple of centimeters to allow the bevel of the needle to lead. The needle is then unlocked by loosening the needle lock knob just prior to penetration in the tissue. Once the target is penetrated, the stylet is pushed forward a couple of times to push out the unwanted epithelial cells captured on the way. (f) Suction is applied after removing the stylet with a locking syringe.

procedure. At this point, the scope should be advanced to the target lesion, with confirmation of the site on ultrasound. Of note, some lymph node stations may be more challenging to image with the needle assembly in the scope, given that it inhibits scope flexion to an extent. Depending on the station, balloon inflation may be required in order to achieve optimal imaging of the lymph nodes. This is particularly true in the more proximal nodal stations that reside in the larger airways. Once the image is confirmed, the operator should take

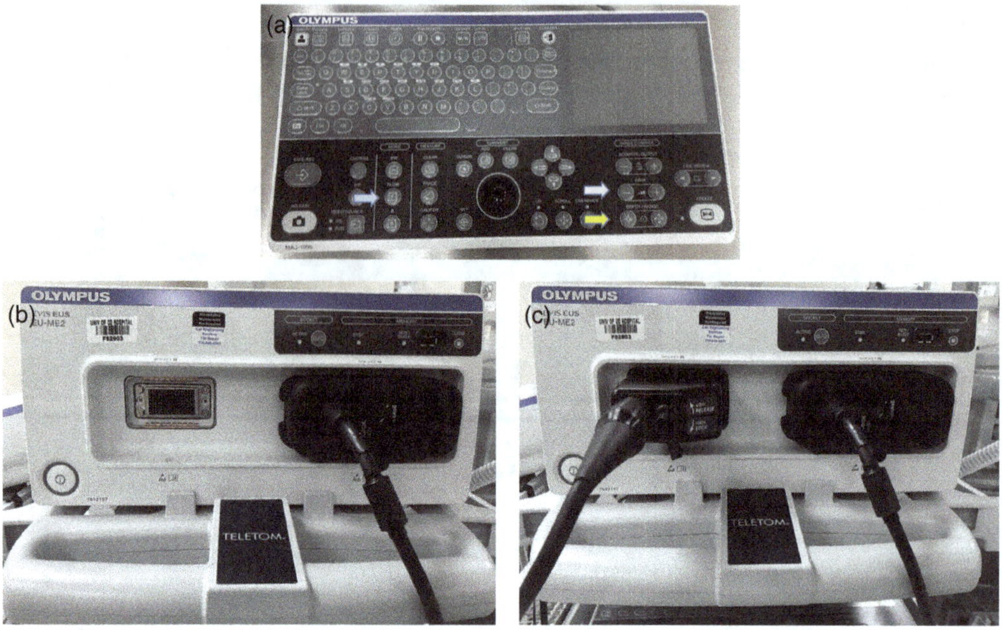

Figure 4.23 (a) Control panel for endobronchial ultrasound processor EU-ME2. Of particular importance are controls for adjusting gain (white arrow), depth (yellow arrow), and flow (i.e. color doppler, blue arrow). (b) Endobronchial ultrasound processor EU-ME2. (c) Endobronchial ultrasound processor EU-ME2 with bronchoscope input attached.

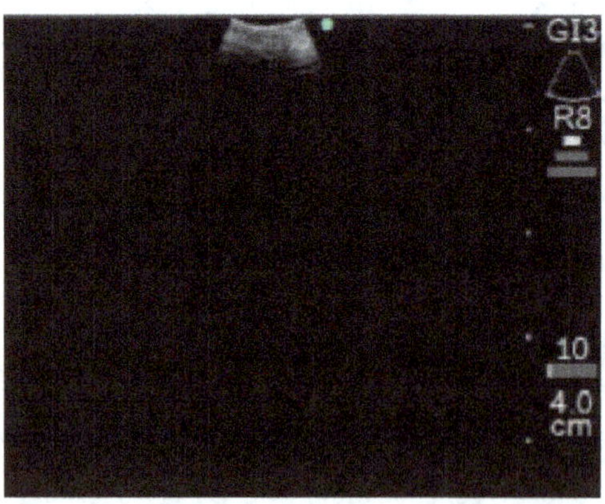

Figure 4.24 Endobronchial ultrasound monitor. The basic settings and format are shown here. The detailed setup is discussed in Chapter 1.

care to keep the target in the center of the screen (see Figure 4.26). The green dot on the ultrasound screen marks the needle insertion site. Doppler ultrasound can be performed on the target site to confirm there are no large vascular structures in the field. At this point respiratory motion should be observed to note how this affects target position. It may help to have an assistant hold the scope in place at this point. Some operators choose to pull the stylet (which is inside the needle) back by 1–2 cm, whereas others keep it completely hubbed in the needle, in order to avoid needle contamination with epithelial cells during insertion.

With the scope held in place, the needle lock is removed. The needle is then advanced into the tissue. An assistant may need to gently push the scope in at this point, given that needle insertion sometimes pushes the scope away from the airway wall, distorting the ultrasound image. When this happens, the ultrasound image may go black due to lack of contact between the balloon and the airway wall. In this case, gently advancing the scope should bring the balloon and wall back into contact and the image should reappear. If significant

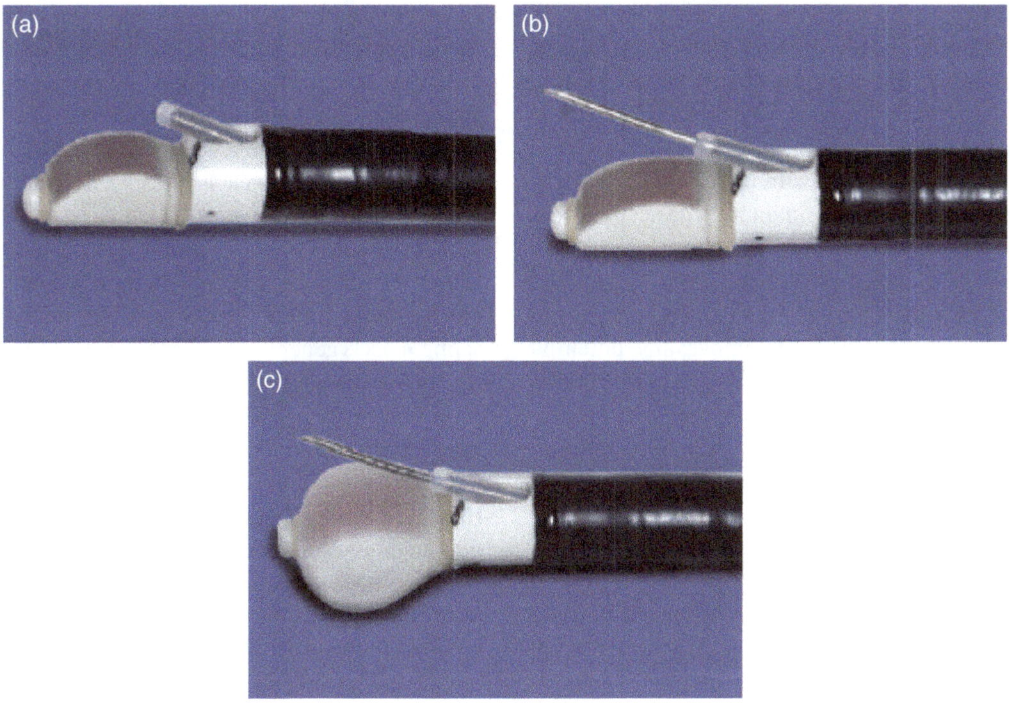

Figure 4.25 (a) Endobronchial ultrasound convex probe with needle sheath pushed out of the working channel. The balloon is deflated to show the safety margin between the catheter and the needle that comes out of it and the probe. (b) Needle pushed out of the catheter pointing at an angle of 45°. Again the balloon is deflated. The angulation of the needle allows for a near perpendicular angle between the target and the needle. (c) Needle pushed out of the catheter pointing at an angle of 45°. The needle stays clear of the inflated balloon.

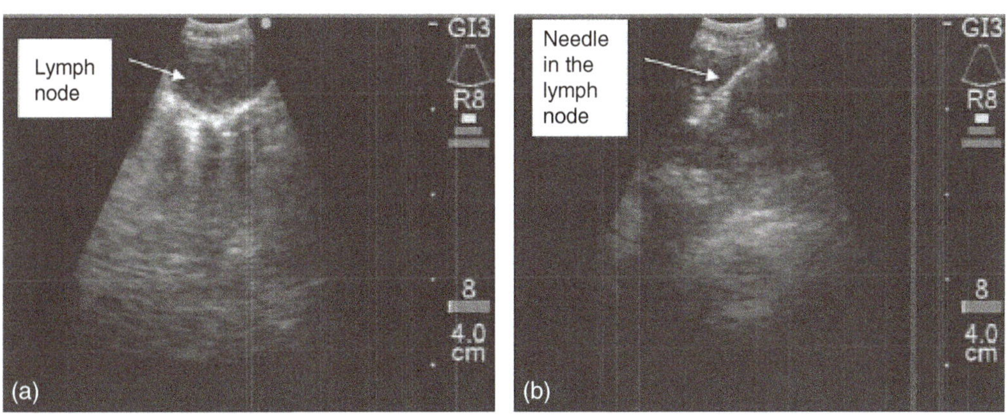

Figure 4.26 (a) A small mediastinal lymph node is seen on the endobronchial ultrasound monitor. (b) A needle is penetrated diagonally across the lymph node. The entry point of the needle is at the green dot on the right upper corner of the ultrasound field.

difficulty is encountered when trying to penetrate the airway wall, the needle may be running into cartilage. If this is the case, an alternative entry site above the cartilage ring is recommended.

Once the needle is in the lymph node, care should be taken to maintain the scope in the same position in order to maintain real-time imaging of the needle within the target. The stylet is then pushed forward once or twice to clean the needle and remove any potential bronchial cells. This can also help to confirm the position of the needle tip on the ultrasound image. The stylet is then removed, and a preloaded suction syringe is connected to the end of the needle assembly, if desired. If no blood is aspirated, then gentle yet steady jabbing is performed, with care taken to keep the needle within the target lymph node to avoid tissue contamination. Five to ten long, smooth passes are made. In order to maximize control of the needle during these passes, the operator should tighten the grip on the fixed portion of the needle assembly, while using the thumb, index, and middle fingers to control the in-and-out motion of the needle. Before removal the needle from the lymph node, the suction is disconnected to avoid collecting unwanted cells in the needle on the way out. The needle is fully retracted, as is the needle locking device. The needle assembly is then unlocked from the scope and removed from the working channel with the scope in the neutral position.

The needle containing the specimen should be taken immediately to the slides, which have been previously laid out, labeled, and numbered. Some bronchoscopists push the specimen out with the stylet onto a filter paper or gauze to absorb blood and separate the core tissue biopsy. The core tissue is then put into formalin for histopathologic examination. Some of the specimen in the needle is pushed out onto the slides for cytologic examination by passing the stylet back into the needle to empty the specimen. The stylet is then cleaned with an alcohol swab to remove blood clots from the surface. Sample remaining in the needle is placed into a tube containing normal saline. This is generally accomplished by flushing the needle with saline, and then air.

If on-site cytology is not available, the specimen retrieved in the needle should be pushed into a tube containing normal saline. However, if on-site cytology is available, the cytologist may help determine whether additional aspirates are needed. If malignant cells, granulomata, or other features reveal a diagnosis, and no more tissue is needed for confirmation, cell block, and molecular studies, the procedure can be concluded. However, if the sample contains lymphoid material but no malignant cells or granulomata, one may proceed to another TBNA of the same site or an additional site. As previously stated, it is now recommended that three TBNA passes are performed at each lymph node station when mediastinal staging is desired, as this has been shown to improve yield [24]. In general, post-procedure chest radiographs are not needed following an uncomplicated TBNA.

Acknowledgments

We would like to acknowledge and thank Barry Silverstein for photographic expertise and Boyd Jacobson for excellent art work.

References

1 Rusch, V.W., Asamura, H., Watanabe, H. et al. (2009). The IASLC lung cancer staging project: a proposal for a new international lymph node map in the forthcoming seventh edition of the TNM classification for lung cancer. *Journal of Thoracic Oncology* 4 (5): 568–577.

2 Nicholson, A.G., Chansky, K., Crowley, J. et al. (2016). The International Association for the Study of Lung Cancer staging project: proposals for the revision of the clinical and pathologic staging of small cell lung cancer in the forthcoming eighth edition of the TNM classification for lung cancer. *Journal of Thoracic Oncology* 11 (3): 300–311.

3 Ost, D.E., Ernst, A., Lei, X. et al. (2011). Diagnostic yield of endobronchial ultrasound-guided transbronchial needle aspiration: results of the AQuIRE bronchoscopy registry. *Chest* 140 (6): 1557–1566.

4 Beaudoin, S., Martel, S., Pelletier, S. et al. (2016). Randomized trial comparing patient comfort between the oral and nasal insertion routes for linear endobronchial ultrasound. *Journal of Bronchology & Interventional Pulmonology* 23 (1): 39–45.

5 Casal, R.F., Lazarus, D.R., Kuhl, K. et al. (2015). Randomized trial of endobronchial ultrasound-guided transbronchial needle aspiration under general anesthesia versus moderate sedation. *American Journal of Respiratory and Critical Care Medicine* 191 (7): 796–803.

6 Stather, D.R., Chee, A., MacEachern, P. et al. (2015). Endobronchial ultrasound learning curve in interventional pulmonary fellows. *Respirology* 20 (2): 333–339.

7 Bonifazi, M., Tramacere, I., Zuccatosta, L. et al. (2017). Conventional versus ultrasound-guided transbronchial needle aspiration for the diagnosis of hilar/mediastinal lymphadenopathies: a randomized controlled trial. *Respiration* 94 (2): 216–223.

8 Wang, D., Shang, B., and Jiang, S. (2014). Diagnostic value of endobronchial ultrasound-guided transbronchial needle aspiration in conventional transbronchial needle aspiration negative paratracheal mediastinal lesions. *Zhonghua Jie He He Hu Xi Za Zhi* 37 (4): 279–282.

9 Um, S.W., Kim, H.K., Jung, S.H. et al. (2015). Endobronchial ultrasound versus mediastinoscopy for mediastinal nodal staging of non-small cell lung cancer. *Journal of Thoracic Oncology* 10: 331–337.

10 Bousema, J.E., Dijkgraaf, M.G.W., Papen-Botterhuis, N.E. et al. (2018). MEDIASTinal staging of non-small cell lung cancer by endobronchial and endoscopic ultrasonography with or without additional surgical mediastinoscopy (MEDIASTrial): study protocol of a multicenter randomized controlled trial. *BMC Surgery* 18: 27.

11 Rintoul, R.C., Glover, M.J., Jackson, C. et al. (2014). Cost effectiveness of endosonography versus surgical staging in potentially resectable lung cancer: a health economic analysis of the ASTER trial from a European perspective. *Thorax* 69: 679–681.

12 Bilaceroglu, S. (2017). Molecular markers in lung cancer: role of EBUS. *Current Opinion in Pulmonary Medicine* 23 (3): 247–253.

13 Moonim, M.T., Breen, R., Fields, P.A., and Santis, G. (2013). Diagnosis and subtyping of de novo and relapsed mediastinal lymphomas by endobronchial ultrasound needle aspiration. *American Journal of Respiratory and Critical Care Medicine* 188 (10): 1216–1223.

14 Grosu, H.B., Illiesiu, M., Caraway, N.P. et al. (2015). Endobronchial ultrasound-guided transbronchial needle aspiration for the diagnosis and subtyping of lymphoma. *Annals of the American Thoracic Society* 12 (9): 1336–1344.

15 Gupta, D., Dadhwal, D.S., Agarwal, R. et al. (2014). Endobronchial ultrasound-guided transbronchial needle aspiration vs conventional transbronchial needle aspiration in the diagnosis of sarcoidosis. *Chest* 146 (3): 547–556.

16 Navasakulpong, A., Auger, M., and Gonzalez, A.V. (2016). Yield of EBUS-TBNA for the diagnosis of sarcoidosis: impact of operator and cytopathologist experience. *BMJ Open Respiratory Research* 3: e000144.

17 Madan, K., Dhungana, A., Mohan, A. et al. (2017). Conventional transbronchial needle aspiration versus endobronchial ultrasound-guided transbronchial needle aspiration, with or without rapid on-site evaluation, for

the diagnosis of sarcoidosis: a randomized controlled trial. *Journal of Bronchology & Interventional Pulmonology* 24 (1): 48–58.

18 Yarmus, L.B., Akulian, J., Lechtzin, N. et al. (2013). Comparison of 21-gauge and 22-gauge aspiration needle in endobronchial ultrasound-guided transbronchial needle aspiration: results of the American College of Chest Physicians quality improvement registry, education, and evaluation registry. *Chest* 143 (4): 1036–1043.

19 Herth, F., Shuler, H., Gompelmann, D. et al. (2012). Endobronchial ultrasound-guided lymph node biopsy with a transbronchial needle forceps: a pilot study. *European Respiratory Journal* 39: 373–377.

20 Kinsey, C.M. and Arenberg, D.A. (2014). Endobronchial ultrasound-guided transbronchial needle aspiration for non-small cell lung cancer staging. *American Journal of Respiratory and Critical Care Medicine* 189 (6): 640–649.

21 Scholten, E.L., Semaan, R., Illei, P. et al. (2017). Stylet use does not improve diagnostic outcomes in endobronchial ultrasonographic transbronchial needle aspiration: a randomized clinical trial. *Chest* 151 (3): 636–642.

22 Gounant, V., Ninane, V., Janson, X. et al. (2011). Release of metal particles from needles used for transbronchial needle aspiration. *Chest* 139 (1): 138–143.

23 Casal, R.F., Staerkel, G.A., Ost, D. et al. (2012). Randomized clinical trial of endobronchial ultrasound needle biopsy with and without aspiration. *Chest* 142 (3): 568–573.

24 Lee, H.S., Lee, G.K., Lee, H.S. et al. (2008). Real-time endobronchial ultrasound-guided transbronchial needle aspiration in mediastinal staging of non-small cell lung cancer: how many aspirations per target lymph node station? *Chest* 134 (2): 368–374.

25 Baram, D., Carcia, R.B., and Richman, P.S. (2006). Impact of rapid on-site cytologic evaluation during transbronchial needle aspiration. *Chest* 128 (2): 869–875.

26 Wang Memoli, J.S., El-Bayoumi, E., Pastis, N.J. et al. (2011). Using endobronchial ultrasound features to predict lymph node metastasis in patients with lung cancer. *Chest* 140 (6): 1550–1556.

5

Endobronchial Ultrasound-Guided Transbronchial Needle Aspiration: Tips and Tricks

David I.K. Fielding

Royal Brisbane and Women's Hospital, Herston, Queensland, Australia

Choice of Sedation Type

Endobronchial ultrasound-guided transbronchial needle aspiration (EBUS-TBNA) is performed either as a conscious sedation or general anesthetic outpatient procedure. For patients with large lymph nodes where a tissue diagnosis is required, the procedure is easily performed under conscious sedation procedure. Randomized clinical studies show no difference in diagnostic rates of EBUS-TBNA comparing the type of anesthetic (general versus conscious sedation) [1]. Öztaş et al. [2] reported a retrospective study comparing sedation with propofol plus midazolam (152 patients) with midazolam alone (122 patients). Diagnosis was obtained in 77.6% versus 85.7% for the two groups with no statistical difference observed.

Franzen et al. [3] showed similar findings, comparing deep sedation versus moderate sedation in 232 patients. The overall diagnostic accuracy for correct diagnosis at the mediastinal, subcarinal, and hilar locations irrespective of the sedation technique was 91%, 93%, and 92%, respectively. At the mediastinal, subcarinal, and hilar locations, overall diagnostic accuracy for deep sedation compared to moderate sedation was not significantly different: 88.5–93.2% and 93.6–95.5%, respectively. In their review of sedation Aswanetmanee et al. [1] showed no difference in procedural complication rates (pneumothorax or bleeding) between deep and moderate sedation. Coughing has been demonstrated in two studies to be more common in moderate sedation. Deep sedation has been shown to require more vasopressor for medication-induced hypotension than moderate sedation. One study assessed patient satisfaction [4]: overall there was no significant difference between deep and moderate sedation groups. More patients in the moderate sedation group recalled the procedure; however, most patients stated that they were willing to undergo the procedure again under the same modality. Some countries allow the use of propofol administered by the proceduralist, but this is not universally sanctioned [5]. With longer procedures such as EBUS-TBNA staging, it may be preferable to do this under general anesthetic, as the procedure can be longer, sometimes up to 45–60 minutes, particularly if, as is recommended, at least two nodes within each station are sampled.

Takakuwa et al. [6] have reported a prospective study of the use of high-flow nasal cannula (HFNC) oxygen during EBUS-TBNA, which might be relevant for more marginal

Endobronchial Ultrasonography, Second Edition. Noriaki Kurimoto, David I.K. Fielding, Ali I. Musani, Christopher Kniese, and Katsuhiko Morita.

Companion website: www.wiley.com/go/kurimoto2e

cases. HFNC use was started at 30% oxygen (O_2) fraction and was titrated to maintain oxygen saturation (SpO_2) over 90%. The mean lowest SpO_2 during the procedure was 93% and remained over 90% throughout, with mean highest cutaneous carbon dioxide ($PcCO_2$) of 39 mmHg (range 30–46 mmHg). This compared to patients who were maintained with a conventional nasal cannula, where the mean lowest SpO_2 was 88%, significantly lower than the HFNC group ($p = 0.005$).

Considerations Regarding Presumed Tissue Type

Some tissue types may render acquiring tissue more difficult due to increased vascularity of nodes, making it potentially difficult to obtain diagnostic material. These include metastatic melanoma and renal carcinoma. Still the procedure is safe and reports do suggest its great feasibility for melanoma [7] and other metastases. Val-Bernal et al. [8] also reported their finding of 14 renal cell carcinoma nodes successfully confirmed on cell block, which were large (mean 2.5 cm, range 1.6–3.8 cm), irregular, inhomogeneous, hypervascular, and hyperechoic. EBUS-TBNA was done safely.

Lymphoma is another situation where there may be difficulties. Korrungruang et al. [9] reported their experience of EBUS-TBNA for lymphoma. From 19 patients histology on cell block was definitive, with subtype classification in 6 cases (32%), and suspicious but not definitive for subtype in 10 (53%). They used a 21 G needle and a mean number of 5 aspirates per case. Cytology was positive or suspicious in 12 cases (63%). Further sampling was by transbronchial biopsy (2 cases) and surgical biopsy in 7 cases. Four of the suspicious cases did not undergo further biopsy, meaning that approximately half of the cases were managed by results of EBUS-TBNA alone. The authors commented that even though the definitive diagnostic rate was relatively low, the sampling of hilar masses which might have a possible diagnosis of lymphoma allows alternative diagnoses to be easily made by EBUS-TBNA, such as lung cancer and sarcoidosis.

Jin et al. [10] reviewed the place of EBUS-TBNA in lymphoma diagnosis. They commented that most studies are favorable and that the addition of ancillary techniques, particularly flow cytometry, increases diagnostic yield. It can be particularly useful to establish recurrent disease in cases where subtype has been determined. There are, however, diagnostic limitations for Hodgkin's lymphoma, grading of follicular lymphoma, and some T-cell lymphomas. This may possibly improve with the use of larger needles or a combination with core biopsy needles. Furukawa et al. [11] have reported on this: an endobronchial ultrasound-guided fine-needle aspiration (EBUS-FNA) was performed using a 22 G EchoTip ProCore EBUS needle (Cook Medical, Bloomington, IN), which produced a cellular aspirate suspicious for lymphoma on rapid on-site evaluation (ROSE). Core samples were fixed in formalin and histology confirmed classical Hodgkin's lymphoma, with scattered Reed–Sternberg cells that were positive for CD15, CD30, PAX-5, CD 20, CD 45, and Epstein–Barr virus-encoded RNA (EBER) on immunohistochemical staining. Also it may be that next-generation sequencing on TBNA specimens may improve the ability to make such diagnoses.

Where non-malignant conditions are suspected, EBUS-TBNA has an important role: Eickhoff et al. [12] reported 111 out of 315 (35%) of their consecutive patients with neither primary signs nor history of a malignant disease. From 245 lymph nodes, pathology revealed non-specific inflammation (n = 81; 70%), carcinoma (n = 7; 6%), and epithelioid cell granulomas (n = 20; 17%). Microbiologic testing of lymph nodes identified three infections (*Mycobacterium tuberculosis* [MTB], n = 2, and *Nocardia nova*, n = 1). Therefore, EBUS-TBNA revealed a specific cause for suspected non-malignant lymphadenopathy in one-third of cases with excellent specificity.

The importance of confirming a benign diagnosis where positron-emission tomography–computed tomography (PET-CT) may be false positive was reported recently by Lee et al. [13]. From 247 cases where PET-CT showed a suspicious positive node, 189 had malignancy confirmed, while 58 patients had negative benign, particularly in older patients (age >65 years), pneumoconiosis, and patients with squamous cell carcinoma as the primary tumor diagnosis. Age ≥65, squamous cell carcinoma as the histologic type, and pneumoconiosis were related with false-positive lymph node involvement on imaging studies such as chest CT and PET-CT.

Other Causes of PET-Positive Nodes with Negative EBUS-TBNA (False-Positive PET)

Anthracosis is well described as a false-positive cause of PET positivity of hilar and mediastinal nodes [14]. In a series of 133 patients having EBUS-TBNA staging for lung cancer, 279 mediastinal lymph nodes were sampled, including 100 malignant nodes. Microscopic anthracotic pigment (MAP) was detected in 61 (21.7%) lymph nodes, and among these only 3 had malignant cells ($p<0.001$). These nodes had only slightly lower (non-significant) standardized uptake values (SUVs) on fluorodeoxyglucose positron-emission tomography (FDG-PET; 4.4 vs. 4.7, $p = 0.256$). Therefore, where there is a question about the final N status of a particular station after PET-CT and EBUS-TBNA, the presence of MAP can help in confirming benign disease.

Pattison et al. [15] have discussed a means of reporting cell block from aspirates of patients with a high pre-test likelihood of anthracosis by way of occupational exposure. Three groups of patients with bilateral hilar and mediastinal adenopathy were studied based on pathologic and clinical follow-up: dust-exposed cases, clinical sarcoidosis cases, and non-specific inflammatory cases. EBUS-TBNA cytology in patients with occupational dust exposure showed a significant increase in the presence of birefringent fibers (60.7% vs. 19.2%, $p = 0.001$) and intracellular carbon pigment (75.0% vs. 28.9%, $p = 0.001$) compared with patients without exposure (Figure 5.1). The presence of these two features together yielded a sensitivity of 53.6% and a specificity of 88.5%. This may assist in confirming a diagnosis of lymphadenopathy due to occupational dust exposure, particularly as an alternative cause of adenopathy by CT or PET.

Sarcoidosis can cause PET false-positive lymph nodes: detection of non-caseating granulomas on EBUS-TBNA smears and cell blocks is straightforward and a commonplace indication for the procedure [16]. Tuberculosis tends to have more asymmetric PET positivity, but can be a cause of PET false-positive lymph nodes [17].

Boongsarauk et al. [18] reported EBUS-TBNA rinse fluid tuberculosis (TB) polymerase chain reaction (PCR) assay for the diagnosis of intrathoracic TB lymphadenitis. Rinse fluid of the needle underwent acid-fast bacillus (AFB) staining, mycobacterial culture, and TB PCR using the Anyplex™ MTB/NTM (non-tuberculous mycobacteria) real-time detection kit (Seegene, Seoul, South Korea). The sensitivity, specificity, positive predictive value, and negative predictive value of rinse fluid TB PCR assay were 56.2%, 100.0%, 100.0%, and 92.5%, respectively. TB PCR had the highest diagnostic utility as a single test, compared with mycobacterial culture, AFB smear, and finding of necrotizing granulomatous inflammation. Combining TB PCR with culture and cytopathology improved the diagnosis performance.

Technical Aspects Including Balloons, Stylet, Use of the Sheath

These factors have recently been reviewed in a guideline paper by Wahidi and co-authors [19]. Many proceduralists vary their practice to suit

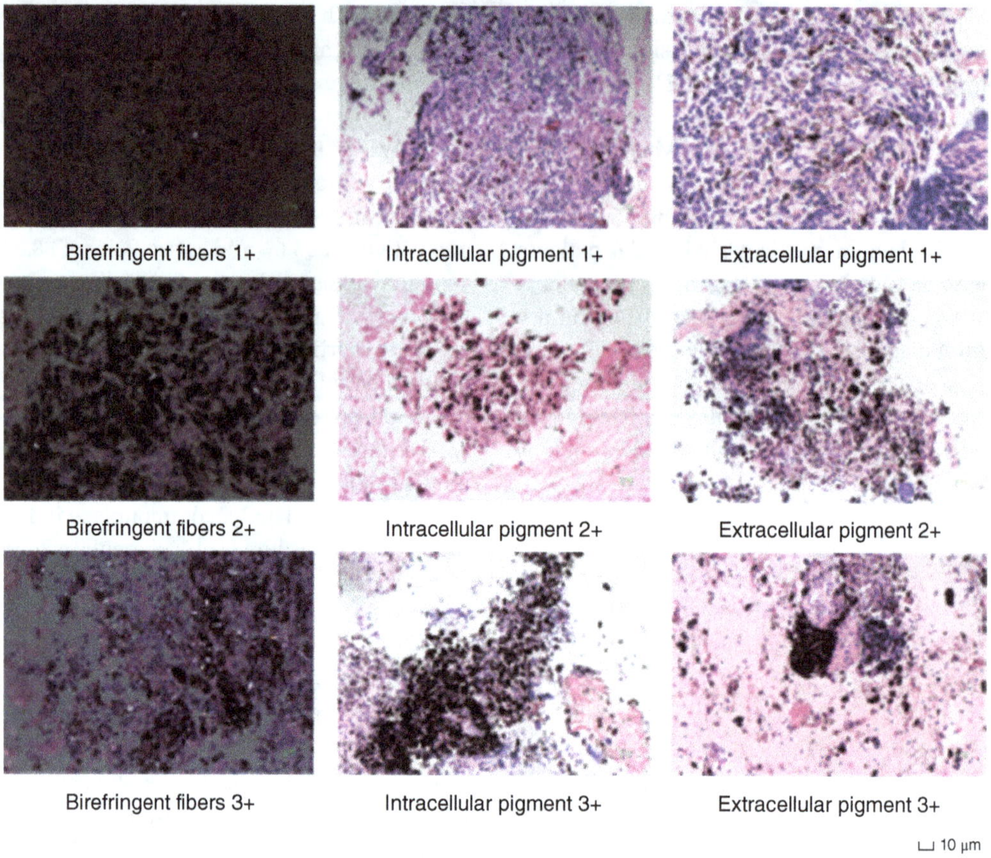

Figure 5.1 Examples of cytology scoring system used for birefringent fibers (polarized light 40× magnification), intracellular pigment (hematoxylin and eosin [H&E] 20× magnification), and extracellular pigment (H&E 20× magnification). *Source:* Pattison et al. [15]. Reprinted with permission from Lippincott Williams & Wilkins, Inc.

conditions. For example, if an initial aspirate is bloody, many proceduralists would perform the subsequent aspirates without suction. Regarding balloons, some node stations (10R, 4L) require more angulation to oppose the ultrasound surface of the scope onto the bronchial wall. Experience suggests that where such nodes are the focus of a procedure, balloon application on the scope tip would be warranted. There is variation in how these various parts of the apparatus are applied: some operators always use a balloon, always leave the stylet in when they enter the lymph node, and always apply suction. Others find the procedure more inexpensive and streamlined without balloons.

Needle Size

Needle size is of some relevance in the diagnosis of lung cancer. Typically a 21 gauge needle has been marginally favored over a 22 gauge needle in previous studies. One relatively small series divided 56 cases into either 21 or 22 G needle sampling [20]. In malignant cases sensitivities for cytology were 88.9% versus 52.2% ($p = 0.01$), and for histology 100% versus 82.6% ($p = 0.09$). In another study of 45 lesions [21], tumor cell abundance was equal between 21 and 22 G needles. However, with the pathologists blinded to needle type, histology was better preserved in five lesions from the 21 G needle, hence it was considered that the 21 G might be better for sampling nodes of unknown etiology. Conversely, there was more blood contamination with the 21 G needle ($p < 0.0001$).

New core needles are available in 22 and 25 G and their place in lung cancer diagnosis remains to be determined. Some proceduralists manually select what appear to be cores from the saline pot and place these directly in formalin, leaving the remainder for cell block preparation. It is unclear at this time whether there is any need to do this, as generally cell block preparations are highly sensitive for the diagnosis of lung cancer. In a study of 270 lung cancer samples, cell block was compared to cytology analysis [22]. Cell blocks could be obtained from 48% of aspirates and added diagnostic material to that from cytology smears in 8%.

Recently a 19 G EBUS-TBNA needle has become available which combines a large caliber with flexibility due to nitinol construction [23]. Tremblay et al. [24] reported the use of a 19 G needle in 297 individual lymph nodes or lesions sampled by 10 bronchoscopists. On average the node sizes were relatively large (mean diameter of nodes was 20.4 mm, and lung lesions 33.5 mm). Procedure sample adequacy was 88.6% in suspected malignant cases, 91.0% in suspected sarcoidosis/lymphadenopathy cases, and 85.7% in cases with suspected lymphoma. Only one case (0.6%) of intra-procedure bleeding was noted.

For sarcoidosis, Balwan [25] has reported the use of a 19 G needle (ViziShot FLEX 19-G) in a series of patients with suspected sarcoidosis. The procedure confirmed sarcoidosis in 14 of 15 (93.3%) patients. Of 33 lymph nodes, 28 (85%) were positive for non-caseating granulomas. By comparison the yields of transbronchial lung biopsy and endobronchial lung biopsy were 38% (5/13) and 43% (6/14), respectively. Overall the high diagnostic rate points to the role of the larger needle in this condition.

Miniami et al. [26] have reported a comparative study of 19 G versus 21 and 22 G needles in EBUS-TBNA. From 11 patients, definitive diagnoses were made using the 19 G needle in 9 patients, including one case of retinal hemangioblastoma, one tuberculous lymphadenitis, one lung adenocarcinoma, one lymphoma, and one sarcoidosis. Programmed death-ligand 1 (PD-L1) expression was confirmed by 19 G following initial negative findings after a 21 or 22 G biopsy. Three patients were diagnosed with sarcoidosis using both the 19 G and 21 or 22 G needles.

Needle Techniques

In the early experience of operators, a common reason for a false-negative test is inability to pass the needle through the cartilages in a lymph node. Many authorities have described the basic principles of the use of the sheath to facilitate the placement of the apparatus between cartilage rings, so the sharp needle can be advanced unopposed. A very elegant refinement of this aspect of the procedure described by Inoue et al. ("the outer sheath method") starts with the plastic outer sheath extended and in view at the top of the ultrasound image. The scope is very slowly pulled back and the sheath is carefully watched for a "drop" into a space between cartilages [27]. In a comparative study of 340 patients divided into before and after the introduction of this outer sheath method, there was a significant improvement in diagnostic yield from 93 to 98%. Other reasons for false-negative tests include bloody aspirates (particularly in metastatic malignancies such as renal cell carcinoma and melanoma) as well as large necrotic nodes. In the latter cases some authorities paradoxically recommend sampling the more vascular parts of a node, as these are more viable. Finally, it is important for the needle not to be passed distal to the node, so early training focuses on starting the needle insertion at the near (head) end of the node.

Diagnosing Primary Masses

EBUS-TBNA can be used to make the diagnosis on primary lung cancers and masses situated centrally in a peri-bronchial position in the inner third of the lung. Almeida et al. [28] reported on EBUS-TBNA for intrapulmonary lesions not able to be visualized by white-light bronchoscopy. From 108 procedures, when EBUS-TBNA could visualize intrapulmonary lesions the diagnostic yield was 87%. EBUS-TBNA was non-diagnostic in 14 (13%), most of which (9 cases) had benign disease based on clinical and follow-up imaging. The sensitivity and the negative predicted value was 94.7% and 75%, respectively. There was one case of major bleeding requiring bronchial artery embolization and one pneumothorax requiring chest tube drainage. In one retrospective study of 32 cases, the diagnostic yield for malignancy overall for EBUS-TBNA was 94%; 13 patients had a transbronchial lung biopsy, yield 61%, and 8 patients could have endobronchial biopsy, yield 75%. In another study of 60 patients [29], EBUS-TBNA was able to make the diagnosis of primary central lung cancer in 46 cases (77%) after a prior negative standard bronchoscopy. Other diagnostic procedures such as CT-FNA or surgical biopsy could be canceled in 47% and 30% of patients, respectively.

Rapid On-Site Evaluation (ROSE)

ROSE by a cytologist or technician examining smears of TBNA material is a well-established adjunct to the procedure. Jain et al. have recently reviewed the role of ROSE [30] (Figure 5.2, which can minimize repeat procedures for additional desired testing (i.e. molecular studies). It does not adversely affect the number of aspirations, total procedure time of

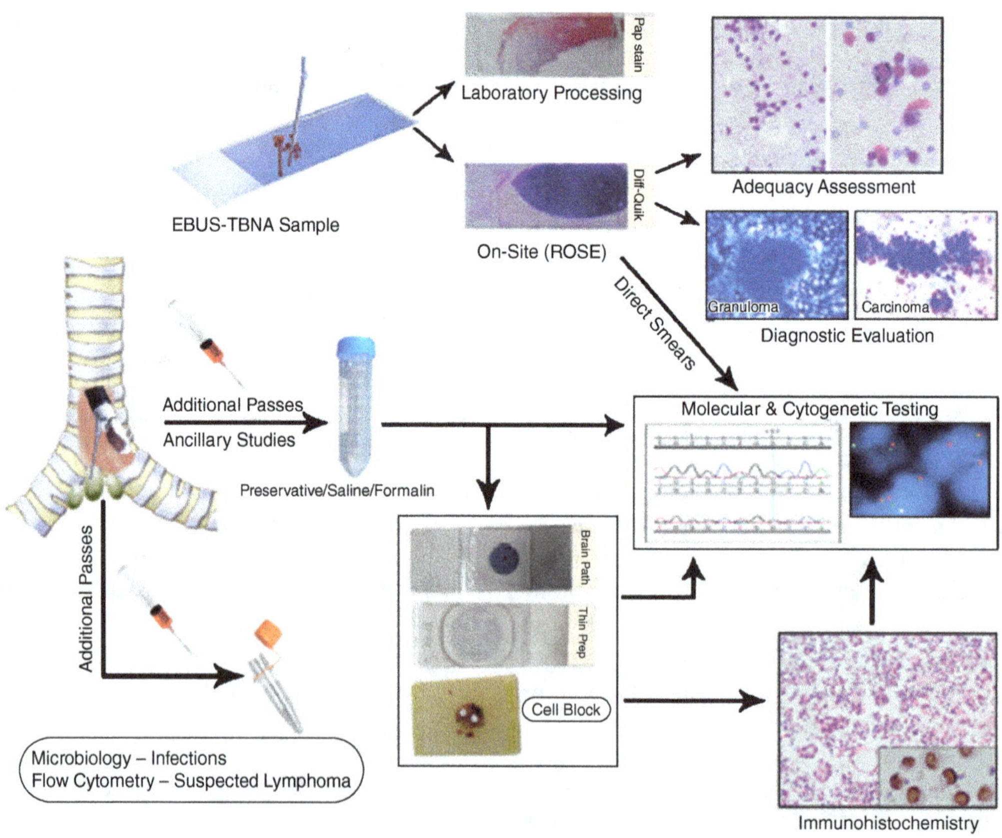

Figure 5.2 Schematic diagram to show purpose and algorithmic flow of rapid on-site evaluation (ROSE) for endobronchial ultrasound-guided transbronchial needle aspirate (EBUS-TBNA) specimens. Pap, Papanicolaou. *Source:* Jain et al. [30]. Reprinted with permission from Elsevier, American Medical Association.

EBUS-TBNA, or the rate of post-procedure complications. The role of ROSE is likely to grow and evolve with roles in next-generation sequencing (NGS) and even PD-L1 testing.

One prospective study of 108 patients showed a significant reduction in the ROSE group of the requirement for other forms of bronchoscopic biopsy. There were significantly fewer passes required to make a diagnosis in the ROSE group (2.2 vs. 3.1 punctures in the non-ROSE group, $p < 0.001$) [31]. This study did not show a significant reduction in procedure time, although others have. ROSE facilitates the division of EBUS-TBNA samples into that which is used for pathologic diagnosis and that for molecular testing, without limiting the ability to make a pathologic diagnosis [19, 24]. One prospective randomized study of 126 patients [32] showed that ROSE reduces the need for repeat diagnostic procedures (for additional material for genetic testing) when lung cancer is known or suspected: for epidermal growth factor receptor (EGFR), Kirsten rat sarcoma viral oncogene (KRAS), and anaplastic lymphoma kinase (ALK), 91% success in the ROSE group compared to 80% in the non-ROSE group. The ROSE group could stop the procedure after sampling just one site (58.9% vs. 44.1%, $p = 0.01$) Importantly, these authors also showed that there were fewer instances where the samples were insufficient for molecular analysis (0 cases vs. 6 in the non-ROSE group, $p = 0.05$).

NGS on Diff-Quik Smears from EBUS-TBNA

ROSE smears often have abundant malignant cells, which can become a source of DNA for molecular analysis. Stoy et al. [33] have shown this utility in NGS panel testing from 54 subjects which had abundant cellularity from 22 and 25 G needles: cytology smears provided the testing material in 85% of cases and it was successful in over 97% of cases. They concluded that NGS can be reliably performed on EBUS-TBNA cytology smears and that needle size did not affect the ability to do NGS.

Fielding et al. [34] have also shown the utility of ROSE Diff-Quik smears for NGS. Overall there was significantly more abundant DNA on smears compared to matched cell blocks, and indeed more mutations were detectable by smear samples compared to the cell blocks. The impact of formalin fixation on the cell blocks was considered the most likely reason for the difference. Triaging of samples is easier because the cellularity can be directly quantitated, and this study showed how simple cellularity quantitation can directly predict DNA content and NGS success (Figure 5.3). Such a process is easier than the requirement to identify tumor in cell block sections, which also may ultimately have a lower yield of DNA.

Elastography

Elastography is a non-invasive adjunct to EBUS-TBNA to characterize nodes based on their degree of stiffness; malignant tissues are more rigid due to increased cellularity and vascularity. The electronic imaging target is tissue strain, the effect of compression and decompression on tissues. Compression can either be the result of the imaging probe, or more subtly the impact of pulsations from cardiac and vascular structures. It has been utilized in breast cancer imaging in particular over the last seven years or so. The electronic measurement of different degrees of strain can be represented in red, green, and blue color format: blue represents the greatest strain and most likely malignant tissue. The tissues can be characterized by region of interest (ROI; by color quantitation) or by comparing a known benign structure and calculating ratios. Nakajima et al. [35] first studied EBUS-TBNA nodes by dividing images into three groups: (i) predominantly non-blue, (ii) partly blue and partly non-blue, and (iii) predominantly blue (Figure 5.4). From this they calculated a stiff area ratio. Live EBUS images were taken from 49 lymph nodes as well as elastography of surgically resected nodes in 11 cases, using the known distribution of

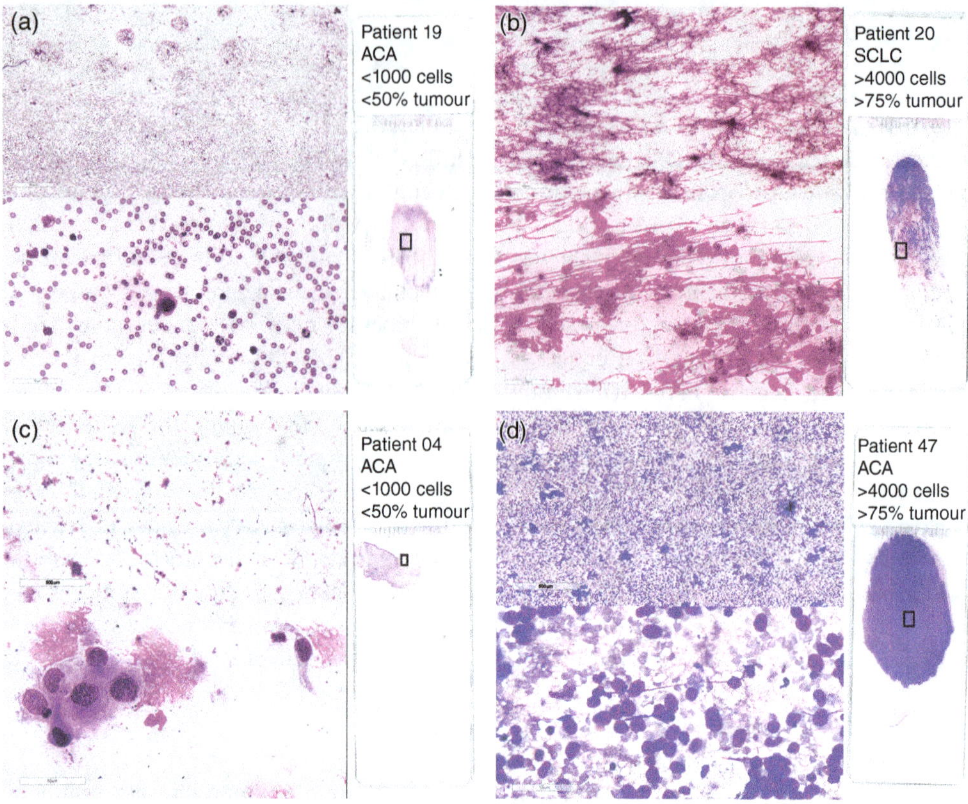

Figure 5.3 Tumour cell density observations for cytology smears of four patients (data reported in Table 1, Fielding et al., *Respiration*, in press). Composite figures of low power (whole slide), 4× and 40× magnification scans of the cytology smears for patients 19 (a), 20 (b), 04 (c), and 47(d). *Source:* Fielding et al. [34]. Reprinted with permission from Karger Publishers.

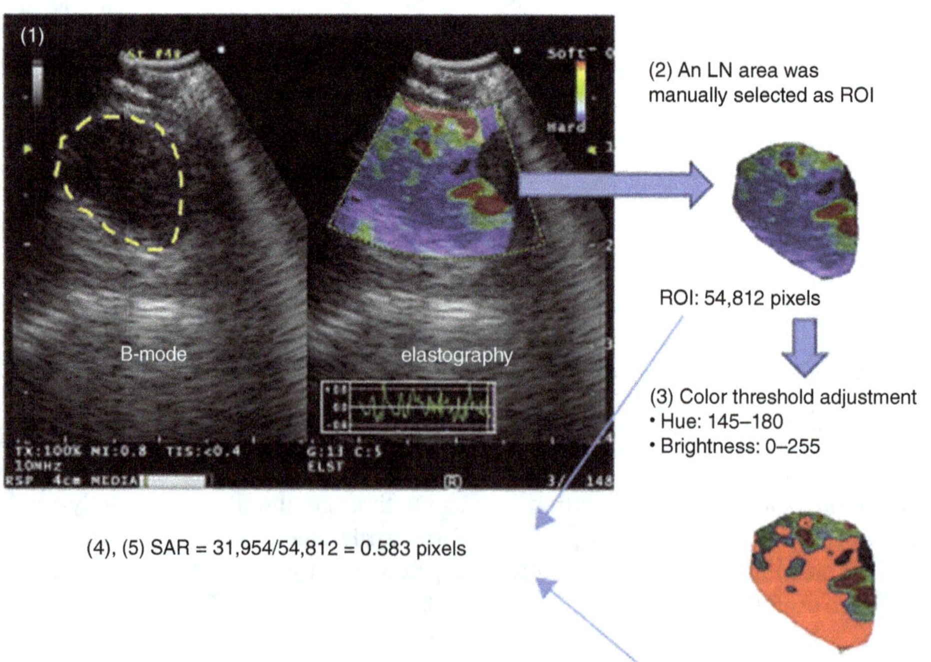

Figure 5.4 Quantification of the stiff area ratio (SAR) using ImageJ. For the quantitative analysis of stiffer areas (blue area) within a lymph node (LN), we defined the SAR as the relatively stiffer area (blue pixel area) per region of interest (ROI; LN area) on an endobronchial elastography image. *Source:* Nakajima et al. [35]. Reprinted with permission from S. Karger AG.

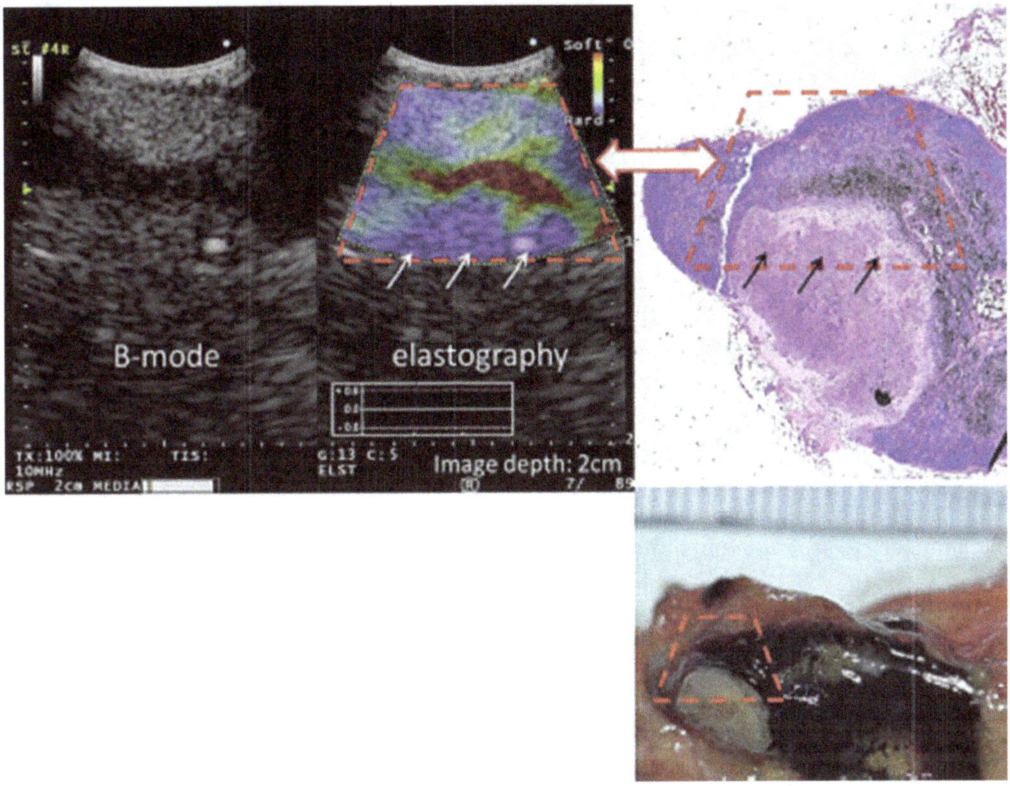

Figure 5.5 Elastography of surgically removed lymph nodes (LNs). The area surrounded by dashes is compatible with the elastography scanning area (the ultrasound image depth was adjusted to 2 cm). The metastatic area displayed a "relatively hard" sign, shown in blue in the elastography image (arrow), and the normal LN exhibited a "relatively soft" sign, shown in green, yellow, and red in the elastography image. *Source:* Nakajima et al. [35]. Reprinted with permission from S. Karger AG.

malignant cells within nodes to directly compare stiff regions as shown by elastography (Figure 5.5). Mean stiff area ratios were significantly greater for metastatic lymph nodes (0.478; that is, showing more predominantly blue) than for benign nodes (0.216; $p = 0.0002$). Using a cutoff value of 0.311 for stiff area ratios, the sensitivity and specificity for predicting metastatic disease was 0.81 and 0.85, respectively. The stiff area was histologically compatible with metastatic distribution in surgically resected lymph nodes. This study was retrospective and subsequent prospective data are now available.

Rozman et al. [36] in the same year studied the ratios of abnormal tissues (the largest possible area of a lymph node selected manually as an ROI) to adjacent normal mediastinal tissue between the lymph node and bronchial cartilage or lateral to the lymph node. The "strain ratio" was calculated for 80 lymph nodes: combining sensitivity and specificity in a receiver operator characteristic curve, the area under the curve was 0.87 ($p < 0.0001$). Strain ratio values higher than 8 represented a probability of malignant involvement with an accuracy of 89.39%: sensitivity 88.24%, specificity 90.61%, positive predictive value (PPV) 90.91%, negative predictive value (NPV) 87.88%. Technical challenges were noted: obtaining consistent measurements was more problematic in the right paratracheal region, possibly because the heart and vascular pulsations were less pronounced on the right side of the trachea, and thus less tissue compression could impair strain calculation. In several patients, calcified cartilage cast intense acoustic shadows and narrowed the field of vision. The third challenge was a scarceness of tissue in the mediastinum from which to select the normal comparator and the presence of large vessels, which sometimes impeded on the image despite attempts to exclude them. While four false-negative cases were observed, overall these authors commented on the high NPV (96.15%) in normal-sized nodes, which represented a new way of thinking about the difficulties of having to sample multiple nodes in a staging procedure. They commented that elastography would not replace sampling, but could supplement it where sampling was difficult or inconclusive, and potentially reduce the number of aspirates on difficult small nodes.

Korrungruang and Boonsargsuk [37] have recently reported a prospective series of 120 lymph nodes from 72 patients using the blue quantitation method. To assess interobserver agreement in qualitative color elastography, still images of all selected lymph nodes undergoing elastography were captured and reviewed independently by an operator not present at the initial procedure. Results showed that malignant nodes had a higher median strain ratio than benign nodes (73.50, range 2.93–305.00, vs. 1.29, range 0.03–194.00, $p < 0.001$). The area under the curve (AUC) for the strain ratio was 0.85 (95% confidence interval [CI]: 0.74–0.97). Importantly, lymph node size did not affect elastography results; however, the study was for cases needing a tissue diagnosis, hence studies of staging procedures might have predominantly more small nodes (and lower pre-test likelihood of involvement), which the authors commented should be the subject of further study. While no case classified as predominantly non-blue had malignant cells, there were six false-positive cases (predominantly blue but benign on cytopathology). For interobserver variability in elastography interpretation, the kappa value was 0.88. There were no cases of disagreement in interpretation from Type 1 to Type 3 and vice versa.

Huang et al. [38] reported a retrospective study of 45 benign and 33 malignant nodes. Using the ROI color scheme, Type 1 nodes were benign in 26/27 (96.3%) and malignant in 1/27 (3.7%); for Type 2 lymph nodes, 15/20 (75.0%) were benign and 5/20 (25.0%) were malignant; Type 3 lymph nodes were benign in 4/31 (12.9%) and malignant in 27/31 (87.1%). In classifying Type 1 as "benign" and Type 3 as "malignant," the sensitivity, specificity, PPV, NPV, and diagnostic accuracy rates were 96.43%, 86.67%, 87.10%, 96.30%, and 91.38%, respectively.

A recent meta-analysis [39] pooled the results of seven studies of elastography at EBUS-TBNA. The pooled sensitivity, specificity, positive likelihood ratio, negative likelihood ratio, and diagnostic odds ratio were 0.93 (95% CI: 0.85–0.97), 0.85 (95% CI: 0.78–0.90), 6.3 (95% CI: 4.2–9.2), 0.08 (95% CI: 0.04–0.18), and 74 (95% CI: 33–168), respectively. The summary receiver operating characteristic curve was 0.93 (95% CI: 0.91–0.95).

Overall there is promise with elastography and most data present the color quantitation method. Some technical questions remain, particularly the need for varying amounts of pressure at different node locations (even noting that the pressure measurements come from the patient's own vascular pulsations), although it is generally considered that the ratio of color overcomes this issue. It is possible that more data will emerge in the difficult procedures of staging where many smaller nodes and groups of nodes within the same station need to be sampled. It is likely its strongest application will be in assisting confirmation of the benign status of nodes, particularly in small nodes where there is limited aspirate material, such that elastography supplements the cytology.

Other Methods of Image Analysis

Spectral analysis of lymph node tissue at EBUS-TBNA has been tested by Nakajima et al. [40]. Spectral features of the raw data of the ultrasound images (mid-band fit, slope, and intercept) were analyzed using techniques previously tested in gastroenterology. They found that these data gave high NPV and fair sensitivity results from a training set of 362 nodes and a testing set of 264 nodes. In the testing set two features (intercept and slope) gave the highest diagnostic accuracy, 83.1%, with PPV and NPV of 64.1% and 92.2%, respectively. The important potential of this technique is that it requires no training and is purely a digital analysis.

Nguyen et al. [41] studied the application of the grayscale features of ultrasound images (pixel values, entropy, energy, and homogeneity, all digitally derived). From a training set and prediction set of 52 and 51 nodes, respectively, ROIs of the nodes were examined. Malignant nodes had a greater difference in the maximal and minimal pixel values, scanning electron microscope (SEM) pixel value, entropy, and correlation, and a lower energy ($p < 0.0001$ for all values). In the validation set, 44 of 51 (86.3%) were classified correctly. When 18 of these lymph nodes also had FDG-PET-CT scan assessment, it correctly classified 14 of 18 nodes (77.8%), compared with grayscale texture analysis, which correctly classified 16 of 18 nodes (88.9%). Potentially the technique could be improved by analyzing multiple images of the same node rather than a single frame, and it holds the possibility of real-time analysis during the procedure.

Genetics on EBUS-TBNA Lung Cancer Samples

During the past decade, substantial progress has been made in the characterization of molecular abnormalities in non-small cell lung carcinoma (NSCLC) tumors that are being used as molecular targets and predictive biomarkers for the selection of targeted therapy [42, 43]. These recent advances in NSCLC-targeted therapy require the analysis of a panel of molecular abnormalities in tumor specimens, including gene mutations (e.g. EGFR, KRAS, B-raf proto oncogene [BRAF], discoidin domain receptor tyrosine kinase 2 [DDR2]), gene amplifications (e.g. MET, fibroblast growth factor receptor 1 [FGFR1]), and fusions (e.g. EML4-ALK) by applying different methods to tumor tissue (biopsy) and cell (cytology) samples. A recent meta-analysis of studies on this subject was published by Labarca et al. [44]. A total of 33 studies including 2698 participants were analyzed. In 28 studies that evaluated EBUS-TBNA for the identification of EGFR mutations, the pooled probability of obtaining a sufficient sample was 94.5% (95% CI: 93.2–96.4%). For identification of ALK mutations, the pooled probability was 94.9% (95% CI: 89.4–98.8%). Finally, the prevalence of EGFR mutation was 15.8% (95% CI: 12.1–19.4%), and the prevalence of ALK mutation was 2.77% (95% CI: 1.0–4.8%). Data for ROS1 and PD-L1 mutations were not suitable for meta-analysis.

While the efficacy of single gene testing was confirmed, more research was called for regarding NGS.

Next-Generation Sequencing (NGS)

Targeted NGS allows for the detection of multiple gene mutations on pre-selected panels [45, 46]. NGS can be done with tiny amounts of material without the need for extra biopsies. A number of authors have reported NGS findings from formalin-fixed paraffin-embedded (FFPE) samples of NSCLC. Takeda studied transbronchial lung biopsy and resected tumor specimens from 110 patients with NSCLC using a gene sequencing panel which covered 22 mutational hotspots as well as 72 major variants of ALK, RET, ROS1, and neurotrophic receptor tyrosine kinase 1 (NTRK1) transcripts [47]. The most common mutations were TP53 (42 patients), EGFR (25 patients), serine/threonine kinase 11 (STK11; 12 patients), and KRAS (10 patients). Potentially actionable mutations were found in 50% of those with adenocarcinomas and 14% of those with squamous cell carcinomas. Deeb et al. reported NGS on FFPE material from 23 primary and metastatic lung cancers with known EGFR and KRAS mutations from previous routine diagnostic evaluation [48]. When needed, micro or macro dissection of blocks was performed to achieve at least 25% tumor cell content. Of the 25 EGFR and KRAS mutations detected by 454 deep sequencing tests, 24 (96%) were correctly identified by pyrosequencing. In addition, four other non-synonymous mutations were detected, including one sample with multiple EGFR mutations and a PIK3CA mutation.

Recently, Roy-Chowdhuri et al. examined cytology preparations for DNA yield and NGS in 207 samples from a range of sites including EBUS-TBNA samples [49]. NGS was possible in over 70% of cases; all cases in their study had high cellularity (60–70% tumor percentage on slides). An earlier study from the same group reported 61 tumor FNA specimens for adequacy of DNA yield for NGS [50]. From 33 smears and 28 FFPE cell blocks, they found that 31 specimens yielded sufficient DNA: 10 ng, for a 46-gene Ion Personal Genome Machine™ (PGM™) sequencer (Ion Torrent, Waltham, MA, USA). This was after excluding specimens with tumor percentage estimated at <20%.

Studies confirming the role of NGS on EBUS-TBNA specimens have established this as an important part of specimen processing. Studies on cell blocks show its feasibility not only for adenocarcinomas, but for a range of cancer types. Fielding et al. [51] showed the successful feasibility of NGS on a prospective series of diagnostic EBUS-TBNA procedures without changing the number of needle passes using sections of cell blocks in 67 cases. Sung et al. studied adenocarcinoma cases and showed that ROSE was important in improving the quality of specimens to allow NGS. Specifically, the presence of at least one cytopathologist from the commencement of the procedure confirmed the adequacy of aspirates on ROSE, meaning that additional passes could directly be placed in media (CytoLyt®, Cytyc, Marlborough, MA, USA) for genetic testing. This factor was positively correlated with successful NGS.

Turner et al. [52] explored massively parallel sequencing, a comprehensive hybrid capture-based assay (MSK-IMPACT™, Memorial Sloan Kettering Cancer Center, New York, USA) of 340 genes. In total, MSK-IMPACT was requested for 115 malignant samples and was successful for 99 (86.1%), using paraffin-embedded cell blocks in 93 cases (93.9%) and needle rinse fluid in 6 cases. The success rate of the assay improved significantly from the first one-third of cases (76.3%), to 92.3% for the final one-third of cases ($p < 0.05$). This may have related to refinements in EBUS-TBNA technique and increased experience with ROSE in the operating room. In addition, the introduction of mineral oil as a solvent, and modification of cell block preparation technique, may have improved the outcome over time.

Doxtader and Jain [53, 54] have reviewed the role of cytology specimens in molecular analysis of lung cancer. The emphasis is on the cytology specimens. Smears are taken for Papanicolaou (Pap) and Diff-Quik staining, while residual aspirate material can be placed in CytoLyt (methanol) solution from which a cell pellet is made by centrifugation. This pellet can be used for cell block and thin prep slides for fluorescence in situ hybridization (FISH) and ALK gene rearrangements), while the residual from the pellet can be sent for NGS (Figures 5.6 and 5.7).

EBUS-TBNA and PD-L1 Staining

It is technically possible to perform PD-L1 staining on cell block specimens from EBUS [55, 56]. Sakata et al. [57] retrospectively analyzed patients who underwent EBUS-TBNA followed by surgical resection of NSCLC. The archived specimens were retrieved and assessed

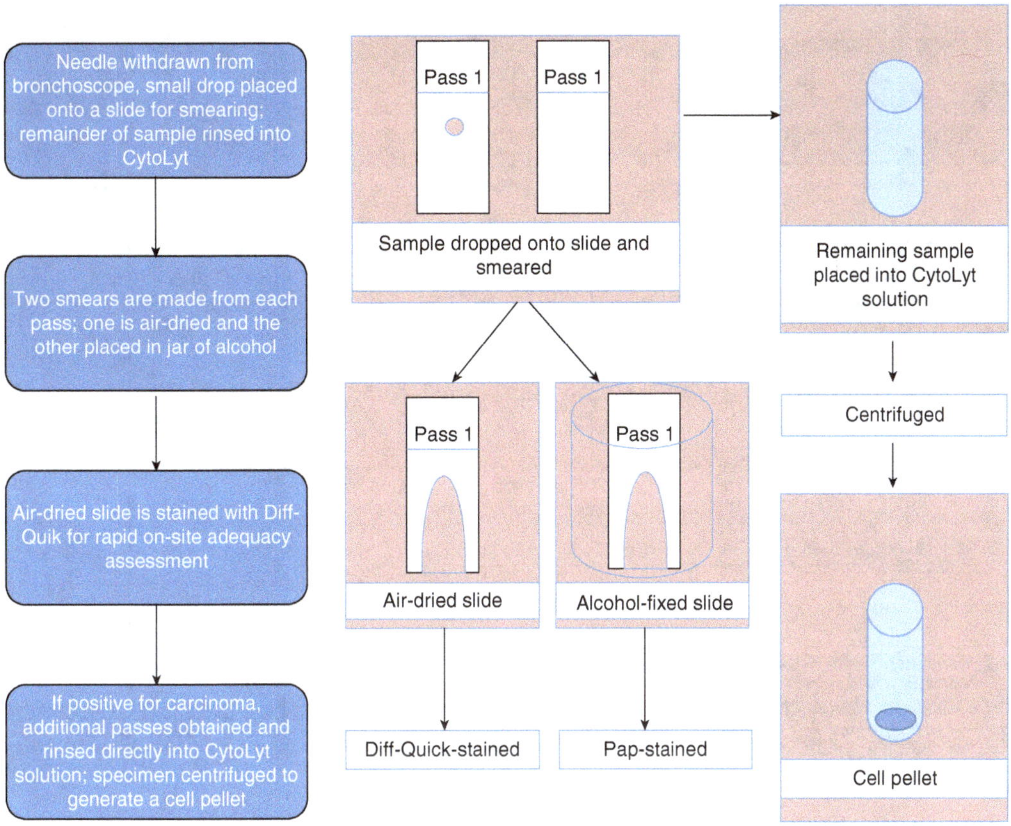

Figure 5.6 Specimen handling at the time of endobronchial ultrasound-guided transbronchial fine-needle aspiration. The cytopathologist is available for rapid on-site assessment to render a preliminary interpretation. A portion of the sample is smeared and then stained with Diff-Quik. If the slide is positive for non-small cell carcinoma, additional passes are requested and directly placed into CytoLyt solution to enrich the specimen for tumor DNA for downstream molecular analysis, if needed. Pap, Papanicolaou. *Source:* Doxtader et al. [53].

for PD-L1. A positive PD-L1 stain was defined using two separate cutoff points: ≥1% and ≥50% of tumor cell positivity. EBUS-TBNA aspirates were compared with the surgically resected specimen to calculate test parameters. From 61 patients, for PD-L1 ≥1%, the sensitivity, specificity, PPV, and NPV were 72%, 100%, 100%, and 80%, respectively. For PD-L1 ≥50%, the sensitivity, specificity, PPV, and NPV were 47%, 93%, 70%, and 84%, respectively. The concordance rates for PD-L1 ≥1% and ≥50% were 87% and 82%, respectively. Overall a cutoff of ≥1% on EBUS-TBNA strongly correlated with resected tumor specimen. However, for PD-L1 ≥50%, there was a significant decrease in the sensitivity and PPV of EBUS-TBNA specimens when compared with resected tumor.

Noll et al. [58] have shown that smears (Pap and Diff-Quik) give similar results on PD-L1 staining to core biopsy samples, and this will undoubtedly be a further area of exploration for ROSE at EBUS-TBNA. Further work is needed along these lines, in particular collecting more samples with higher staining percentages, as these are often the cases most suited to first-line systemic therapy. The temporal changes in node lymphocyte activity compared to the primary tumor require further investigation.

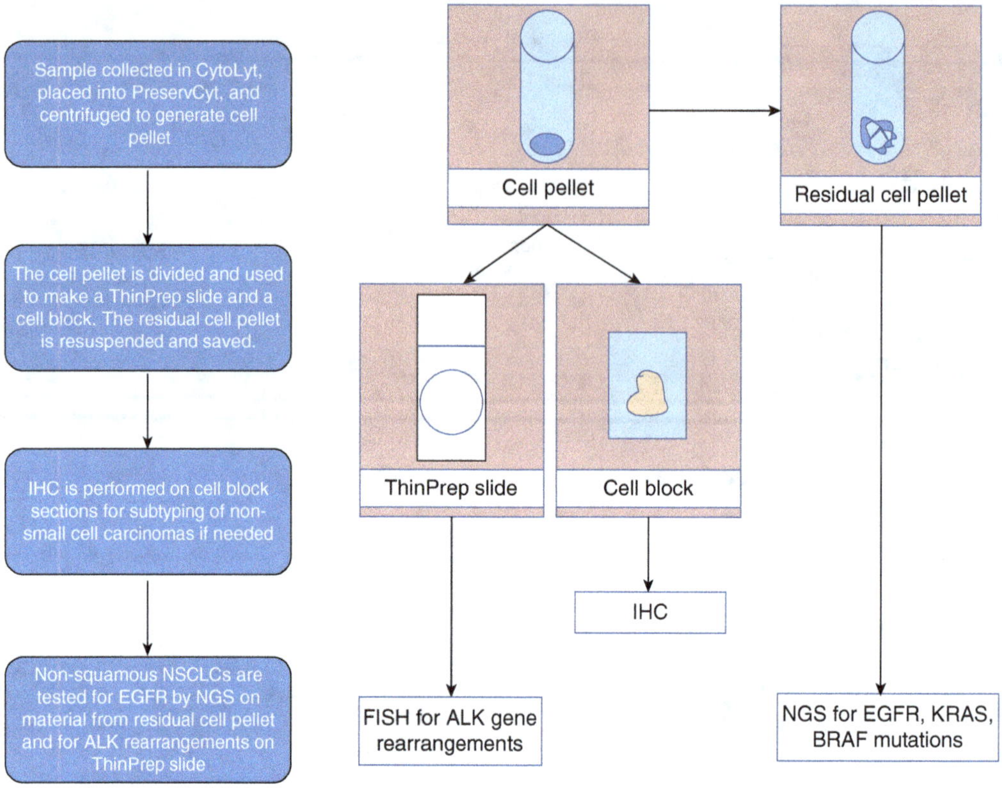

Figure 5.7 Processing of endobronchial ultrasound-guided transbronchial fine-needle aspiration cytology specimens at the Cleveland Clinic. Cytopathology specimens are collected in CytoLyt solution, placed into PreservCyt® (Hologic, Marlborough, MA, USA), and then centrifuged to generate a cell pellet. The cell pellet is divided to make a ThinPrep® slide (Hologic) and a cell black. Residual cell pellet material is saved and used for next-generation sequencing (NGS) for epidermal growth factor receptor (EGFR), Kirsten rat sarcoma viral oncogene homolog (KRAS), and B-raf proto oncogene (BRAF) mutations if needed; the ThinPrep slide is used for anaplastic lymphoma kinase (ALK) fluorescence in situ hybridization (FISH) testing. IHC, immunohistochemistry; NSCLC, non-small cell lung carcinoma. *Source:* Doxtader et al. [53].

References

1 Aswanetmanee, P., Limsuwat, C., Kabach, M. et al. (2016). The role of sedation in endobronchial ultrasound-guided transbronchial needle aspiration: systematic review. *Endoscopic Ultrasound* 5: 300–306.

2 Öztaş, S., Aka Aktürk, Ü., Alpay, L.A. et al. (2017). A comparison of propofol-midazolam and midazolam alone for sedation in endobronchial ultrasound-guided transbronchial needle aspiration: a retrospective cohort study. *Clinical Respiratory Journal* 11: 935–941.

3 Franzen, D., Schneiter, D., Weder, W., and Kohler, M. (2017). Impact of sedation technique on the diagnostic accuracy of endobronchial ultrasound-guided transbronchial needle aspiration. *Endoscopic Ultrasound* 6: 257–263.

4 Casal, R.F., Lazarus, D.R., Kuhl, K. et al. (2015). Randomized trial of endobronchial ultrasound-guided transbronchial needle aspiration under general anesthesia versus moderate sedation. *American Journal of Respiratory and Critical Care Medicine* 191: 796–803.

5 Khemasuwan, D., Teerapuncharoen, K., and Griffin, D.C. (2018). Diagnostic yield and safety of bronchoscopist-directed moderate sedation with a bolus dose administration of propofol during endobronchial ultrasound bronchoscopy. *Journal of Bronchology & Interventional Pulmonology* 25: 181–188.

6 Takakuwa, O., Oguri, T., Asano, T. et al. (2018). Prevention of hypoxemia during endobronchial ultrasound-guided transbronchial needle aspiration: usefulness of high-flow nasal cannula. *Respiratory Investigation* 56: 418–423.

7 Val-Bernal, J.-F., Martino, M., Yllera, E. et al. (2019). Endobronchial ultrasound-guided transbronchial needle aspiration in the diagnosis of hilar and mediastinal lymph node metastases of melanoma. *Turk Patoloji Dergisi* 35 (2): 92–101.

8 Val-Bernal, J.-F., Martino, M., Romay, F., and Yllera, E. (2018). Endobronchial ultrasound-guided transbronchial needle aspiration in the diagnosis of mediastinal metastases of clear cell renal cell carcinoma. *Pathology, Research and Practice* 214: 949–956.

9 Korrungruang, P., Oki, M., Saka, H. et al. (2016). Endobronchial ultrasound-guided transbronchial needle aspiration is useful as an initial procedure for the diagnosis of lymphoma. *Respiratory Investigation* 54: 29–34.

10 Jin, M. and Wakely, P.E. Jr. (2016). Endoscopic/endobronchial ultrasound-guided fine needle aspiration and ancillary techniques, particularly flow cytometry, in diagnosing deep-seated lymphomas. *Acta Cytologica* 60: 326–335.

11 Furukawa, B.S., Bernstein, M., Siddiqi, N., and Pastis, N.J. (2016). Diagnosing Hodgkin lymphoma from an endobronchial ultrasound core needle biopsy. *Journal of Bronchology & Interventional Pulmonology* 23: 336–339.

12 Eickhoff, L., Golpon, H., Zardo, P. et al. (2018). Endobronchial ultrasound in suspected non-malignant mediastinal lymphadenopathy. *Pneumologie (Stuttgart, Germany)* 72: 559–567.

13 Lee, J., Kim, Y.K., Seo, Y.Y. et al. (2018). Clinical characteristics of false-positive lymph node on chest CT or PET-CT confirmed by endobronchial ultrasound-guided transbronchial needle aspiration in lung cancer. *Tuberculosis and Respiratory Diseases* 81: 339–346.

14 Park, Y.S., Lee, J., Pang, J.C. et al. (2013). Clinical implication of microscopic anthracotic pigment in mediastinal staging of non-small cell lung cancer by endobronchial ultrasound-guided transbronchial needle aspiration. *Journal of Korean Medical Science* 28: 550–554.

15 Pattison, A., Cook, A., Singh, M. et al. (2018). EBUS-TBNA cytology specimens are predictive of occupational dust exposure in patients with bilateral mediastinal and hilar lymphadenopathy. *Journal of Occupational and Environmental Medicine* 60: 880–885.

16 Plit, M., Pearson, R., Havryk, A. et al. (2012). Diagnostic utility of endobronchial ultrasound-guided transbronchial needle aspiration compared with transbronchial and endobronchial biopsy for suspected sarcoidosis. *Internal Medicine Journal* 42: 434–438.

17 Hata, Y., Sakamoto, S., Otsuka, H. et al. (2013). EBUS-TBNA-related complications in a patient with tuberculous lymphadenopathy. *Internal Medicine (Tokyo, Japan)* 52: 2553–2559.

18 Boonsarngsuk, V., Saengsri, S., and Santanirand, P. (2017). Endobronchial ultrasound-guided transbronchial needle aspiration rinse fluid polymerase chain reaction in the diagnosis of intrathoracic tuberculous lymphadenitis. *Infectious Diseases (London, England)* 49: 193–199.

19 Wahidi, M.M., Herth, F., Yasufuku, K. et al. (2016). Technical aspects of endobronchial ultrasound-guided transbronchial needle aspiration: CHEST guideline and expert panel report. *Chest* 149: 816–835.

20 Saji, J., Kurimoto, N., Morita, K. et al. (2011). Comparison of 21-gauge and 22-gauge needles for endobronchial ultrasound-guided transbronchial needle aspiration of mediastinal and hilar lymph nodes. *Journal of Bronchology & Interventional Pulmonology* 18: 239–246.

21 Nakajima, T., Yasufuku, K., Takahashi, R. et al. (2011). Comparison of 21-gauge and 22-gauge aspiration needle during endobronchial ultrasound-guided transbronchial needle aspiration. *Respirology (Carlton, Vic)* 16: 90–94.

22 Sanz-Santos, J., Serra, P., Andreo, F. et al. (2012). Contribution of cell blocks obtained through endobronchial ultrasound-guided transbronchial needle aspiration to the diagnosis of lung cancer. *BMC Cancer* 12: 34–34.

23 Herth, F.J., Gompelman, D., Shah, P.L., Eberhardt, R. (2015). Endobronchial ultrasound-guided TBNA (EBUS-TBNA) with a 19 gauge needle – first experience. B103 Fixing a Hole: Advances in Diagnostic and Therapeutic Bronchoscopy, poster discussion session. *American Thoracic Society International Conference* (15–20 May 2015). p. A3726.

24 Tremblay, A., McFadden, S., Bonifazi, M. et al. (2018). Endobronchial ultrasound-guided transbronchial needle aspiration with a 19-G needle device. *Journal of Bronchology & Interventional Pulmonology* 25: 218–223.

25 Balwan, A. (2018). Endobronchial ultrasound-guided transbronchial needle aspiration using 19-G needle for sarcoidosis. *Journal of Bronchology & Interventional Pulmonology* 25: 260–263.

26 Minami, D., Ozeki, T., Okawa, S. et al. (2018). Comparing the clinical performance of the new 19-G ViziShot FLEX and 21- or 22-G ViziShot 2 endobronchial ultrasound-guided transbronchial needle aspiration needles. *Internal Medicine (Tokyo, Japan)* 57 (24): 3515–3520.

27 Inoue, T., Kurimoto, N., Furuya, N. et al. (2013). New technique for endobronchial ultrasound-guided transbronchial needle aspiration to improve diagnostic yield. *Journal of Bronchology & Interventional Pulmonology* 20: 28–32.

28 Almeida, F.A., Salam, S., Mehta, A.C. et al. (2018). Sampling utility of the convex probe endobronchial ultrasound visible intrapulmonary lesion. *Journal of Bronchology & Interventional Pulmonology* 25: 290–299.

29 Tournoy, K.G., Rintoul, R.C., van Meerbeeck, J.P. et al. (2009). EBUS-TBNA for the diagnosis of central parenchymal lung lesions not visible at routine bronchoscopy. *Lung Cancer (Amsterdam, Netherlands)* 63: 45–49.

30 Jain, D., Allen, T.C., Aisner, D.L. et al. (2018). Rapid on-site evaluation of endobronchial ultrasound-guided transbronchial needle aspirations for the diagnosis of lung cancer: a perspective from members of the pulmonary pathology society. *Archives of Pathology & Laboratory Medicine* 142: 253–262.

31 Oki, M., Saka, H., Kitagawa, C. et al. (2013). Rapid on-site cytologic evaluation during endobronchial ultrasound-guided transbronchial needle aspiration for diagnosing lung cancer: a randomized study. *Respiration; International Review of Thoracic Diseases* 85: 486–492.

32 Trisolini, R., Cancellieri, A., Tinelli, C. et al. (2015). Randomized trial of endobronchial ultrasound-guided transbronchial needle aspiration with and without rapid on-site evaluation for lung cancer genotyping. *Chest* 148: 1430–1437.

33 Stoy, S. and Murgu, S. (2017). The use of endobronchial ultrasound guided transbronchial needle aspiration specimens for next generation sequencing in non-small cell lung cancer: a clinical perspective. *Journal of Thoracic Disease* 9: E398–E401.

34 Fielding, D., Dalley, A.J., Bashirzadeh, F. et al. (2019). Diff-Quik Cytology Smears from Endobronchial Ultrasound Transbronchial Needle Aspiration Lymph

Node Specimens as a Source of DNA for Next-Generation Sequencing Instead of Cell Blocks. *Respiration* 97: 525–539.

35 Nakajima, T., Inage, T., Sata, Y. et al. (2015). Elastography for predicting and localizing nodal metastases during endobronchial ultrasound. *Respiration; International Review of Thoracic Diseases* 90: 499–506.

36 Rozman, A., Malovrh, M.M., Adamic, K. et al. (2015). Endobronchial ultrasound elastography strain ratio for mediastinal lymph node diagnosis. *Radiology and Oncology* 49: 334–340.

37 Korrungruang, P. and Boonsarngsuk, V. (2017). Endobronchial ultrasound elastography for the differentiation of benign and malignant lymph nodes – reply. *Respirology (Carlton, Vic.)* 22: 1038–1038.

38 Huang, H., Huang, Z., Wang, Q. et al. (2017). Effectiveness of the benign and malignant diagnosis of mediastinal and hilar lymph nodes by endobronchial ultrasound elastography. *Journal of Cancer* 8: 1843–1848.

39 Chen, Y.-F., Mao, X.-W., Zhang, Y.-J. et al. (2018). Endobronchial ultrasound elastography differentiates intrathoracic lymph nodes: a meta-analysis. *Annals of Thoracic Surgery* 106: 1251–1257.

40 Nakajima, T., Shingyoji, M., Anayama, T. et al. (2016). Spectrum analysis of endobronchial ultrasound radiofrequency of lymph nodes in patients with lung cancer. *Chest* 149: 1393–1399.

41 Nguyen, P., Bashirzadeh, F., Hundloe, J. et al. (2015). Grey scale texture analysis of endobronchial ultrasound mini probe images for prediction of benign or malignant aetiology. *Respirology (Carlton, Vic.)* 20: 960–966.

42 Reck, M., Heigener, D.F., Mok, T. et al. (2013). Management of non-small-cell lung cancer: recent developments. *Lancet* 382: 709–719.

43 Rosell, R., Bivona, T.G., and Karachaliou, N. (2013). Genetics and biomarkers in personalisation of lung cancer treatment. *Lancet* 382: 720–731.

44 Labarca, G., Folch, E., Jantz, M. et al. (2018). Adequacy of samples obtained by endobronchial ultrasound with transbronchial needle aspiration for molecular analysis in patients with non-small cell lung cancer. Systematic review and meta-analysis. *Annals of the American Thoracic Society* 15: 1205–1216.

45 Wistuba, I.I. (2012). Molecular testing of non-small cell lung carcinoma biopsy and cytology specimens. *American Society of Clinical Oncology Educational Book / ASCO American Society of Clinical Oncology Meeting* 2012: 459–464.

46 Ghigna, M.-R., Crutu, A., Florea, V. et al. (2018). Endobronchial ultrasound-guided fine-needle aspiration for pulmonary carcinomas genotyping: experience with 398 cases including rapid EGFR/KRAS analysis in 43 cases. *Journal of Thoracic Disease* 10: 4653–4658.

47 Takeda, M., Sakai, K., Terashima, M. et al. (2015). Clinical application of amplicon-based next-generation sequencing to therapeutic decision making in lung cancer. *Annals of Oncology* 26: 2477–2482.

48 Deeb, K.K., Hohman, C.M., Risch, N.F. et al. (2015). Routine clinical mutation profiling of non-small cell lung cancer using next-generation sequencing. *Archives of Pathology & Laboratory Medicine* 139: 913–921.

49 Roy-Chowdhuri, S., Chow, C.-W., Kane, M.K. et al. (2016). Optimizing the DNA yield for molecular analysis from cytologic preparations. *Cancer Cytopathology* 124 (4): 254–260.

50 Kanagal-Shamanna, R., Portier, B.P., Singh, R.R. et al. (2014). Next-generation sequencing-based multi-gene mutation profiling of solid tumors using fine needle aspiration samples: promises and challenges for routine clinical diagnostics. *Modern Pathology* 27: 314–327.

51 Fielding, D., Dalley, A.J., Bashirzadeh, F. et al. (2017). Next-generation sequencing of endobronchial ultrasound transbronchial needle aspiration specimens in lung cancer.

American Journal of Respiratory and Critical Care Medicine 196: 388–391.

52 Turner, S.R., Buonocore, D., Desmeules, P. et al. (2018). Feasibility of endobronchial ultrasound transbronchial needle aspiration for massively parallel next-generation sequencing in thoracic cancer patients. *Lung Cancer (Amsterdam, Netherlands)* 119: 85–90.

53 Doxtader, E.E., Cheng, Y.-W., and Zhang, Y. (2019). Molecular testing of non-small cell lung carcinoma diagnosed by endobronchial ultrasound-guided transbronchial fine-needle aspiration. *Archives of Pathology & Laboratory Medicine* 143 (6): 670–676.

54 Jain, D. and Roy-Chowdhuri, S. (2018). Molecular pathology of lung cancer cytology specimens: a concise review. *Archives of Pathology & Laboratory Medicine* 142: 1127–1133.

55 Stoy, S., Rosen, L., and Murgu, S. (2017). The use of endobronchial ultrasound-guided transbronchial needle aspiration cytology specimens for programmed death ligand 1 immunohistochemistry testing in non-small cell lung cancer. *Journal of Bronchology & Interventional Pulmonology* 24: 181–183.

56 Biswas, A., Leon, M.E., Drew, P. et al. (2018). Clinical performance of endobronchial ultrasound-guided transbronchial needle aspiration for assessing programmed death ligand-1 expression in nonsmall cell lung cancer. *Diagnostic Cytopathology* 46: 378–383.

57 Sakata, K.K., Midthun, D.E., Mullon, J.J. et al. (2018). Comparison of programmed death ligand-1 immunohistochemical staining between endobronchial ultrasound transbronchial needle aspiration and resected lung cancer specimens. *Chest* 154: 827–837.

58 Noll, B., Wang, W.-L., Gong, Y. et al. (2018). Programmed death ligand 1 testing in non-small cell lung carcinoma cytology cell block and aspirate smear preparations. *Cancer Cytopathology* 126: 342–352.

6

Endoscopic Ultrasound-Guided Mediastinal Lymph Node Aspiration for Lung Cancer Diagnosis and Staging

Christopher Kniese[1] *and Ali I. Musani*[2]

[1] *Indiana University School of Medicine, Indianapolis, IN, USA*
[2] *Division of Pulmonary Sciences & Critical Care Medicine, University of Colorado School of Medicine, Denver, CO, USA*

Introduction

Endoscopic ultrasound-guided fine-needle aspiration (EUS-FNA) of mediastinal lymph nodes to stage lung cancer has been performed since the 1990s. The different anatomic orientation of the esophagus allows for visualization and sampling of lymph nodes that are not readily accessible via endobronchial ultrasound-guided aspiration (EBUS). The purpose of this chapter is to acknowledge the role of EUS in sampling mediastinal lymph nodes and to compare EBUS and EUS for this particular indication. An in-depth discussion of EUS for sampling mediastinal lymph nodes is beyond the scope of this book. To learn more about mediastinal sampling with EUS, one should review the gastroenterology literature.

Because they can access different mediastinal lymph node stations, EUS-FNA and EBUS-TBNA (transbronchial needle aspiration) should be considered complementary to each other. When used together, EUS-FNA and EBUS-TBNA allow access to almost all of the mediastinal nodes during one session of conscious sedation. However, when lymph nodes are potentially accessible by both modalities, the EBUS approach is preferred because it also allows examination of the airways for endobronchial disease, which may be easily missed on chest computed tomography (CT) scans. Both EUS-FNA and EBUS-TBNA carry a very low risk of complications.

Technique

As is evident from its name, EUS is performed via a transesophageal approach (Figure 6.1). The EUS scope, like its counterpart the EBUS scope, allows for real-time ultrasound-guided needle aspiration (Figures 6.2 and 6.3). Like EBUS-TBNA, EUS-FNA may be performed as an outpatient procedure. It is usually carried out with the patient under conscious sedation. The needle used for EUS-FNA is typically 19 or 22 gauge (G). The 19 G needle provides the benefit of allowing a core biopsy, which may improve diagnostic accuracy in diseases such as sarcoidosis and lymphoma, although recent literature in endobronchial ultrasound has demonstrated that the overall yield may be similar across various needle sizes [1].

Endobronchial Ultrasonography, Second Edition. Noriaki Kurimoto, David I.K. Fielding, Ali I. Musani, Christopher Kniese, and Katsuhiko Morita.

Companion website: www.wiley.com/go/kurimoto2e

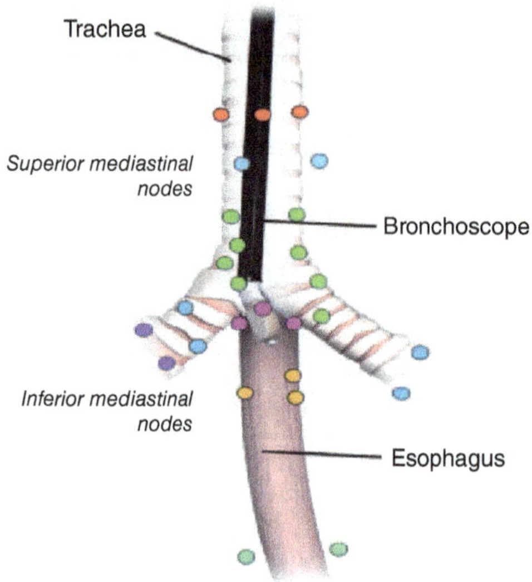

Figure 6.1 Endoscopic ultrasound scope in the esophagus behind the trachea. The subcarinal and para-esophageal lymph nodes are easily accessible by endoscopic approach with ultrasound-guided fine-needle aspiration.

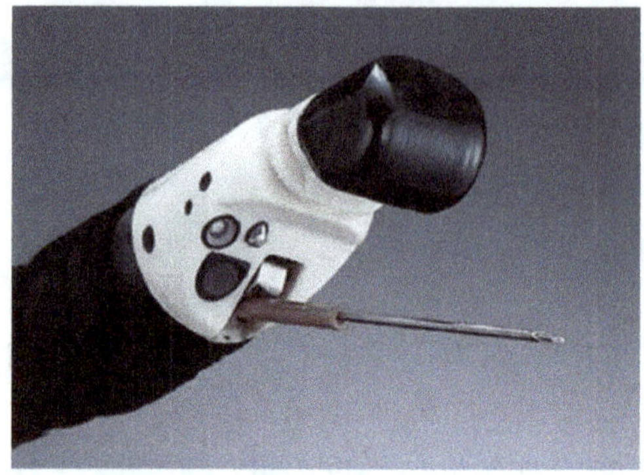

Figure 6.2 Endoscopic ultrasound scope (GF-UC140P-AL5, Olympus America). *Source:* Picture obtained with permission from http://medical.olympusamerica.com/products/curved-linear-array-gf-uc140p-al5.

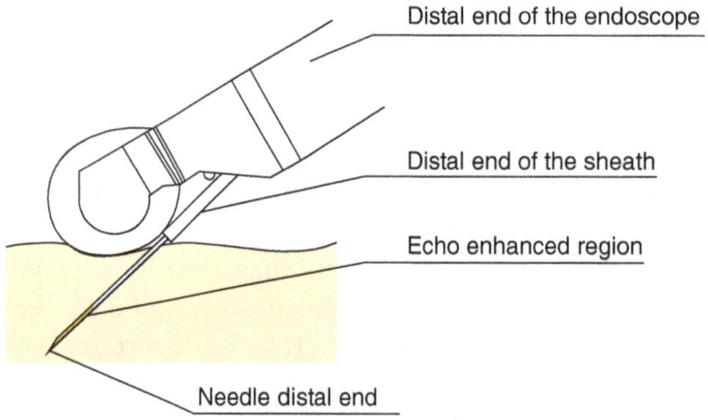

Figure 6.3 Endoscopic ultrasound via the esophagus. The real-time images of a mass or node outside the walls of the esophagus allow fine-needle aspiration.

Posterior and inferior mediastinal nodes are easily accessible by EUS-FNA (Tables 6.1 and 6.2). Mediastinal lymph node stations accessible by EUS-FNA include stations 4L (left lower paratracheal), 7 (subcarinal), 8 (para-esophageal), and station 9 (inferior pulmonary ligament). Superior mediastinal stations (1, 2, 3, and 4R), N1 stations (10, 11, 12, 13, regardless of side), subaortic (station 5), and the para-aortic (station 6) nodes are not accessible by EUS-FNA. In comparison, the lymph node stations accessible by EBUS-TBNA include stations 1, 2, 3, 4, 7, 10, 11, and 12. EBUS-TBNA for lung cancer staging has been performed since the early 2000s.

Role of EUS in Lung Cancer Staging

As previously stated, EUS-FNA can be used to sample mediastinal lymph nodes not readily accessible via EBUS-TBNA for the diagnosis and staging of lung cancer. In a meta-analysis, the sensitivity of EUS-FNA was 81–97% and

Table 6.1 Lymph node stations.

Location	Station
Superior mediastinal nodes	
Highest mediastinal	1
Upper paratracheal	2
Pre-vascular and retrotracheal	3
Lower paratracheal	4
Aortic nodes	
Subaortic (aortopulmonary [A-P] window)	5
Para-aortic (ascending aorta or phrenic)	6
Inferior mediastinal nodes	
Subcarinal	7
Para-esophageal	8
Pulmonary ligament	9
N1 nodes	
Hilar	10
Interlobar	11
Lobar	12
Segmental	13
Subsegmental	14

Adapted from: Mountain and Dresler [2].

Table 6.2 Accessibility of lymph node stations by different modalities.

Modality	Accessible lymph node stations
Standard	Superior mediastinal, subcarinal
mediastinoscopy	Stations 1, 2, 3, 4, and 7
Extended	Aortic nodes
mediastinoscopy	Stations 5 and 6
Anterior	Aortic nodes
mediastinoscopy[a]	Stations 5 and 6
VATS	Superior mediastinal (right), subcarinal, and aortic nodes
	Stations 1, 2R, 3, 4R, 7, 5, and 6
TBNA	Superior mediastinal, subcarinal, N1 nodes
	Stations 1, 2, 3, 4, 7, 10, 11, and 12
TTNA	Superior mediastinal (anterior)
	Stations 4L, 7, 8, and 9
EUS-FNA	Left lower paratracheal, subaortic, inferior mediastinal
	Stations 4L, 7, 8, and 9
EBUS-TBNA	Superior mediastinal, subcarinal, and N1 nodes
	Stations 1, 2, 3, 4, 7, 10, 11, and 12

[a] Chamberlain procedure. EBUS-TBNA, endobronchial ultrasound-guided transbronchial needle aspiration; EUS-FNA, endoscopic ultrasound-guided fine-needle aspiration; TBNA, transbronchial needle aspiration; TTNA, transthoracic needle aspiration; VATS, video-assisted thoracoscopic surgery.
Adapted from: Mountain and Dresler [2].

specificity was 83–100% for the diagnosis of posterior mediastinal lymphadenopathy in non-small cell carcinoma of the lung [3]. The major limitation of EUS-FNA was its high false-negative rate. Studies comparing positron-emission tomography (PET) scan with EUS-FNA for posterior mediastinal adenopathy have shown that EUS-FNA is better than PET in staging lung cancer [4]. These studies suggest a high false-positive rate for the PET scan; therefore, EUS-FNA can be used to confirm whether PET-avid lymph nodes are benign or malignant.

EBUS-TBNA appears to have greater sensitivity and specificity than EUS-FNA. In a case series of 70 patients with mediastinal (n = 58) and hilar (n = 12) adenopathy, EBUS-TBNA had a sensitivity of 95.7%, specificity of 100%, and accuracy of 97.1% for differentiating benign from malignant lymph nodes [5].

A multicenter trial of more than 500 patients showed EBUS-TBNA to be a very sensitive and specific diagnostic modality for sampling mediastinal adenopathy (sensitivity 94% and specificity 100%) [6]. Other studies comparing the sensitivity of PET, CT, and EBUS-TBNA for staging of lung cancer showed a higher yield with EBUS-TBNA [7]. The sensitivity of CT, PET, and EBUS-TBNA for diagnosing lung cancer in mediastinal and hilar lymph nodes was 76.9%, 80%, and 92.3%, respectively. The specificities were 55.3%, 70.1%, and 100%, respectively. The diagnostic accuracies were 60.8%, 72.5%, and 98%, respectively, for the three modalities [7]. Therefore, EBUS-TBNA has better sensitivity and specificity than either CT or PET scanning in staging mediastinal disease in lung cancer.

Combination of EUS and EBUS for Mediastinal Lymph Node Sampling

Given their complementary nature, and the ability to sample the entire spectrum of mediastinal lymph nodes in a non-invasive fashion, recent studies have assessed the combination of EUS-FNA and EBUS-TBNA as a diagnostic modality. Given that both procedures can be performed under moderate sedation, it is feasible to do both in a single procedure, potentially expediting diagnosis and staging in patients in whom either approach in isolation is felt to be inadequate.

A single-center study in 2008 compared traditional (i.e. non-ultrasound-guided) TBNA, EBUS-TBNA, and EUS-FNA [8]. The authors found that while EBUS-TBNA was more sensitive than traditional TBNA, the combination of EBUS-TBNA and EUS-FNA yielded the best results, with estimated sensitivity of 93% and negative predictive value of 97%, both of which were superior to either EBUS-TBNA or EUS-FNA alone. A more recent meta-analysis of the combination approach showed excellent results, with reported sensitivity of 86%, specificity of 100%, and an area under the curve (AUC) of 0.99 for diagnosis and staging of lung cancer [9].

One additional study assessed the combination approach in a staged fashion, comparing an EBUS-centered approach (EBUS, then EUS-FNA) to an EUS-centered approach (EUS-FNA, then EBUS-TBNA). While the overall yields between the two groups were similar, the authors noted that EBUS following EUS-FNA improved rates of diagnosis more than when EUS-FNA was added to EBUS, suggesting that EBUS may be a better primary option if only one of the two methods is employed [10]. Based on these recent studies, in many centers pulmonologists are performing both EBUS-TBNA and EUS-FNA. While most pulmonologists are not conventionally trained in gastrointestinal endoscopy, recent data has suggested that EBUS proceduralists can quickly gain competency in EUS-FNA at experienced centers [11].

References

1 Yarmus, L.B., Akulian, J., Lechtzin, N. et al. (2013). Comparison of 21-gauge and 22-gauge aspiration needle in endobronchial ultrasound-guided transbronchial needle aspiration: results of the American College of Chest Physicians quality improvement registry, education, and evaluation registry. *Chest* 143 (4): 1036–1043.

2 Mountain, C.F. and Dresler, C.M. (1997). Regional lymph node classification for lung cancer staging. *Chest* 111: 1718–1723.

3 Kramer, H. and Groen, H.J.M. (2003). Current concepts in the mediastinal lymph node staging of non-small cell lung cancer. *Annals of Surgery* 238: 180–188.

4 Eloubeidi, M.A., Cerfolio, R.I., Chen, V.K. et al. (2005). Endoscopic ultrasound-guided fine needle aspiration of mediastinal lymph node in patients with suspected lung cancer after positron emission tomography and computed tomography scans. *Annals of Thoracic Surgery* 79: 263–268.

5 Yasufuku, K., Chiyo, M., Sekine, Y. et al. (2004). Real-time endobronchial ultrasound-guided transbronchial needle aspiration of mediastinal and hilar lesions. *Chest* 126: 122–128.

6 Herth, F.J., Eberhart, R., Vilmann, P. et al. (2006). Real-time endobronchial ultrasound-guided transbronchial needle aspiration for sampling mediastinal lymph nodes. *Thorax* 61: 795–798.

7 Yasufuku, K., Nakajima, T., Motoori, K. et al. (2006). Comparison of endobronchial ultrasound, positron emission tomography, and CT for lymph node staging of lung cancer. *Chest* 130: 710–718.

8 Wallace, M.B., Pascual, J.M., Raimondo, M. et al. (2008). Minimally invasive endoscopic staging of lung cancer. *JAMA* 299 (5): 540–546.

9 Zhang, R., Ying, K., Shi, L. et al. (2013). Combined endobronchial and endoscopic ultrasound-guided fine needle aspiration for mediastinal lymph node staging of lung cancer: a meta-analysis. *European Journal of Cancer* 49: 1860–1867.

10 Kang, H.J., Hwangbo, B., Lee, G.-K. et al. (2014). EBUS-centred vs. EUS-centred mediastinal staging in lung cancer: a randomised controlled trial. *Thorax* 69: 261–268.

11 Leong, P., Deshpande, S., Irving, L.B. et al. (2017). Endoscopic ultrasound fine-needle aspiration by experienced pulmonologists: a cusum analysis. *European Respiratory Journal* 50: 1701102.

7

How to Accurately Identify the Bronchial Pathway to a Peripheral Pulmonary Lesion

Noriaki Kurimoto

Department of Internal Medicine, Division of Medical Oncology and Respiratory Medicine, Shimane University Faculty of Medicine, Izumo, Japan

Introduction

Just as a map is needed when driving in an unfamiliar city, a bronchoscopist needs a bronchial map for inserting a bronchoscope and obtaining specimens from peripheral pulmonary lesions. There are two methods for obtaining such a map: by manually tracing the bronchus leading to the peripheral pulmonary lesions on computed tomographic (CT) images, or by using a navigation system (Figure 7.1). In recent years, a navigation system has become available in many countries; however, it is expensive and sometimes unable to establish the peripheral bronchial pathway around the visceral pleura. Therefore, in this chapter, we explain how to trace the bronchus leading to peripheral pulmonary lesions on CT images.

Reading CT Anatomy versus Virtual Bronchoscopic Navigation

Currently, the best diagnostic imaging modality for accurately following the distal bronchial lumen is chest CT. It is often possible to visually follow the bronchial lumen from the trachea, via the main bronchus, the lobar bronchus, and the segmental bronchus to a bronchiole about 2–3 cm from the pleura; however, it can be difficult to follow the bronchial lumen around the pleura, so the pulmonary artery beside the bronchus can be followed instead.

In virtual bronchoscopic navigation (VBN) using a computer workstation navigation system, it is possible to establish the exact branching form and branching angle of the hilar bronchus. However, in areas close to the pleura, VBN can be somewhat inferior for tracing the bronchial lumen compared with a doctor reading the CT anatomy, who can trace the thinner bronchus and the pulmonary artery where the bronchial lumen becomes invisible, thereby completing the bronchial branch diagram in the peripheral pulmonary area.

VBN can establish the accurate direction and location of bronchial branching along the bronchial route. However, as you enter the periphery using VBN, the image of the bronchi is expanded on the monitor, and it can become difficult for the operator to judge which bronchial generation the bronchoscope is currently looking at, sometimes requiring a return to the proximal bronchus to re-enter the distal bronchus. Conversely, in a bronchial branch diagram, the branches of the bronchus to the periphery are depicted in a single diagram, making it easy to

Endobronchial Ultrasonography, Second Edition. Noriaki Kurimoto, David I.K. Fielding, Ali I. Musani, Christopher Kniese, and Katsuhiko Morita.

Companion website: www.wiley.com/go/kurimoto2e

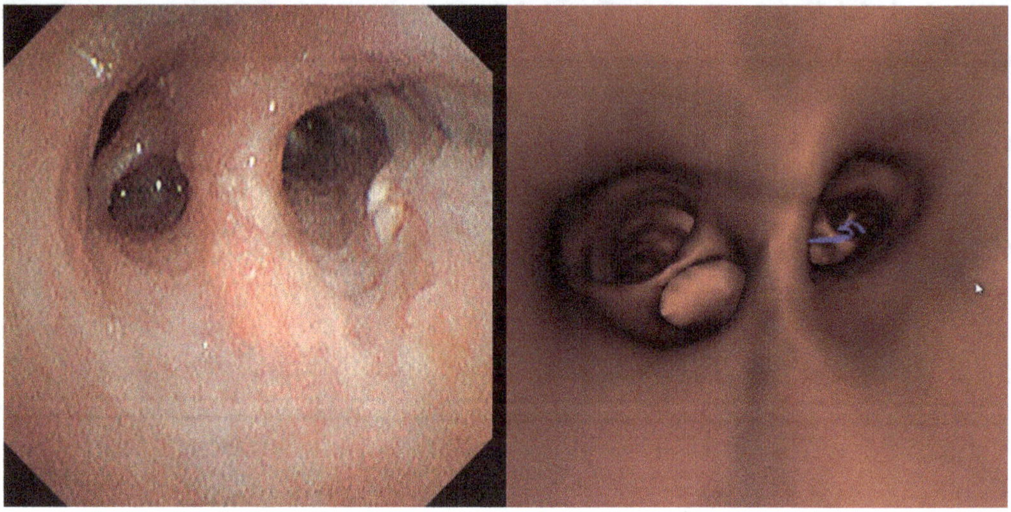

Figure 7.1 The image of virtual bronchoscopic navigation corresponding to the bronchoscopic image.

identify the current bronchus and bronchial generation at all times. The entire bronchial branch diagram from the lobar bronchus to the peripheral bronchus is easy to understand.

Doctors specializing in respiratory medicine commonly diagnose pulmonary lesions from chest CT images. It is easy to trace the bronchi that lead to a peripheral pulmonary lesion. While doing so, it would be useful to be able to illustrate the condition of the bronchial branch leading to the lesion. In addition, it would be of great benefit for the doctor to have confidence in the bronchoscopic procedure as this reading technique becomes available. VBN is expensive, whereas there is no direct cost to reading CT anatomy, although it requires some training. In Japan, the standard textbook about reading CT anatomy is readily available; because doctors have become accustomed to the bronchoscopic approach to peripheral pulmonary lesions over many years, reading CT anatomy is widespread.

Step-by-Step Guide to Reading CT Anatomy

1) Take the CT images. Prepare thin, 1 mm slices in the lung field condition of the chest CT. With 2 mm slices, it is difficult to trace all the branches of the peripheral lung tissue.
2) Rotate or reverse the CT images. Tracing the bifurcation of the bronchial lumen in the CT image is usually similar to advancing the bronchoscope tip through the bronchial lumen. In other words, we image the bronchial lumen on the CT image in the same way as the bronchoscope visualizes the bronchus. The CT image is observed from the caudal side, so when the lesion is in the right middle or lower lobe or left lingular segment or lower lobe, reverse the image from left to right so that it can be observed from the cranial side (Figure 7.2a). When the lesion is on the right upper lobe, rotate the CT image by 90° in the counterclockwise direction (Figure 7.2b). This is because the bronchoscope is rotated by 90° in the clockwise direction at the carina and advances to the right upper lobe when guiding the bronchoscope tip to the right upper lobe bronchus. When the lesion is located in the left superior segment, rotate the CT image by 90° in the clockwise direction (Figure 7.2c). This is because the bronchoscope is rotated counterclockwise by 90° at the carina and advanced to the left superior segment when guiding the bronchoscope tip to the left superior segmental bronchus.
3) Classify the bronchi into vertical and horizontal branches on the axial CT images.

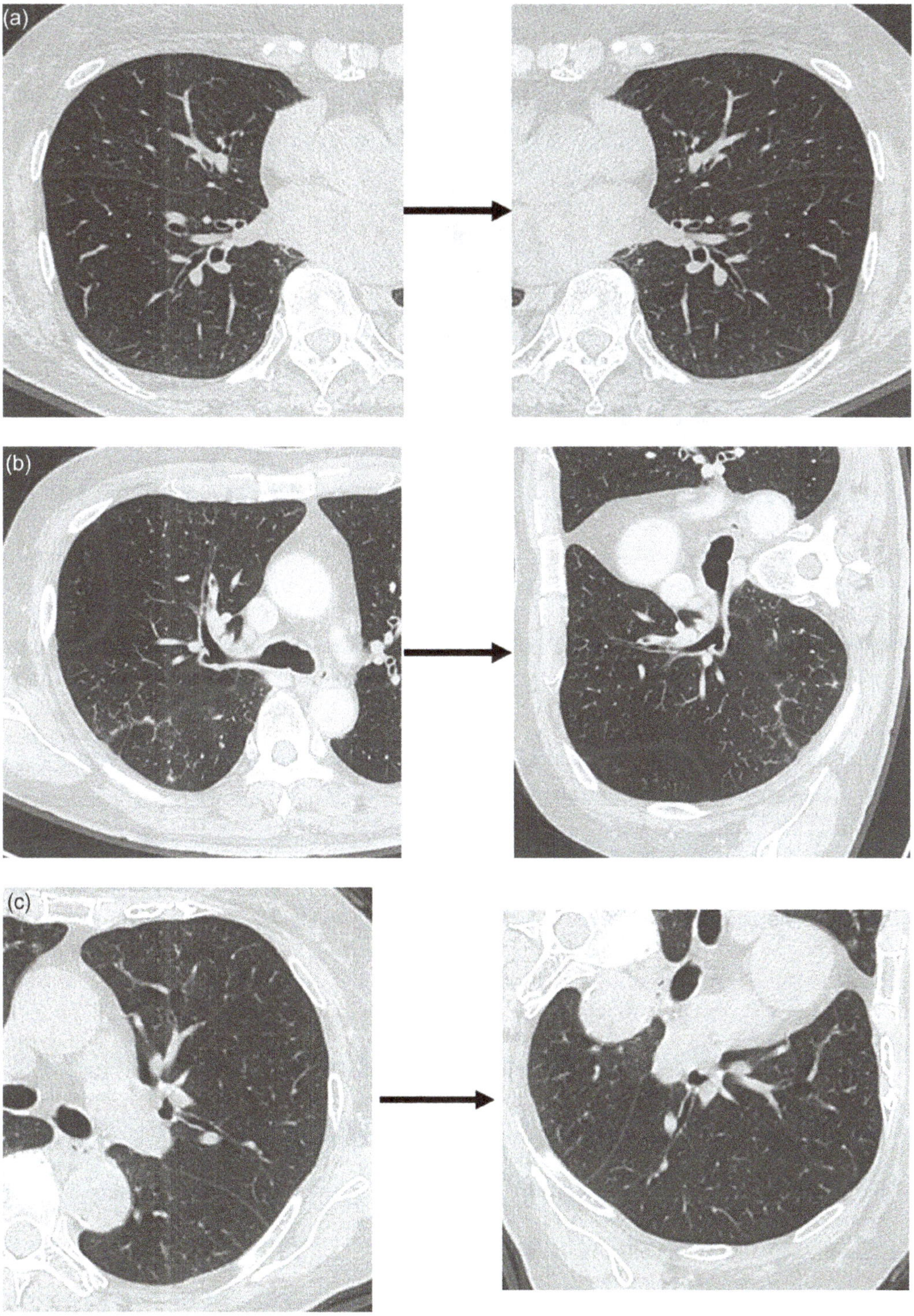

Figure 7.2 (a) Reverse of computed tomographic (CT) images. (b) Rotation of computed tomographic (CT) images by 90° in the counterclockwise direction for a lesion in the right upper lobe. (c) Rotation of computed tomographic (CT) images by 90° in the clockwise direction for a lesion in the left superior segment.

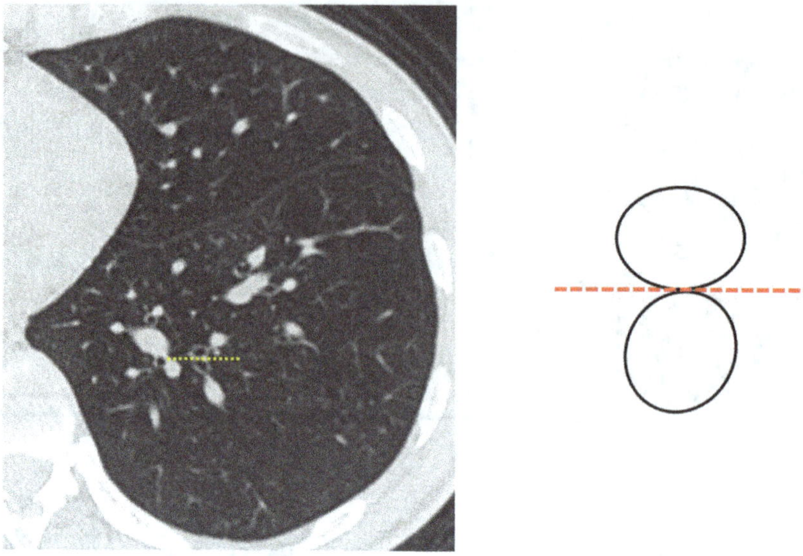

Figure 7.3 Vertical branch.

Based on the angle of the bronchus in the axial CT images, classify each as a vertical branch if at an angle close to vertical on the image or a horizontal branch if at an angle close to horizontal on the image. Thus, B^1, B^7, B^8b, B^9b, B^{10}b, and B^{10}c on the right and B^{1+2}a, B^{1+2}b, B^8b, B^9b, B^{10}b, and B^{10}c on the left are considered to be vertical branches, whereas B^2, B^3, B^4, B^5, B^6, B^8a, B^9a, and B^{10}a on the right and B^{1+2}c, B^3, B^4, B^5, B^6, B^8a, B^9a, and B^{10}a on the left are usually considered to be horizontal branches.

4) In a vertical branch, draw the bronchial branch according to the CT image. With the CT image reversed from right to left or rotated by 90° in the counterclockwise or clockwise direction, draw the bifurcation angle of the vertical branch in the same location as on the CT image (Figure 7.3). The bronchial branch diagram is similar to the bronchial branches observed with the bronchoscope.
5) In a horizontal branch, consider the direction of its long axis. With the CT image reversed from right to left or rotated by 90° in the counterclockwise or clockwise direction, confirm the longitudinal line of the horizontally running bronchus and put the viewpoint at the proximal site of the longitudinal line of the horizontally running bronchus. When the horizontal branch leads to further horizontal branches in the distal generation (horizontal–horizontal branch), horizontal branches are seen branching right and left on a bronchoscope. Go back to the viewpoint of the proximal site of the horizontal bronchus, and draw these left and right branches in the horizontal bronchus on the bronchial branching diagram (Figure 7.4a). When the horizontal branch leads to vertical branching in the distal generation (horizontal–vertical branch), the horizontal branch is seen branching in the up (cranial) and down (caudal) directions on a bronchoscope. Go back to the viewpoint of the proximal site of the horizontal bronchus, and draw these up and down branches in the horizontal bronchus on the bronchial branching diagram (Figure 7.4b).

Representative Cases

To illustrate the branch reading technique, here are three representative cases (Cases 1–3).

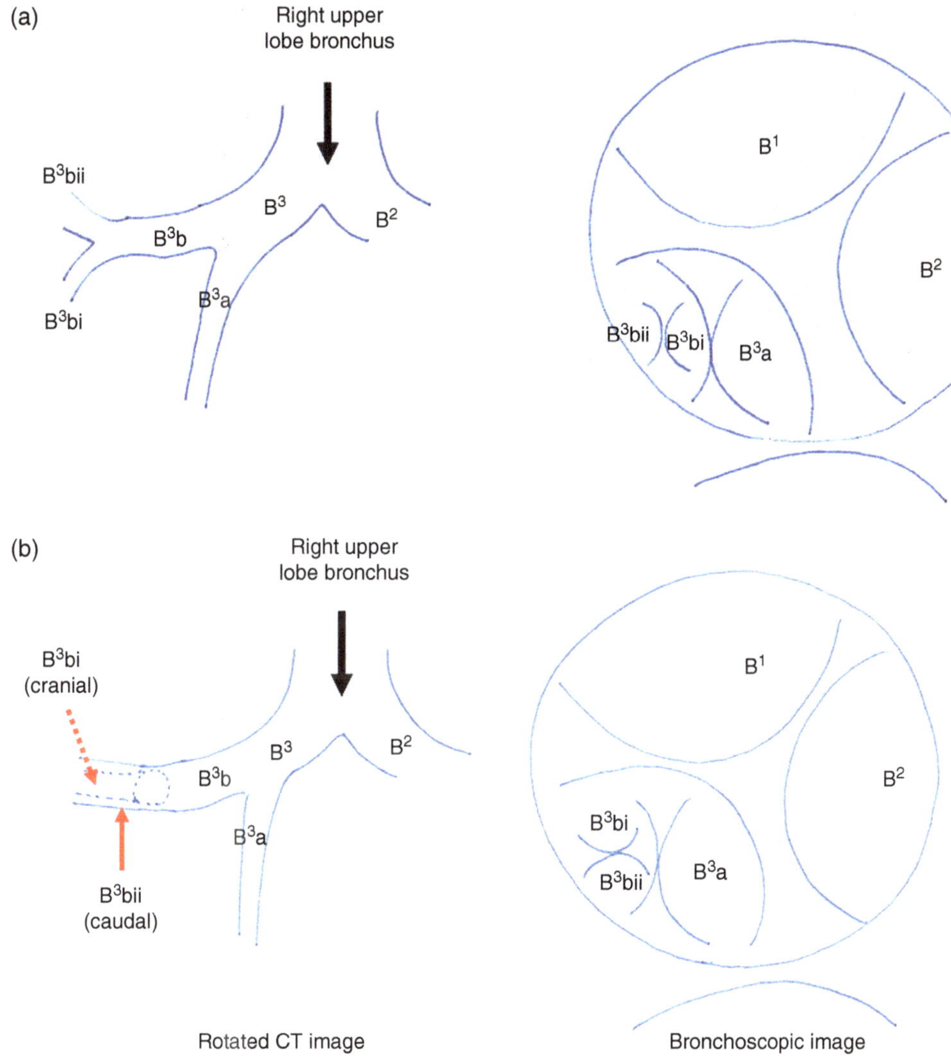

Figure 7.4 (a) Horizontal–horizontal branch. (b) Horizontal–vertical branch.

Case 1 Vertical pattern: Right B^1biiβ.

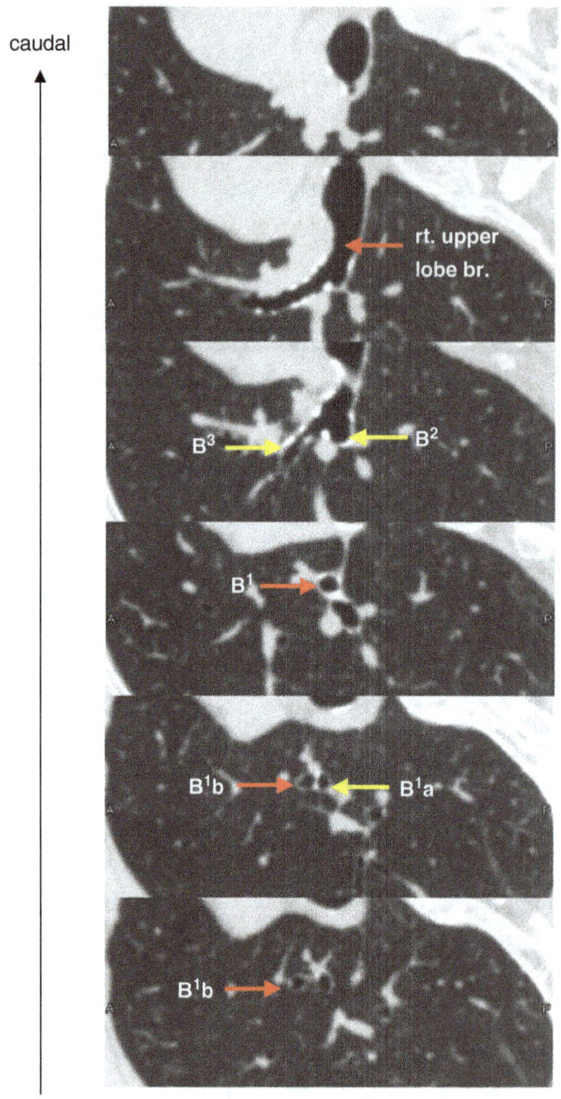

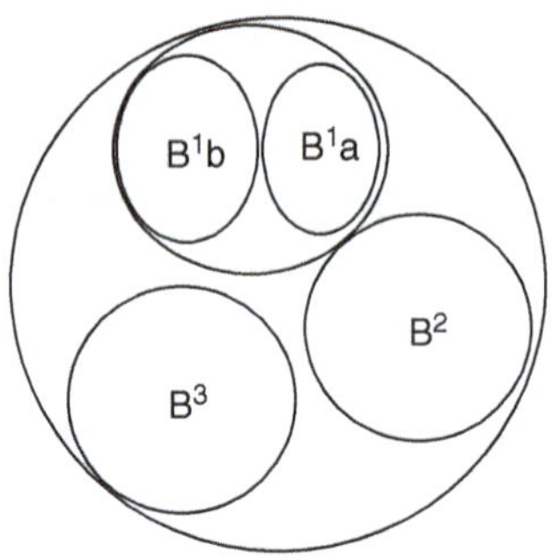

The right upper lobe bronchus branched into B^1, B^2, and B^3. B^1 branched into B^1a (dorsal) and B^1b (ventral).

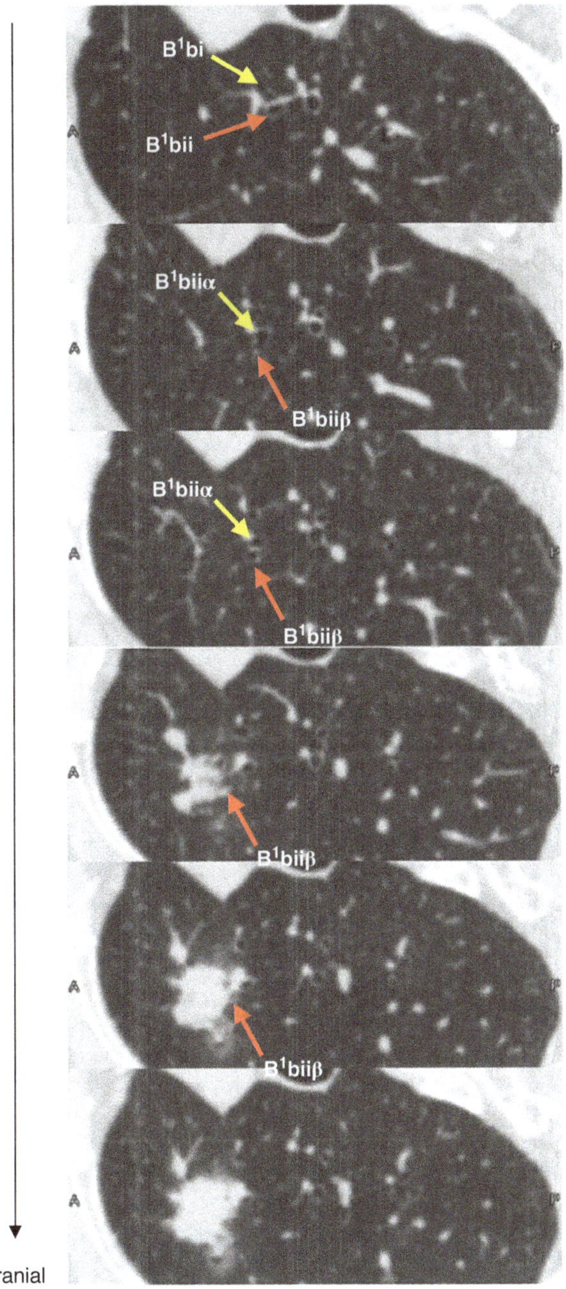

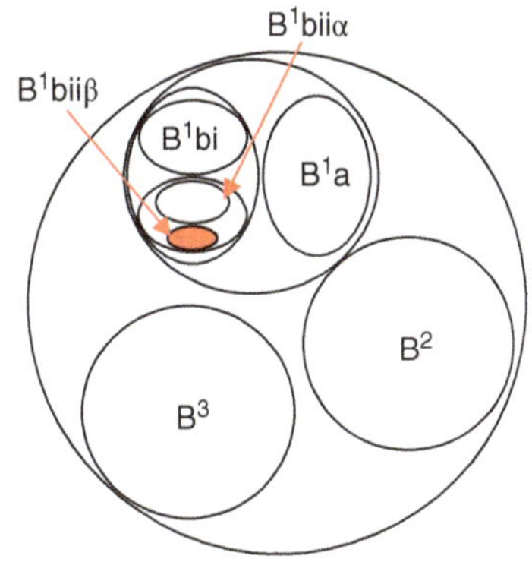

B^1b branched into B^1bi (cranial) and B^1bii (lateral). B^1bii branched into $B^1bii\alpha$ (cranial) and $B^1bii\beta$ (lateral).

(*Continued*)

Case 1 *(Continued)*

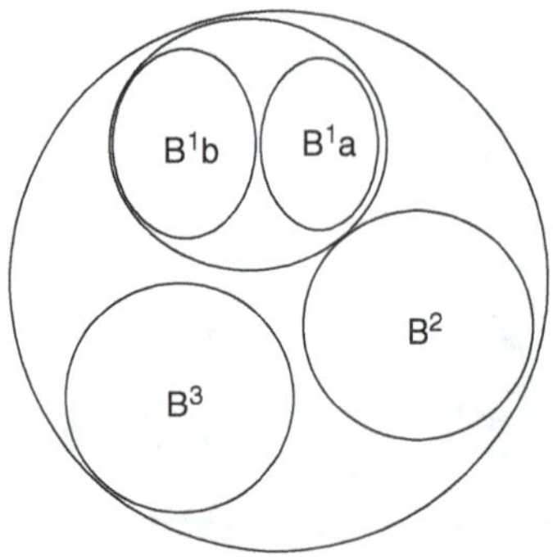

The right upper lobe bronchus branched into B^1, B^2, and B^3. B^1 branched into B^1a (dorsal) and B^1b (ventral).

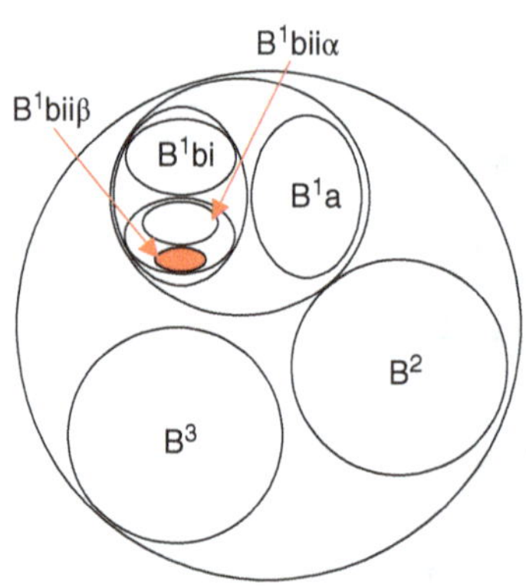

B^1b branched into B^1bi (cranial) and B^1bii (lateral). B^1bii branched into $B^1bii\alpha$ (cranial) and $B^1bii\beta$ (lateral).

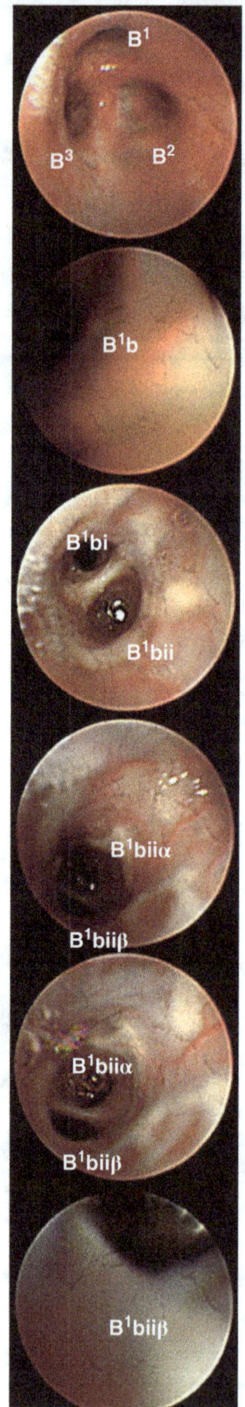

Case 2 Vertical pattern: Left B^{1+2}biiβxyy.

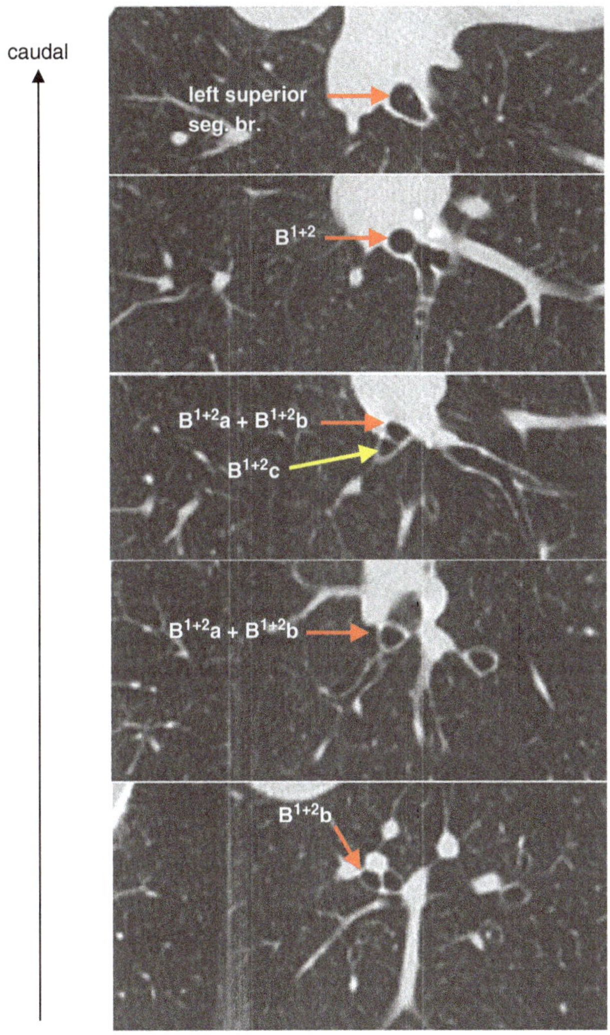

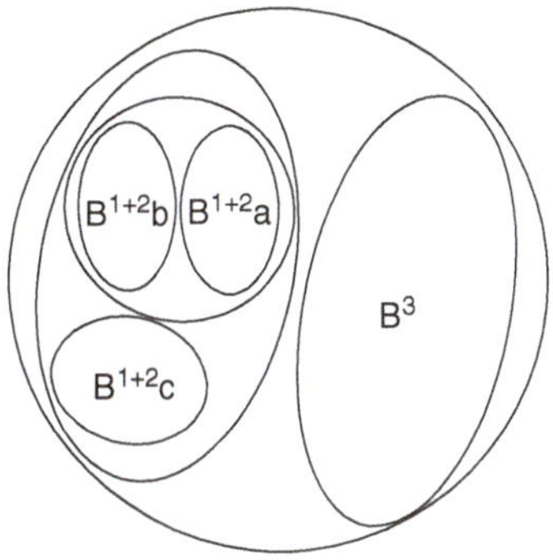

The left superior segment bronchus branched into B^{1+2} and B^3. B^{1+2} branched into B^{1+2}a, B^{1+2}b, and B^{1+2}c.

(*Continued*)

Case 2 (*Continued*)

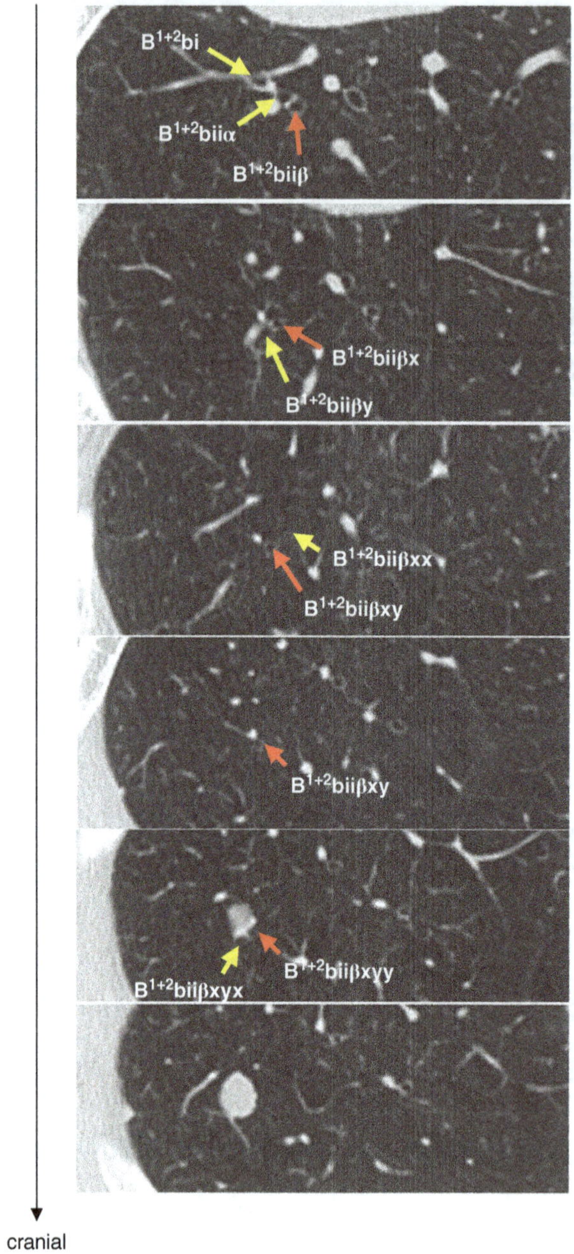

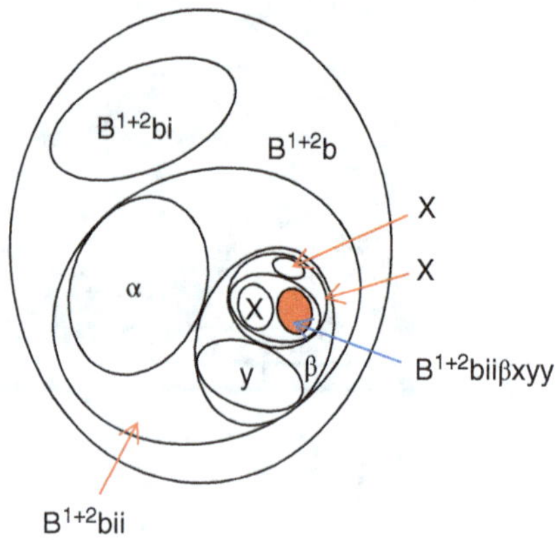

B^{1+2}b branched into B^{1+2}bi (dorsal and medial) and B^{1+2}bii (lateral). B^{1+2}bii branched into B^{1+2}biiα (dorsal) and B^{1+2}biiβ (ventral). B^{1+2}biiβ branched into B^{1+2}biiβx (cranial) and B^{1+2}biiβy (lateral). B^{1+2}biiβx branched into B^{1+2}biiβxx (cranial) and B^{1+2}biiβxy (lateral and dorsal). B^{1+2}biiβxy branched into B^{1+2}biiβxyx (dorsal) and B^{1+2}biiβxyy (ventral). B^{1+2}biiβxyy was adjacent to the lesion.

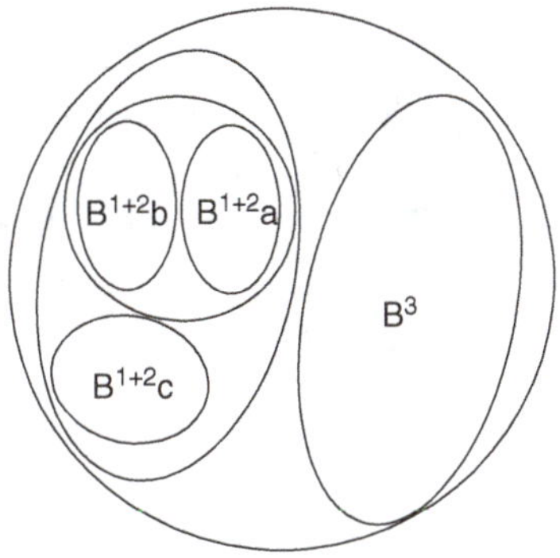

The left upper segment bronchus branched into $B^{1+2}$and B^3. B^{1+2}branched into B^{1+2}a, B^{1+2}b, and B^{1+2}c.

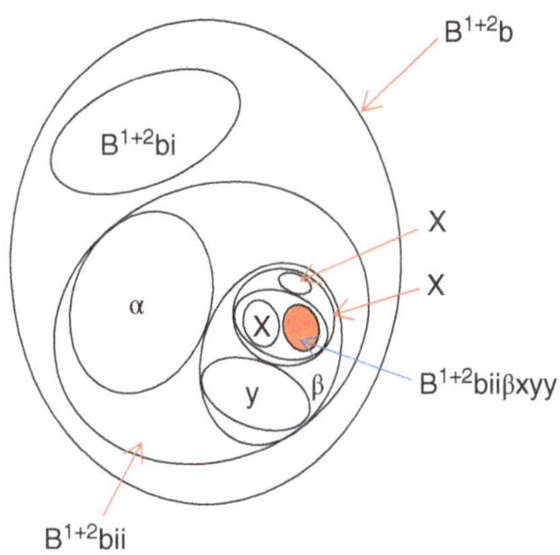

B^{1+2}b branched into B^{1+2}bi (dorsal and medial) and B^{1+2}bii (lateral). B^{1+2}bii branched into B^{1+2}biiα (dorsal) and B^{1+2}biiβ (ventral). B^{1+2}biiβ branched into B^{1+2}biiβx (cranial) and B^{1+2}biiβy (lateral). B^{1+2}biiβx branched into B^{1+2}biiβxx (cranial) and B^{1+2}biiβxy (lateral and dorsal). B^{1+2}biiβxy branched into B^{1+2}biiβxyx (dorsal) and B^{1+2}biiβxyy (ventral). B^{1+2}biiβxyy was adjacent to the lesion.

The ultra-thin bronchoscope (BF-XP290; Olympus Optical, Tokyo, Japan; outer diameter, 3.2 mm) reached B^{1+2}biiβxy.

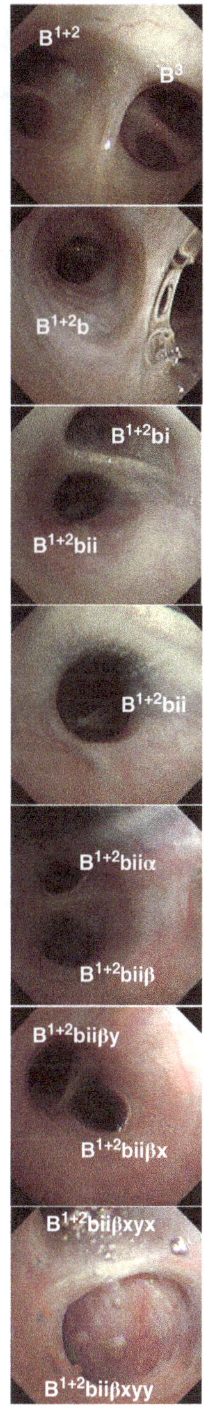

(*Continued*)

Case 2 (*Continued*)

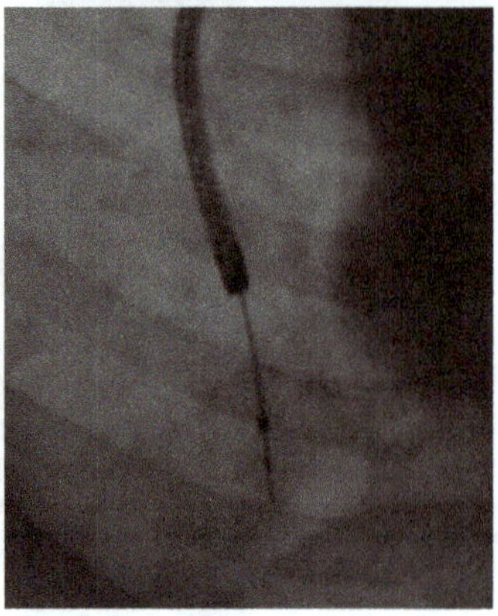

The fluoroscopic image was rotated by 180°. The bronchoscope (BF-P290; Olympus; outer diameter, 4.2 mm) reached the left B^{1+2}biiβ. The ultrasonic probe covered by a guide sheath approached the lesion.

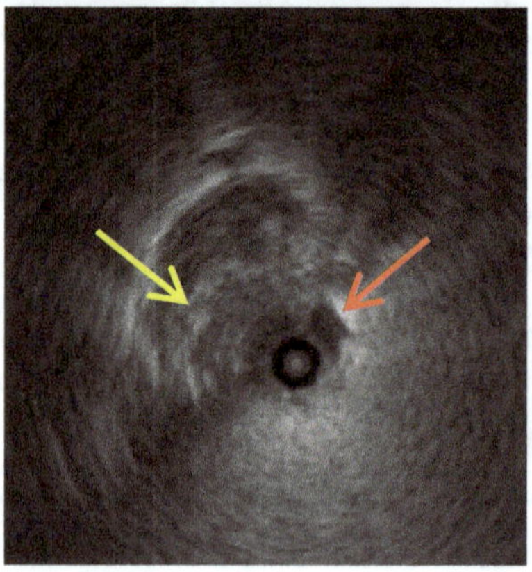

The ultrasonic probe was finally located adjacent to the lesion. The pulmonary artery (red arrow) was located next to the probe, and a hyperechoic lines (yellow arrow) were detected in the lesion

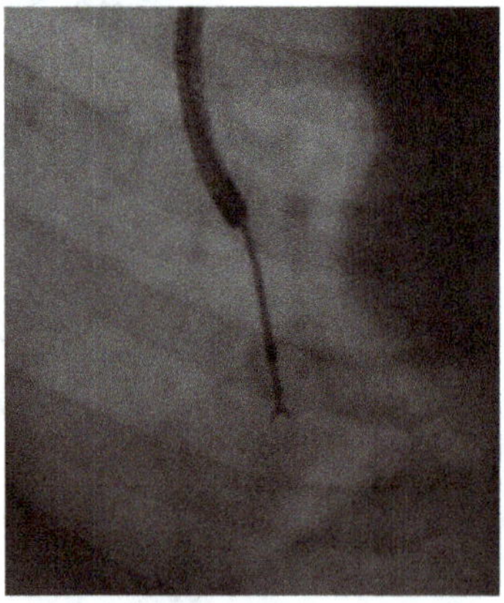

The biopsy forceps inserted through the guide sheath were opened against the target lesion and then closed to obtain a specimen.

Case 3 Horizontal pattern: Left B^3 aiαx.

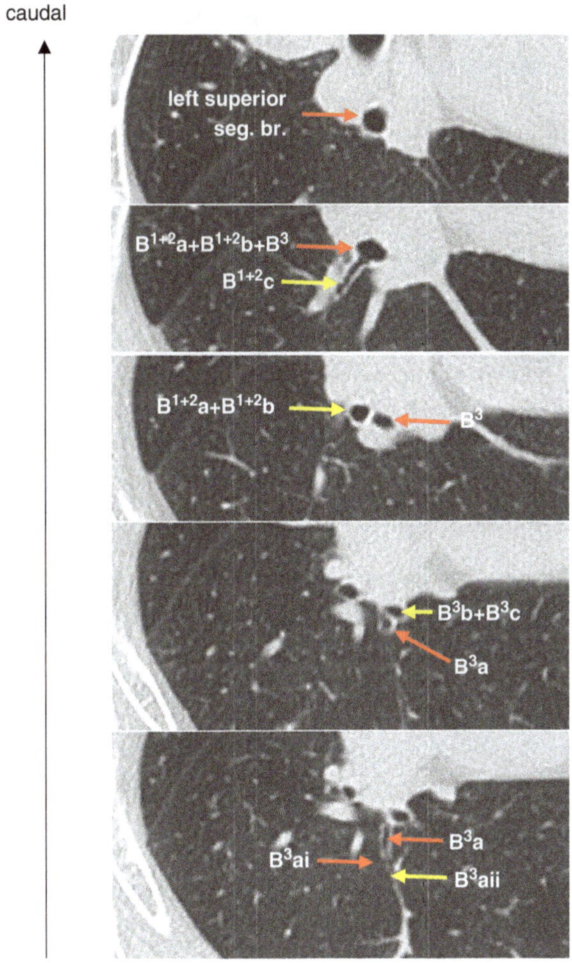

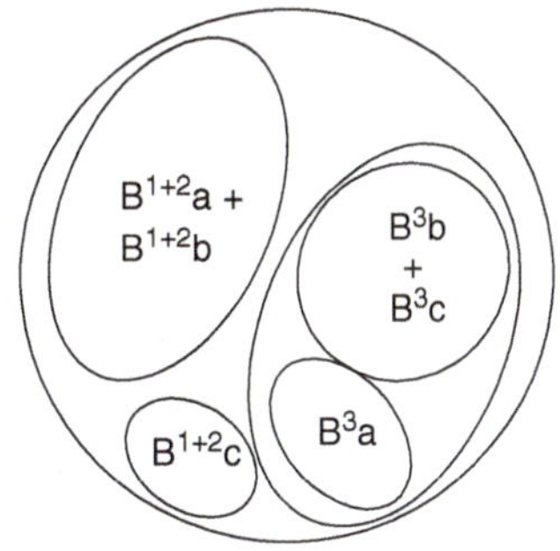

The left superior segment bronchus branched into $B^{1+2}a+B^{1+2}b$, $B^{1+2}c$, B^3a, and B^3b+B^3c.

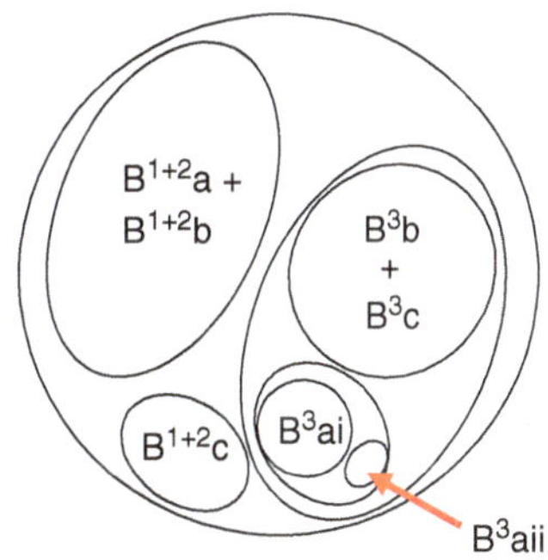

B^3a branched into B^3ai (cranial and dorsal) and B^3aii (caudal and ventral). Viewed B^3a (horizontal branch) from $B^{1+2}a$ (vertical branch) on the axial CT image, branching between B^3ai (cranial and dorsal) and B^3aii (caudal and ventral) was in a horizontal–oblique pattern.

(Continued)

Case 3 (*Continued*)

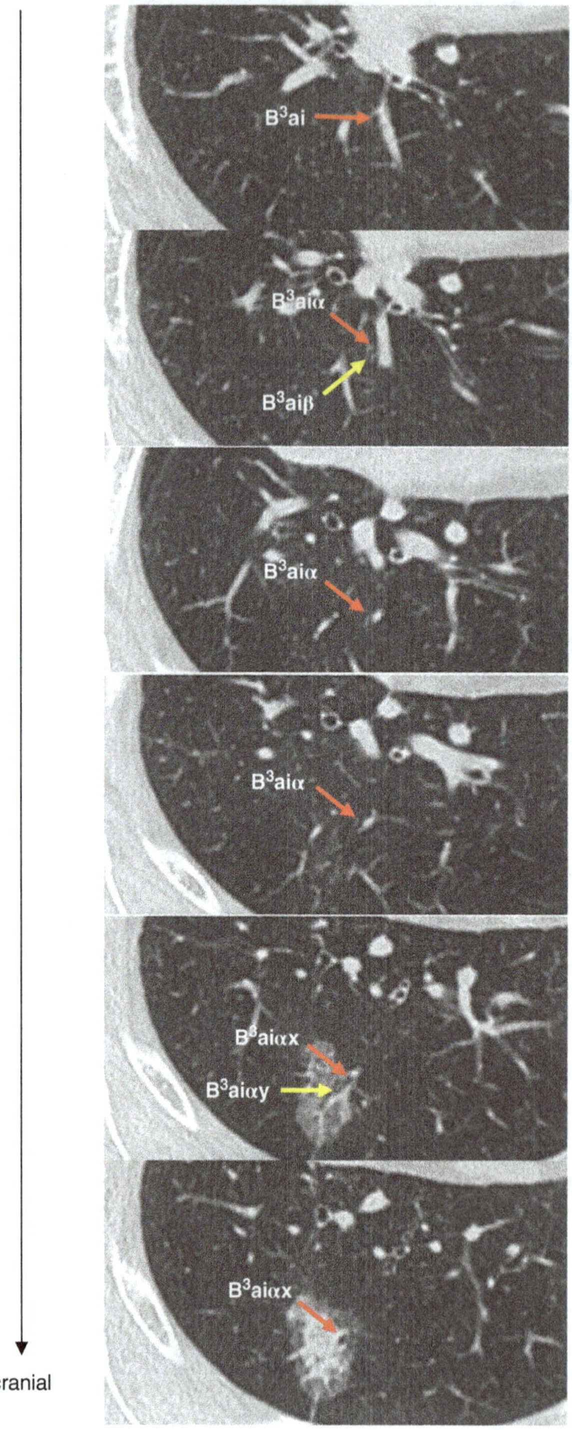

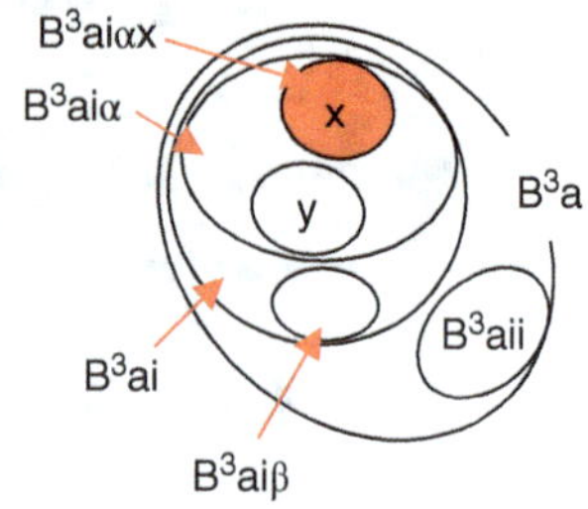

B^3ai branched into B^3aiα (cranial) and B^3aiβ (caudal and lateral). B^3aiα branched into B^3aiαx (cranial) and B^3aiαy (lateral). B^3aiαx entered the lesion.

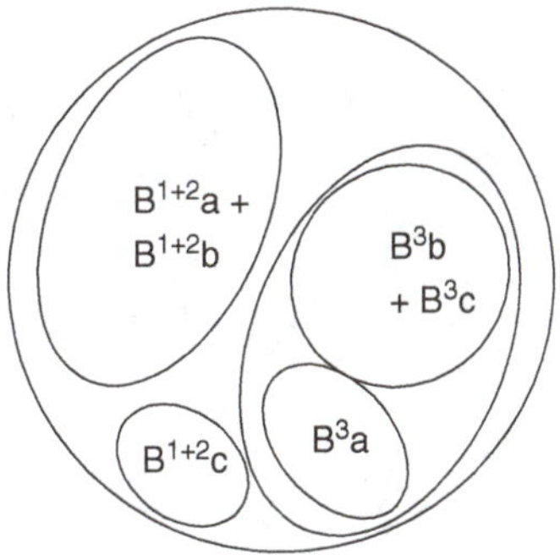

The left superior segment bronchus was branched into $B^{1+2}a$+$B^{1+2}b$, $B^{1+2}c$, $B^{3}a$, and $B^{3}b$+$B^{3}c$.

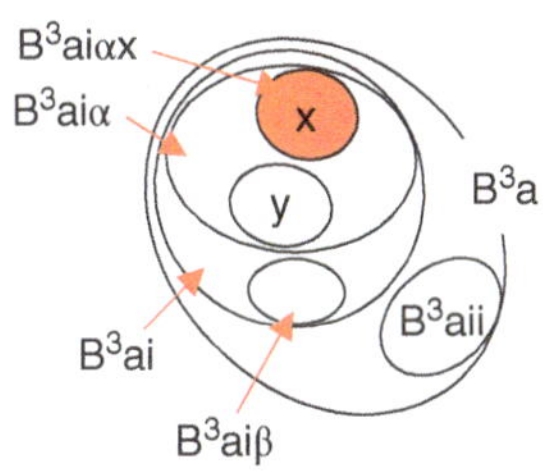

$B^{3}a$ branched into $B^{3}ai$ (cranial and dorsal) and $B^{3}aii$ (caudal and ventral). Viewed $B^{3}a$ (horizontal branch) from $B^{1+2}a$ (vertical branch), branching between $B^{3}ai$ (cranial and dorsal) and $B^{3}aii$ (caudal and ventral) on the axial CT image was in a horizontal–oblique pattern. $B^{3}ai$ branched into $B^{3}ai\alpha$ (cranial) and $B^{3}ai\beta$ (caudal and lateral). $B^{3}ai\alpha$ branched into $B^{3}ai\alpha x$ (cranial) and $B^{3}ai\alpha y$ (lateral). $B^{3}ai\alpha x$ entered the lesion.

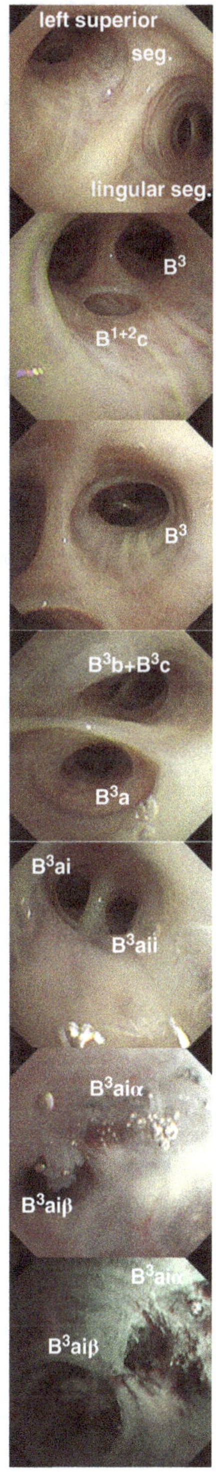

(*Continued*)

Case 3 (*Continued*)

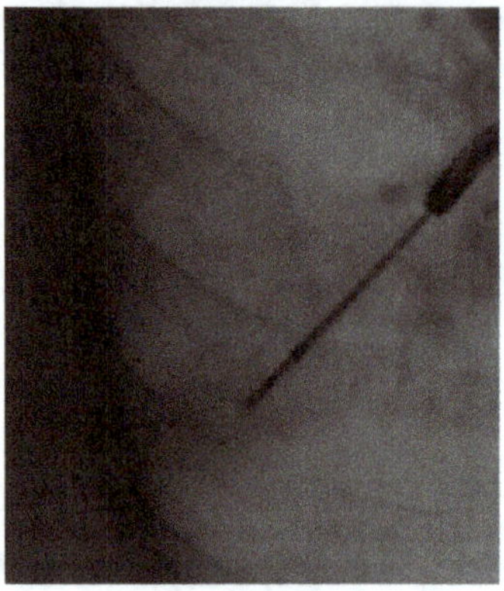

The fluoroscopic image was rotated by 180°. The bronchoscope (BF-P290; Olympus; outer diameter, 4.2 mm) reached the left B3. The ultrasonic probe covered with a guide sheath approached the lesion.

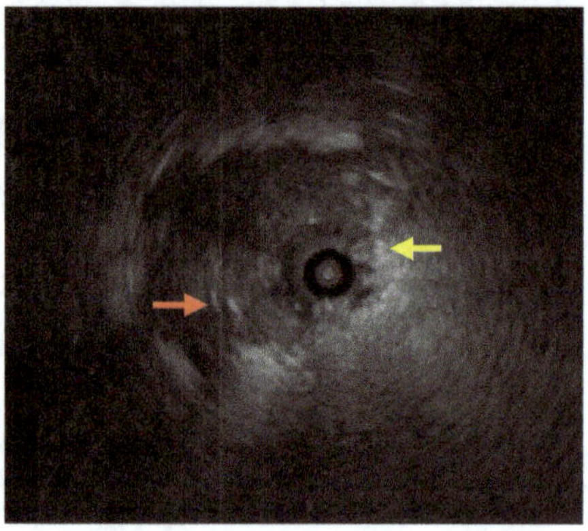

The ultrasonic probe was located "within" the lesion. Hyperechoic points (yellow arrow) and open vessel (red arrow) were detected.

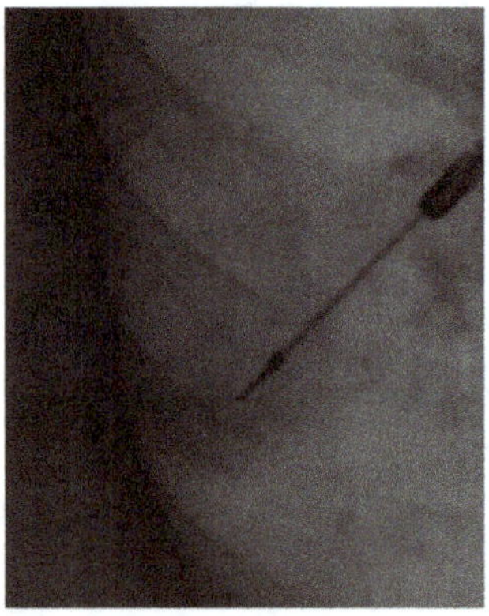

The biopsy forceps inserted through the guide sheath were opened against the target lesion and then closed to obtain a specimen.

Future Directions

Reading CT anatomy is a useful skill for doctors tracing bronchial routes from CT images. To learn this skill, doctors should accumulate representative cases they have experienced or study representative cases in textbooks. Reviewing these cases regularly will help establish and maintain the procedure for reading CT anatomy.

With rapid improvement in computer performance, VBN is likely to improve, with progress in extraction of the bronchial lumen around the pleura, which is currently difficult. Improvements in artificial intelligence should allow VBN performance to match the doctor's skill in reading CT anatomy. We also hope that the cost, which is a big problem for VBN, will decrease.

How can people live with confidence in a world in which computers and artificial intelligence are popular? Is it a good era when bronchoscopic procedures cannot be performed without VBN? When a doctor performs a bronchoscopic procedure with incomplete VBN, they may be able to identify the bronchi that lead to the lesion by using the skill of reading CT anatomy; we hope that this skill will be maintained in the next generation.

8

Qualitative Analysis of Peripheral Pulmonary Lesions Using Endobronchial Ultrasonography

Noriaki Kurimoto

Department of Internal Medicine, Division of Medical Oncology and Respiratory Medicine, Shimane University Faculty of Medicine, Izumo, Japan

Introduction

Numerous studies have shown that high-frequency, two-dimensional ultrasonography is a useful technique for evaluating the depth of invasion of gastrointestinal tumors, detecting lymph node metastasis, and identifying coronary arterial stenosis and thrombosis [1–5]. Since 1994, I have developed endobronchial ultrasonography (EBUS), including the localization of peripheral pulmonary lesions during endobronchial brushing and transbronchial biopsy. In addition to using EBUS to localize a lesion, the analysis of EBUS images can be useful for suggesting the underlying pathology. By comparing EBUS findings with histopathologic findings, it has been possible to develop concepts related to the qualitative analysis of the internal structures of peripheral pulmonary lesions visualized by EBUS. The aim of this chapter is to set out clear criteria for distinguishing between benign and malignant peripheral pulmonary lesions.

EBUS uses high-frequency ultrasound (20 MHz) to create detailed images of the internal structures of lesions, although it cannot delineate any tissues external to the lesion. Endoscopic ultrasonography has been used to examine the internal structures of the pancreas; the results have correlated well with histopathologic findings in cases of cystic tumors, calcification, and pancreatic stones [6, 7]. However, there have been few published analyses of the internal structures of peripheral pulmonary lesions visualized by EBUS; therefore, this chapter is mostly based on our own results.

Internal Structure of Peripheral Pulmonary Lesions Visualized by EBUS

On EBUS images, most cases of well-differentiated adenocarcinoma showed the preservation of blood vessels within the lesion (Figure 8.1, red arrow). Generally, these lesions showed homogeneous internal echoes, but sometimes there were hyperechoic dots (<1 mm in size), which represent residual air in the invaded alveoli. The distribution of these hyperechoic dots was irregular (Figure 8.2, yellow arrow), as were the margins of the lesion. Blood vessels could be seen passing through

Endobronchial Ultrasonography, Second Edition. Noriaki Kurimoto, David I.K. Fielding, Ali I. Musani, Christopher Kniese, and Katsuhiko Morita.

Companion website: www.wiley.com/go/kurimoto2e

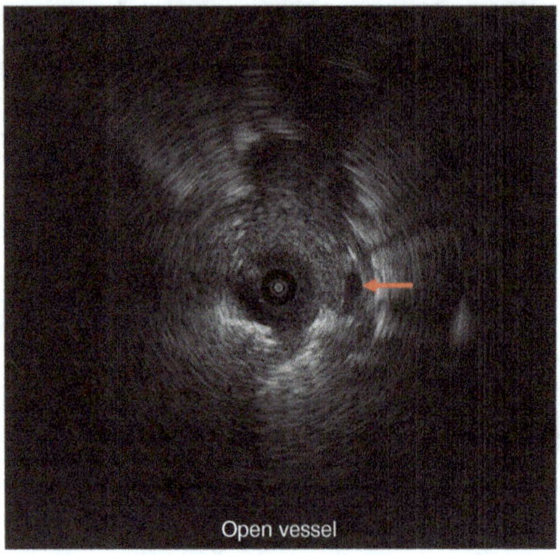

Figure 8.1 Open vessel.

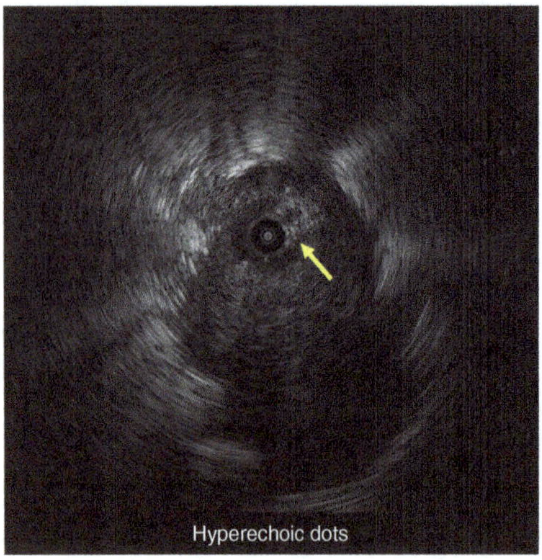

Figure 8.2 Hyperechoic dots.

the lesions. However, in some cases of well-differentiated adenocarcinoma, no blood vessels were visualized. These lesions also presented an irregular distribution of hyperechoic dots or arcs around the probe and had poorly defined borders.

In most cases of moderately differentiated adenocarcinoma and squamous cell carcinoma, EBUS images showed obstruction of the blood vessels within the lesion, obstruction of the bronchi, heterogeneous internal echoes, and irregular margins. In some case of moderately differentiated adenocarcinoma, numerous very small hyperechoic echoes were observed within the lesion, with a distribution identical to that of the multiple calcifications observed histopathologically. In some cases of squamous cell carcinoma, numerous anechoic areas of various sizes were noted with a distribution that corresponded to the areas of necrosis. Squamous cell carcinoma sometimes showed a circumferential hyperechoic line around the probe corresponding to the bronchial wall; this is caused by tumor growth that results in outward compression of the bronchial adventitia (Figure 8.3, yellow arrow). On EBUS images, most cases of poorly differentiated adenocarcinoma showed heterogeneous internal echoes, irregular margins, and few patent blood vessels or bronchi.

In my experience, a small nodular small cell carcinoma directly invaded the pulmonary artery adjacent to the affected bronchus, resulting in stenosis of the pulmonary artery within the lesion. In some carcinoids, the tumor arises in the bronchial wall and grows across the bronchial lumen, resulting in a characteristic snowman-shaped form, with the neck located at the cartilaginous part of the bronchus. Bleeding within the carcinoid appears as mottled hyperechoic areas on the EBUS image. Cases of primary malignant lymphoma of the lung can show homogeneous internal echoes with an appearance similar to that of pneumonia. Large blood vessels remain patent within the lesions, indicating that the lesions are soft. An inflammatory pseudotumor was observed, wherein anechoic areas with star-shaped margins were visible within the lesion, corresponding to the lumen of the dilated bronchus.

Corresponding to histopathology, EBUS enables the visualization of the internal structures of peripheral pulmonary lesions, such as vessels and bronchioles, as well as bleeding, calcifications, bronchial dilatation, and necrosis.

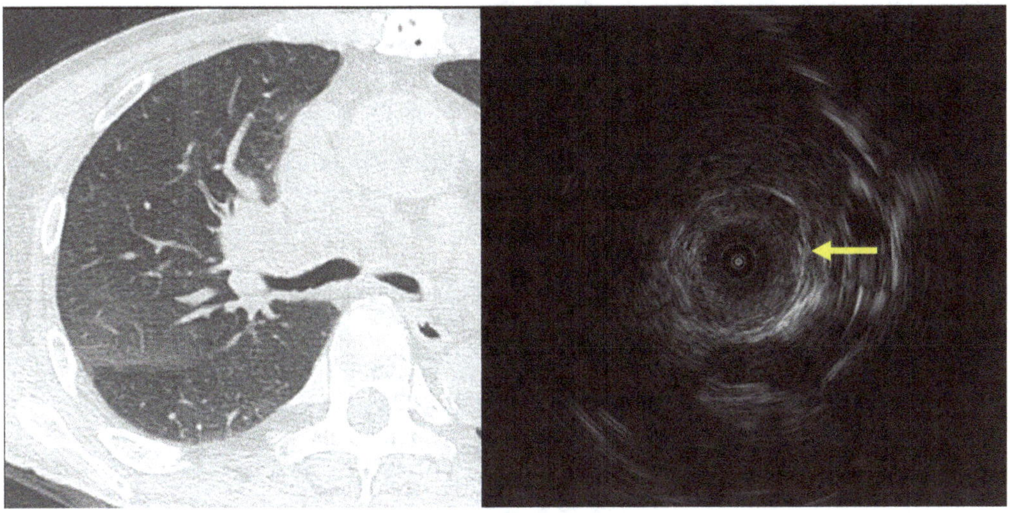

Figure 8.3 Expanded bronchial wall.

Internal Structural Components in EBUS Images of Peripheral Pulmonary Lesions

The focus of an ultrasound probe at 20 MHz is around 5–10 mm from the probe. The analysis of internal structural components on EBUS images should therefore concentrate on the area of the image around 5–10 mm from the probe.

Internal Echo

The homogeneous speckle pattern on EBUS images is a sign of relatively regular structures within the lesion. When the internal structure of the lesion is relatively regular around 5–10 mm from the probe, the ultrasound waves are able to penetrate some distance with little attenuation. This results in a homogeneous echo at around 10–15 mm from the probe. The heterogeneous speckle pattern is relatively irregular. When the internal structure of the lesion is relatively irregular around 5–10 mm from the probe, the ultrasound waves cannot penetrate far and there is high attenuation. Consequently, the EBUS image around 10–15 mm from the probe is dark (Figure 8.4).

Open Vessels

Sometimes when pulling back the ultrasound probe during scanning, a round anechoic area is seen on the EBUS image continuously from a distal site to a proximal site. This is likely to be an open vessel (Figure 8.1). When an anechoic area corresponds with necrosis, it cannot usually be followed continuously as the probe is pulled back.

Hyperechoic Arcs, Short Lines, and Dots

When there is a relatively large amount of air in the bronchus or lung tissue, hyperechoic arcs can be seen (Figures 8.5 and 8.6, yellow arrow). The length of these arcs is usually about ≥2 mm. When there is only a little air in the bronchus or lung tissue, hyperechoic short lines are seen (Figure 8.6, red arrow). These are usually 1–2 mm long. When there is very little air in the lung tissue, hyperechoic dots can be seen (Figure 8.2). Their diameter is usually <1 mm.

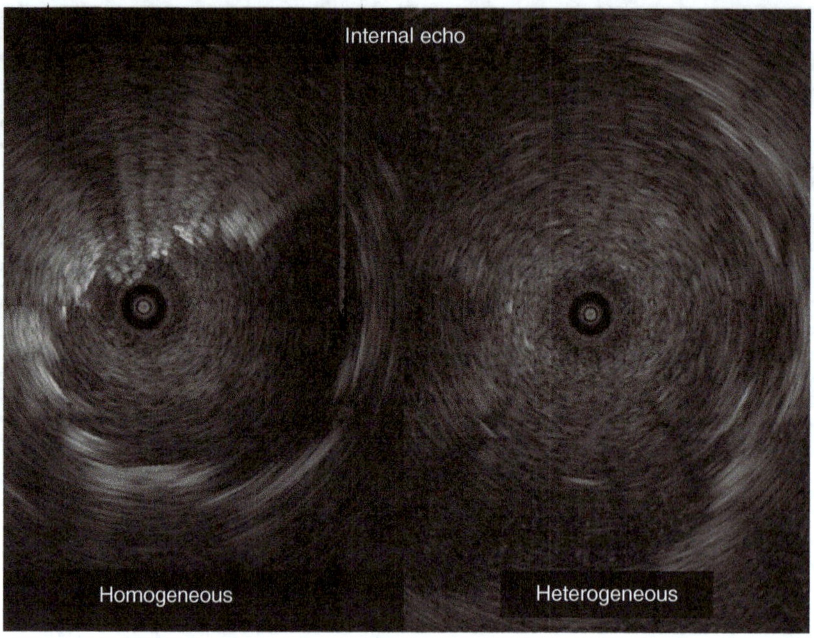

Figure 8.4 Internal echo. Left (homogeneous): the homogeneous speckle pattern is relatively regular on endobronchial ultrasound (EBUS) images. Right (heterogeneous): the heterogeneous speckle pattern is relatively irregular on EBUS images.

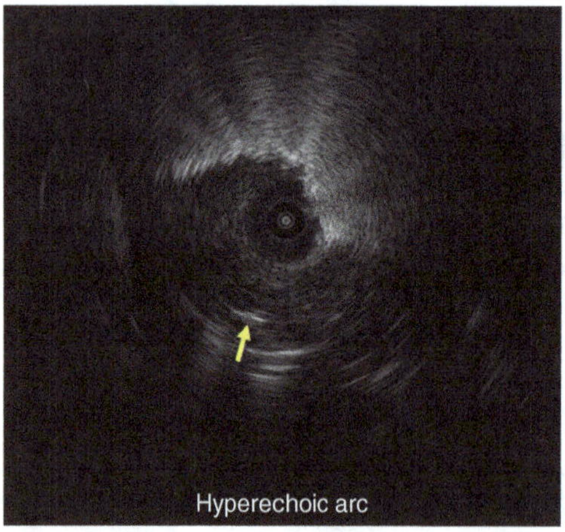

Figure 8.5 Hyperechoic arc.

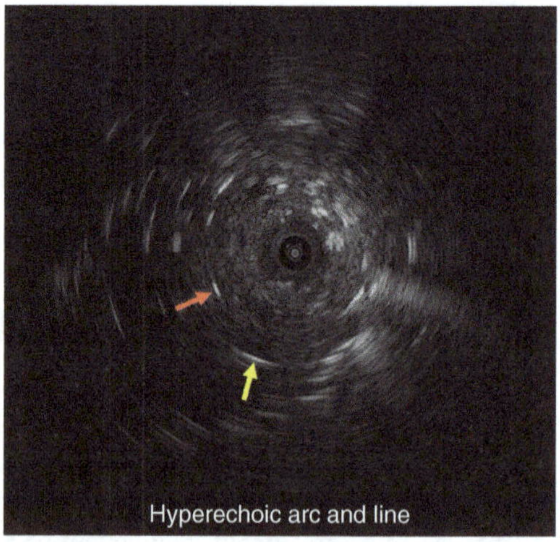

Figure 8.6 Hyperechoic arc and line.

Classifications of Lesions Based on Internal Structures Visualized by EBUS

EBUS can clearly visualize the internal structures of peripheral pulmonary lesions, including vessels and bronchioles, as well as compressed alveolar air within the lesion, calcifications, and necrosis, and it reveals the homogeneity or heterogeneity of the ultrasonic pattern. Tumor typing based on the internal structures visualized by EBUS can assist in distinguishing between benign and malignant tumors and in assessing the degree of differentiation.

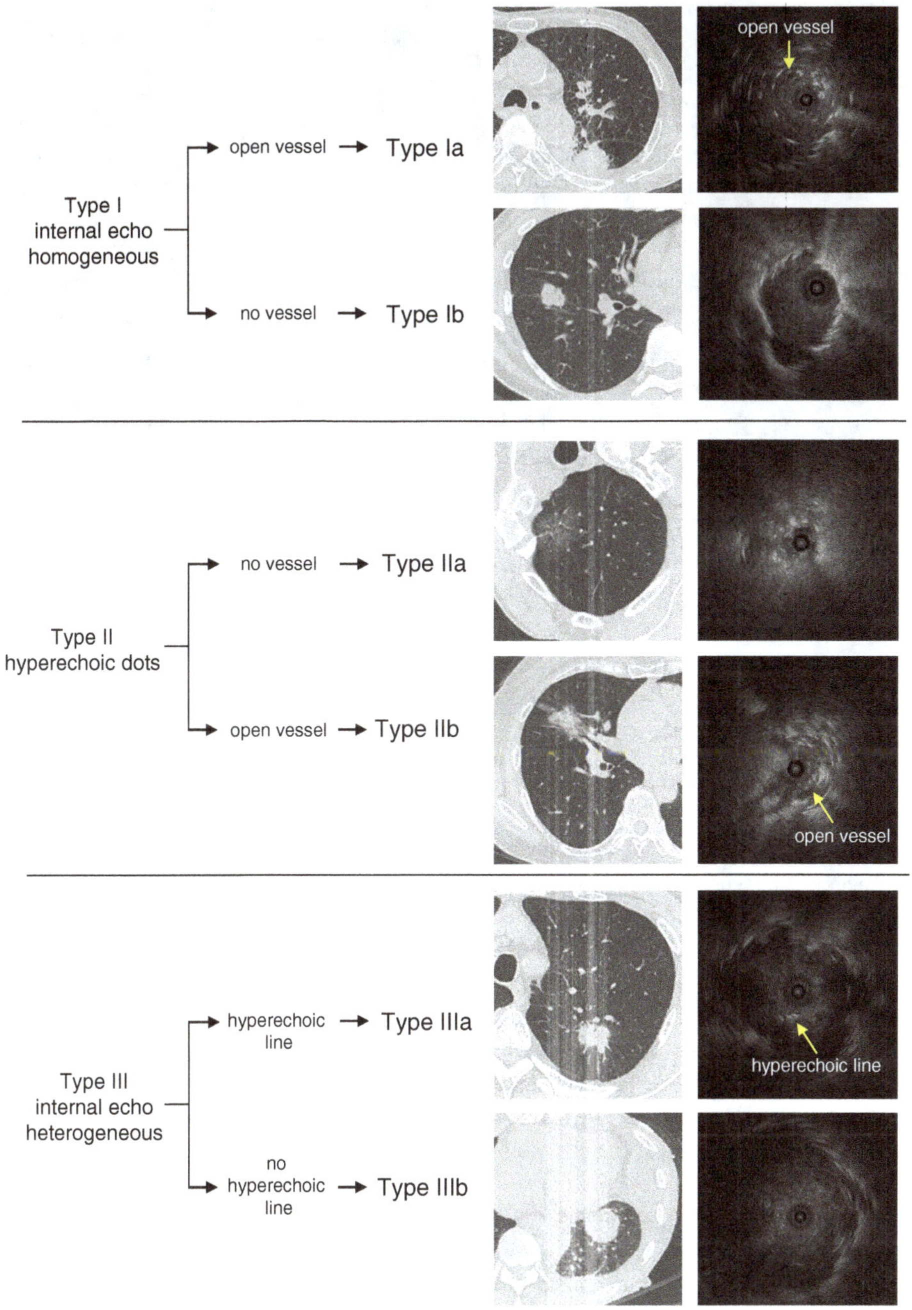

Figure 8.7 Type classification for peripheral pulmonary lesions.

We conducted a study of lesion typing based on the internal structure of lesions as visualized by high-resolution EBUS [8]. The internal structures of these lesions were analyzed, and the lesions were typed according to the internal echo pattern (homogeneous or heterogeneous), the vascular patency, and the morphology of hyperechoic areas (which reflects the presence of air and the state of the bronchi; Figure 8.7).

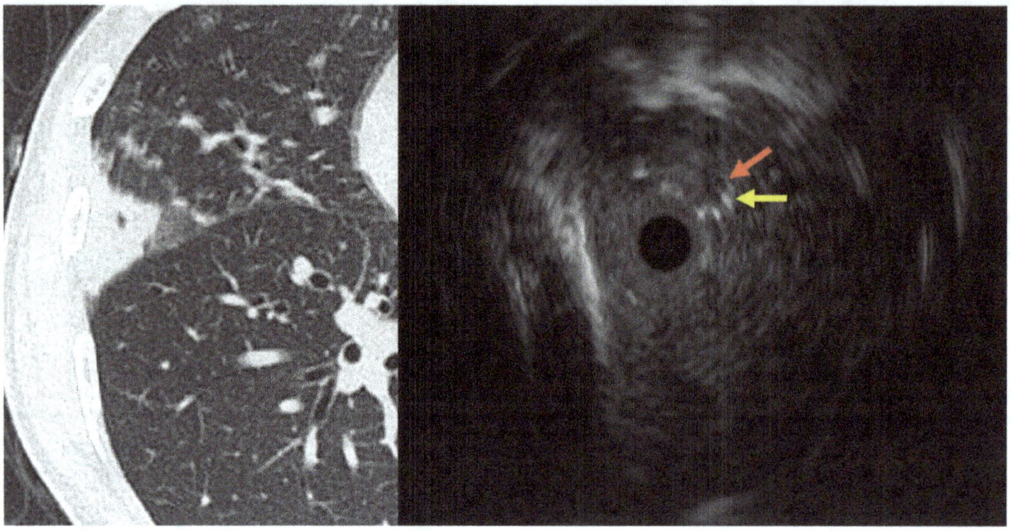

Figure 8.8 Type Ia lesion. This endobronchial ultrasound image of a Type Ia lesion shows normal blood vessels and bronchi within the lesion, free from compression or stenosis. The internal echoes are homogeneous.

Type I: Homogeneous Patterns

Type Ia: Homogeneous Pattern with Patent Vessels and Bronchioles

Most Type Ia cases were associated with pneumonia, characterized by exudate-filled alveoli. EBUS images of this type showed normal blood vessels (Figure 8.8, red arrow) and bronchi (Figure 8.8, yellow arrow) within the lesion, free from compression or stenosis. The internal echoes were homogeneous. There was therefore little ultrasonic attenuation, and even tissue 10–15 mm from the probe could be seen clearly. Because the lesions extended from one lobule to another, the margins were linear in some areas.

Type Ib: Homogeneous Pattern without Vessels or Bronchioles

The Type Ib group (Figure 8.9) mostly included cases of organizing pneumonia and tuberculomas. No blood vessels were seen within the lesions, and mottled or linear hyperechoic areas were scarce. The internal echoes were homogeneous. As with the Type Ia pattern, there was little ultrasonic attenuation, and even tissue 10–15 mm from the probe could be seen clearly.

Type II: Patterns with Hyperechoic Dots and Linear Arcs

Type IIa: Hyperechoic Dots and Linear Arcs without Vessels

Most cases of Type IIa lesions (Figure 8.10) were well-differentiated adenocarcinomas that had replaced the alveolar epithelium. No blood vessels were seen within the lesions on EBUS images. Hyperechoic dots or hyperechoic linear arcs (primarily around the probe) were distributed irregularly within the lesions. The presence of residual air in the alveoli is a characteristic feature of a well-differentiated adenocarcinoma that has grown to replace the alveolar epithelium. The air remaining in the alveoli hampers the visualization of blood vessels within the lesion and obscures the margins of the lesion.

Type IIb: Hyperechoic Dots and Linear Arcs with Patent Vessels

Most cases of Type IIb lesions were well-differentiated adenocarcinomas that had proliferated and replaced the alveolar epithelium while preserving the blood vessels within the lesion. On the EBUS images, the blood vessels showed little or no compression or stenosis

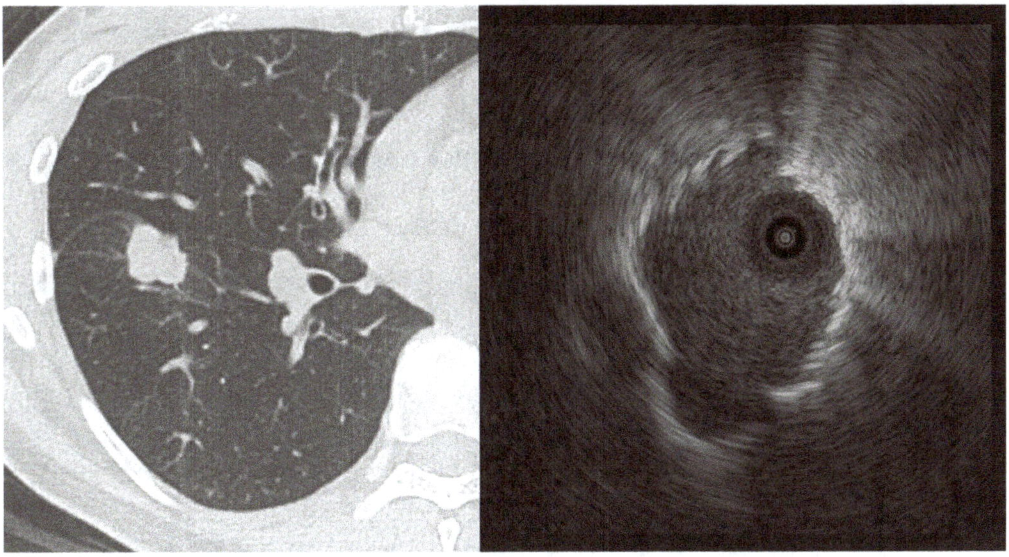

Figure 8.9 Type Ib lesion. In this endobronchial ultrasound image of a Type Ib lesion, no patent blood vessels can be seen within the lesion. The internal echoes are hypoechoic and homogeneous.

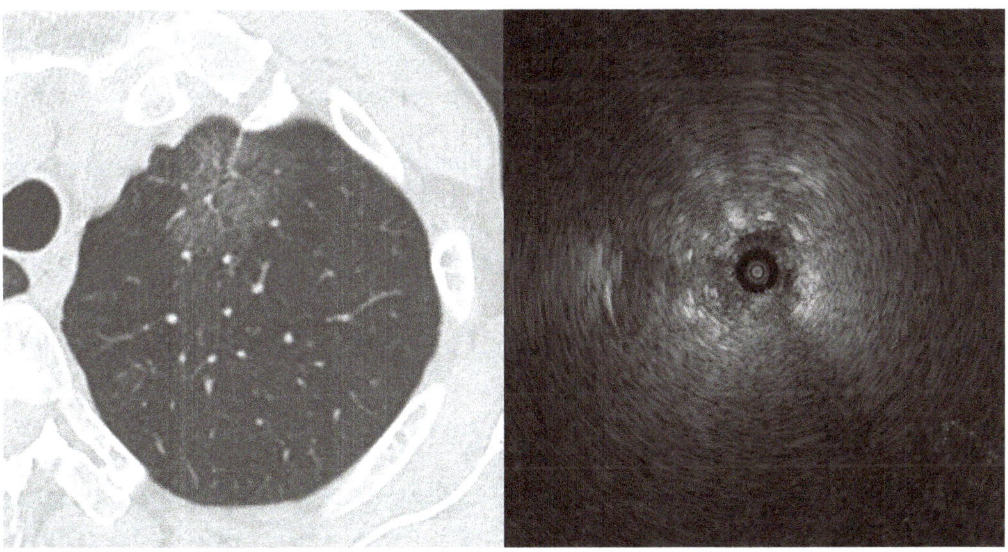

Figure 8.10 Type IIa lesion. In this endobronchial ultrasound image of a Type IIa lesion, no blood vessels can be seen within the lesion. Hyperechoic dots (<1 mm in diameter) and hyperechoic linear arcs are distributed irregularly within the lesion.

within the lesion (Figure 8.11, red arrow), and the internal echoes were relatively homogeneous. Hyperechoic dots, distributed irregularly within the lesions, corresponded to residual air in the alveoli, which is a characteristic feature of well-differentiated adenocarcinomas. Compared with Type IIa lesions, the density of cancer cells was higher in Type IIb lesions and the volume of air remaining in the alveoli was smaller. The margins were irregular because the lesions grew without any relationship to the existing structures.

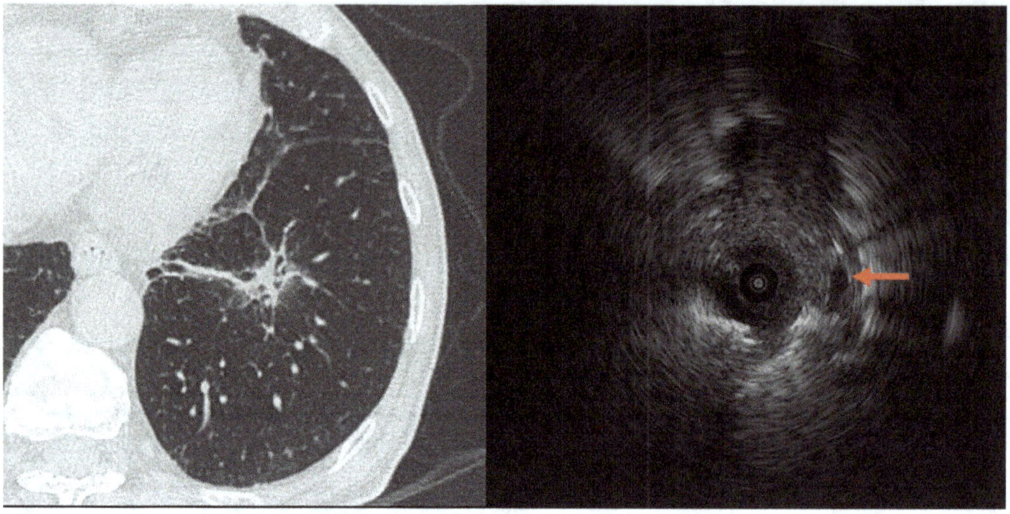

Figure 8.11 Type IIb lesion. In this endobronchial ultrasound image of a Type IIb lesion, blood vessels, almost free from compression or stenosis (red arrow), are visible within the lesion. The internal echoes are relatively homogeneous. Hyperechoic dots (<1 mm in diameter) are distributed irregularly within the lesion, indicating the presence of residual air in the alveoli.

Type III: Heterogeneous Patterns

Type IIIa: Heterogeneous Pattern with Hyperechoic Dots and Short Lines

Most cases of Type IIIa lesions (Figure 8.12) were moderately differentiated adenocarcinoma that had grown with relatively high cell densities and had formed a mass. The EBUS images showed no blood vessels within these lesions. Mottling and linear hyperechoic lines were irregularly distributed within the lesions, corresponding to compressed or stenotic bronchi

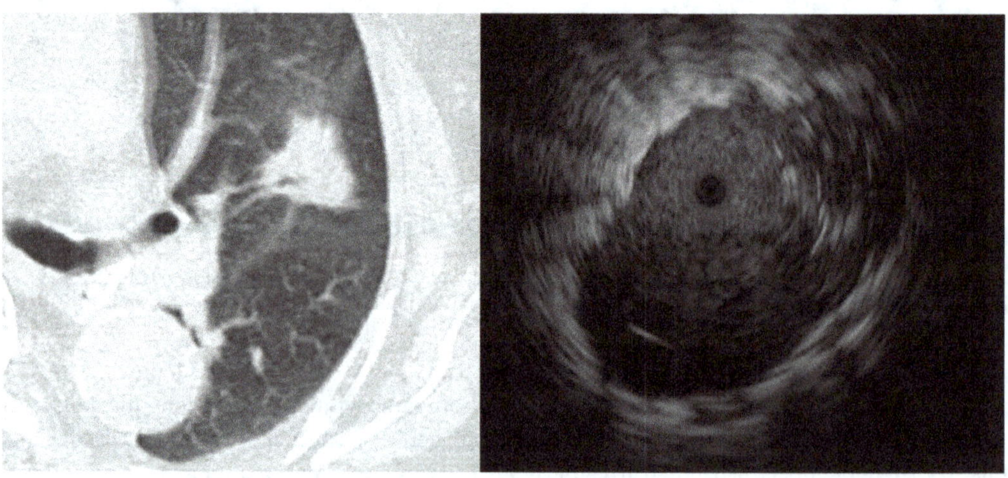

Figure 8.12 Type IIIa lesion. In this endobronchial ultrasound image, no blood vessels are seen within the lesion. Hyperechoic lines are irregularly distributed within the lesion, corresponding to compressed or stenotic bronchi or alveolar air. The internal echoes are heterogeneous.

or alveolar air. The internal echoes were heterogeneous, with markedly attenuated sound wave transmission; therefore, only areas about 6–8 mm from the probe could be visualized clearly. Because the lesions spread in a random manner rather than extending along lung structures, the margins of the lesions were often rounded. Moderately differentiated squamous cell carcinoma presented numerous anechoic areas, which corresponded to areas of necrosis within the tumor; this is a characteristic feature of this carcinoma.

Type IIIb: Heterogeneous Pattern without Hyperechoic Dots and Short Lines

Most cases of Type IIIb lesions (Figure 8.13) were poorly differentiated adenocarcinomas with high cell densities, which had formed a mass. The lesions were avascular and showed only a small amount of mottled or linear hyperechoic lines. The internal echoes were heterogeneous. Because the lesions extended outward, their margins tended to be somewhat rounded.

In our study [8], we were able to visualize lesions in 143 of 168 cases (85%) of a peripheral pulmonary lesion in which EBUS was performed. Of these, a definitive tissue diagnosis was obtained in 124 cases (74%). We found that 92% of the Type I lesions were benign and 99% of the Type II and III lesions were malignant. Well-differentiated adenocarcinomas accounted for 88% of the Type II lesions. All of the Type IIIb cases were malignant; 82% were poorly differentiated adenocarcinomas.

Articles and Discussion

Some investigators have reported that dynamic magnetic resonance imaging (MRI) provides information on the enhancement patterns of peripheral pulmonary lesions [9, 10]. Awaya et al. [11] reported that bronchi and blood vessels can be seen on dynamic MRI as they cross peripheral pulmonary lesions. MRI is less invasive than EBUS, but the images are of poorer quality because the beating heart and breathing introduce motion artifacts.

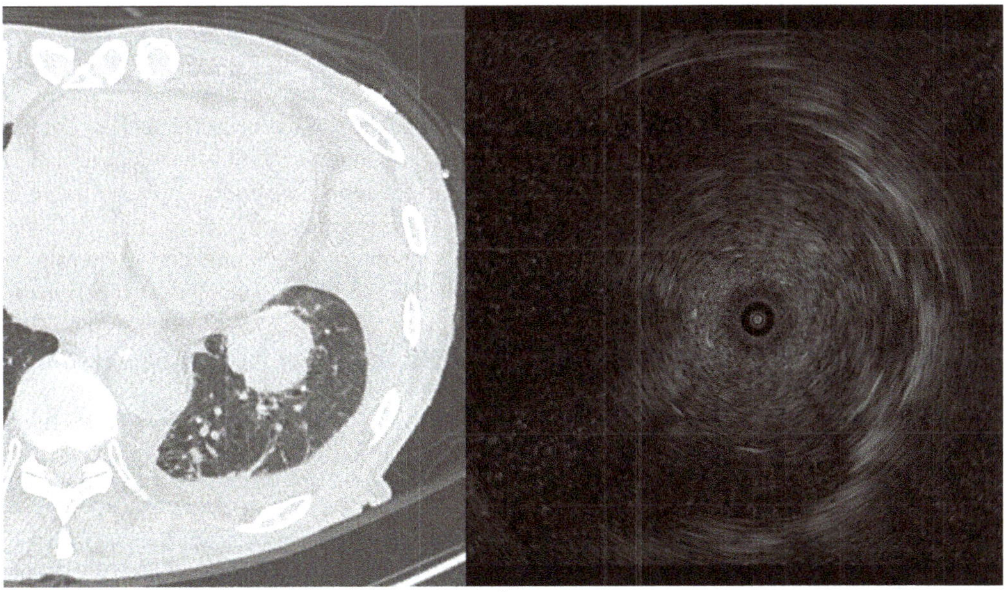

Figure 8.13 Type IIIb lesion. In this endobronchial ultrasound image, the lesion is avascular, and few hyperechoic lines can be seen. The internal echoes are heterogeneous.

There have been reports of using miniature ultrasonic probes for diagnosing peripheral pulmonary lesions. Hürter et al. [12] reported the successful visualization of peripheral lung lesions in 19 of 26 cases, and Goldberg and colleagues [13] reported that EBUS provided unique information that complemented other diagnostic modalities in 18 of 25 cases (which comprised 6 peripheral lesions and 19 hilar tumors).

Hosokawa et al. [14] reported that a typical EBUS pattern for neoplastic disease involves three characteristics: a continuous marginal echo, rough internal echoes, and either no hyperechoic spots associated with bronchi or no longitudinal continuity if such spots are present. Kuo et al. [15] assessed the feasibility of using EBUS for differentiating between benign and malignant lesions, using the following three characteristic ultrasonic features to indicate malignancy: a continuous margin, the absence of a linear-discrete air bronchogram, and heterogeneous echogenicity. When a lesion showed none of these three echoic features, the negative predictive value for malignancy was 93.7%. Conversely, for a lesion with any two of these features, the positive predictive value for malignancy was 89.2%. We developed our classification system with the aims of distinguishing between benign and malignant lesions, identifying the type of lung carcinoma, and determining the degree of differentiation.

Morikawa et al. [16] reported the contribution to the diagnosis of lung cancer of histogram data collected from images obtained using EBUS with a guide sheath. Median values of histogram height, histogram width, height/width ratio, and standard deviation differed significantly between malignant lesions and benign lesions. With a cutoff value for standard deviation of 10.5, lung cancer could be diagnosed with an accuracy of 81.7%.

Although computed tomographic (CT) and MRI scans have been used for the qualitative diagnosis of peripheral pulmonary lesions, ultrasonograms have several advantages. For example, EBUS can be used to determine the following items:

- The patency of the microvasculature within the lesion.
- The distribution of micropneumatosis (small hyperechoic dots) within the lesion.
- The existence of any anechoic areas corresponding to necrosis within the lesion.
- The internal echo within the lesion.

In particular, the internal echo within lesions visualized by high-frequency 20 MHz ultrasonography varies according to factors such as the distribution and density of tumor cells and the presence of mucus and interstitial hyperplasia within the lesion. The internal echo depends on the extent to which the ultrasound waves are reflected at interfaces between tissue types. Bronchioloalveolar carcinoma (a mucinous type), which is difficult to distinguish from pneumonia using CT scanning, produces a stronger echo than pneumonia on high-frequency ultrasonography at 20 MHz. The reason for this is unclear, but it is thought that it may be due to viscous mucus or increased reflection from neoplastic tissue in the alveolar septa.

In summary, EBUS provides a new way to visualize the internal structures of peripheral pulmonary lesions. Classification of the EBUS images can suggest the pathology and histology of the lesion.

References

1 Grimm, H., Binmolleller, K.F., Hamper, K. et al. (1993). Endosonography for preoperative locolesional staging of esophageal and gastric cancer. *Endoscopy* 25: 224–230.

2 Abe, S., Lifhtdale, C.J., and Brennan, M.F. (1993). The Japanese experience with endoscopic ultrasonography in staging of gastric cancer. *Gastrointestinal Endoscopy* 39: 536–541.

3 Murata, Y., Yoshida, M., Akimoto, S. et al. (1988). Evaluation of endoscopic ultrasonography for the diagnosis of submucosal tumors of the esophagus. *Surgical Endoscopy* 2: 51–58.

4 Rosch, T. (1992). Endoscopic ultrasonography. *Endoscopy* 24: 144–153.

5 Murata, Y., Muroi, M., Yoshida, M. et al. (1987). Endoscopic ultrasonography in diagnosis of esophageal carcinoma. *Surgical Endoscopy* 1: 11–16.

6 Yasuda, K., Mukai, H., Nakajima, M. et al. (1993). Staging of pancreatic carcinoma by endoscopic ultrasonography. *Endoscopy* 25: 151–155.

7 Rosch, T., Braig, C., Gain, T. et al. (1992). Staging of pancreatic and ampullary carcinoma by endoscopic ultrasonography. *Gastroenterology* 102: 188–199.

8 Kurimoto, N., Murayama, M., Yoshioka, S. et al. (2002). Analysis of the internal structure of peripheral pulmonary lesions using endobronchial ultrasonography. *Chest* 122: 1877–1894.

9 Kusumoto, M., Kono, M., Yamasaki, K. et al. (1995). Pulmonary nodules: quantitative assessment with contrast-enhanced MR imaging. *Radiology* 197: 232.

10 Guckel, C., Schnabel, K., Deimling, M. et al. (1996). Solitary pulmonary nodules: MR evaluation of enhancement patterns with contrast-enhanced dynamic snapshot gradient-echo imaging. *Radiology* 200: 681–686.

11 Awaya, H., Matsumoto, T., Miura, G. et al. Evaluation of internal characteristic in small adenocarcinoma by MR imaging. *Japanese Journal of Radiology* 45: 47–57.

12 Hürter, T. and Hanarath, P. (1990). Endobronchiale Sonographie zur Diagnostik pulmonaler und mediastinaler Tumoren. *Deutsche Medizinische Wochenschrift* 115: 1899–905 [in German].

13 Goldberg, B., Steiner, R., Liu, J. et al. (1994). US-assisted bronchoscopy with use of miniature transducer-containing catheters. *Radiology* 190: 233–237.

14 Hosokawa, S., Matsuo, K., Watanabe, Y. et al. (2004). Two cases of nodular lesions in the peripheral lung field, successfully diagnosed by endobronchial ultrasonography (EBUS). *Kokyuu* 23: 57–60.

15 Kuo, C., Lin, S., Chen, H. et al. (2007). Diagnosis of peripheral lung cancer with three echoic features via endobronchial ultrasound. *Chest* 132: 922–929.

16 Morikawa, K., Kurimoto, N., Inoue, T. et al. (2015). Histogram-based quantitative evaluation of endobronchial ultrasonography images of peripheral pulmonary lesion. *Respiration* 89: 148–154.

9

Diagnosis of Peripheral Pulmonary Lesions Using Endobronchial Ultrasonography with a Guide Sheath

Noriaki Kurimoto

Department of Internal Medicine, Division of Medical Oncology and Respiratory Medicine, Shimane University Faculty of Medicine, Izumo, Japan

Introduction

Bronchial brushing cytology and transbronchial biopsy (TBB) are used to diagnose peripheral pulmonary lesions (PPLs). In most cases, fluoroscopy is required to assist the operator in directing the brush or biopsy forceps to the site of interest, but it is often difficult to confirm whether the biopsy forceps have reached the lesion. Since 1994, it has been possible to delineate a PPL through introducing a miniature ultrasonic probe into the peripheral bronchus where the lesion is located [1]. This involves withdrawing the probe after obtaining the ultrasound image and then introducing a brush or biopsy forceps to acquire the brushing or tissue sample. However, with this method, it is difficult to ensure that the sample is accurately taken from the site of the lesion. To increase the reliability of sample collection from PPLs, we devised a technique using endobronchial ultrasound with a guide sheath (EBUS-GS).

Equipment

After the commencement of EBUS-GS in 1996, we used a 20 MHz mechanical radial miniature ultrasonic probe (UM-S20-20R, Olympus Corporation, Tokyo, Japan) with an outer diameter of 1.7 mm. Since 2000, we have used a 20 MHz mechanical radial thin ultrasonic probe (UM-S20-17R, Olympus) with an outer diameter of 1.4 mm (see Figure 3.4). The probe is connected to an endoscopic ultrasound system. Guide sheaths are commercially available (Guide Sheath Kit, Olympus).

EBUS-GS Procedure

The preparation of the equipment for EBUS-GS and the techniques used for EBUS-GS were described in Chapter 3. Here, we illustrate the procedure with a representative case.

Representative Case Study

The patient had a 28 × 25 mm nodular lesion in segment B^2a of the right lung (Figure 9.1). We introduced a miniature probe covered by a guide sheath into B^2ai and obtained EBUS images. These revealed homogeneous internal echoes in the lesion that contained open vessels and open bronchial branches. These findings were suggestive of inflammation. The probe was withdrawn, leaving the guide sheath

Endobronchial Ultrasonography, Second Edition. Noriaki Kurimoto, David I.K. Fielding, Ali I. Musani, Christopher Kniese, and Katsuhiko Morita.

Companion website: www.wiley.com/go/kurimoto2e

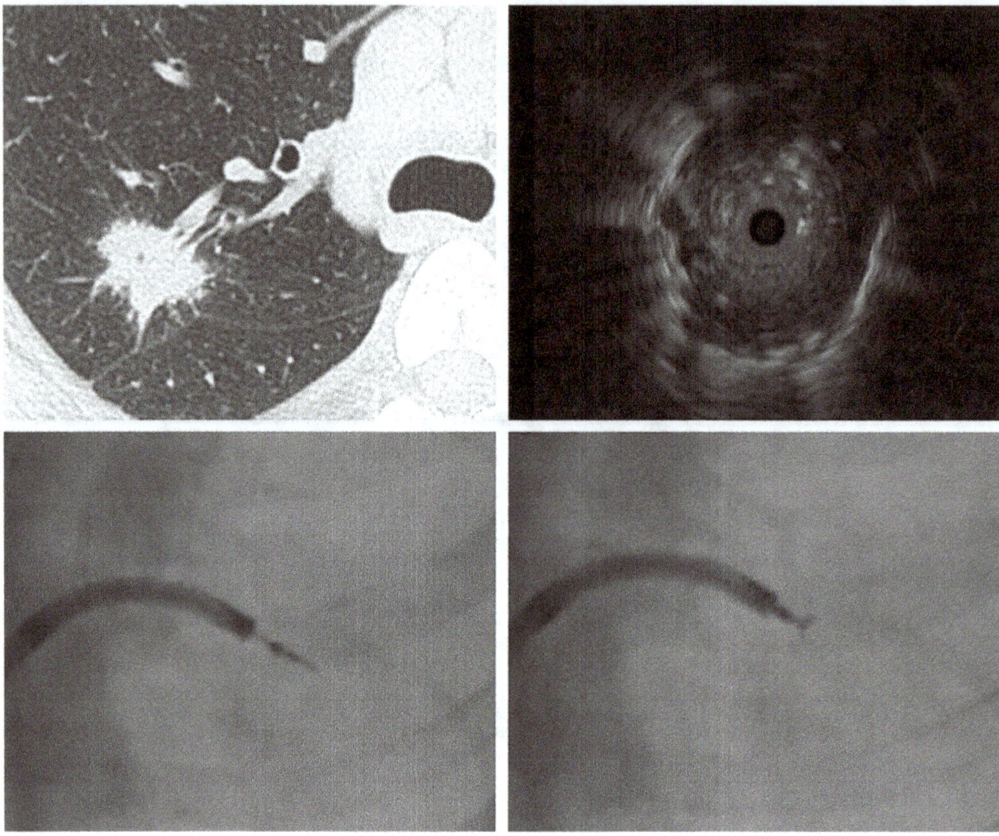

Figure 9.1 A representative case of endobronchial ultrasonography with a guide sheath.

at the site of the lesion identified by EBUS. A bronchial brush and biopsy forceps were introduced into the bronchus.

Effectiveness of Using EBUS-GS to Diagnose PPLs

We previously conducted a study of the effectiveness of EBUS using a thick guide sheath for diagnosing PPLs in 150 patients [2]. The overall diagnostic yield was 77%, with diagnostic yields for malignant and benign lesions of 81% and 69%, respectively. The diagnostic yield was significantly higher for lesions where the EBUS image showed the probe within the lesion (87%) rather than adjacent to the lesion (42%). The diagnostic yield was significantly higher for lesions defined as masses (>30 mm; 92%) than for those defined as nodules (≤30 mm; 74%). However, for lesions ≤30 mm, lesion size did not affect the diagnostic yield, even for lesions ≤10 mm, with similar diagnostic yields observed for lesions ≤10 mm (76%), 10–15 mm (76%), 15–20 mm (69%), and 20–30 mm (77%). In 54/81 lesions ≤20 mm in size, it was impossible to confirm fluoroscopically that the biopsy forceps had reached the lesion. The diagnostic yield for those lesions was 74%, similar to the yield when it was determined fluoroscopically that the forceps had reached the lesion (67%).

Moderate bleeding was seen in 2 (1%) of the 150 patients. There were no deaths, pneumothoraces, or other clinically significant morbidities.

EBUS-GS increases the reliability of specimen collection during bronchoscopy. Reported bronchoscopic diagnostic yields for PPLs ≤2 cm in size have varied from 5 to 28% [3–11]; for example, Radke et al. [5] reported a positive yield of 28%, Stringfield et al. [6] of 27%, Fletcher et al. [7] of 12%, and Wallace et al. [8] of 5%. The diagnostic yield in our study was far superior to those reported by the earlier studies. Lesions that are fluoroscopically undetectable can be visualized using EBUS when the lesion is in contact with the EBUS probe. EBUS-GS is particularly useful for lesions ≤20 mm that are undetectable using fluoroscopy.

We use two terms, “within” and “adjacent to,” for describing the location of the probe at a PPL. “Within” indicates that the probe is located inside the lesion, with the lesion surrounding the probe 360° (Figure 3.5, right). “Adjacent to” indicates that the probe is located beside the lesion (Figure 3.5, left). EBUS-GS is most successful when the probe is placed within the lesion. In our study described earlier [2], the yield for TBB when the probe was adjacent to the lesion was very low. This suggested that for these lesions, the probe was in contact only with the outer surface of the affected bronchus; therefore, the sampling was unlikely to be diagnostic. When this happens, the operator should attempt to delineate the lesion via another bronchus.

An advantage of EBUS-GS is the repeatability of accessing the bronchial lesion for sampling. Without a guide sheath, it is sometimes difficult to be certain that the forceps have been inserted into the same bronchial branch for a second biopsy. In addition, the bronchial mucosa becomes edematous after several attempts at manipulation, making it difficult to introduce the forceps into the bronchus.

Another advantage of EBUS-GS is its ability to protect against bleeding into the bronchus proximal to the biopsy site. Although massive hemorrhages into the bronchus following TBB are infrequent (occurring in <2% of TBB procedures) [9, 10], excessive bleeding may require the tip of the bronchoscope to be wedged against the lumen of the bronchus to obtain hemostasis. Because the outer surface of the sheath is snug against the internal surface of the bronchus during EBUS-GS, if bleeding occurs, the blood drains through the sheath.

The final advantage of EBUS-GS is the ability to obtain short-axis bronchial views of PPLs. Several investigators have reported the successful use of miniature probes [1, 2].

Yoshikawa [12] evaluated the feasibility and efficacy of TBB and bronchial brushing guided by EBUS-GS for diagnosing PPLs without radiographic fluoroscopy. Of 123 PPLs in that study, 76 (62%) were diagnosed by EBUS-GS guidance without fluoroscopy. The diagnostic yield was significantly higher for PPLs >20 mm in diameter (76%) than for PPLs ≤20 mm in diameter. In addition, PPLs located in the middle lobe and the lingular segment had significantly higher diagnostic yields than those in other locations. In multivariate analysis, the diameter and location of the PPL were independent predictors of diagnostic sensitivity by EBUS-GS-guided bronchoscopy.

Further studies are needed to determine the diagnostic yield for transbronchial needle aspiration under EBUS-GS guidance, as well as the usefulness of using a curette via the guide sheath.

Changes in EBUS-GS Techniques

When we began using EBUS-GS in 1996, we used large-bore guide sheaths with an outer diameter of 2.5 mm. Now, for almost all PPLs, we insert narrow-bore guide sheaths with an outer diameter of 2.0 mm down the working channel of a bronchoscope with an outer diameter of 4.0 mm. We use large-bore guide sheaths only for cases where relatively large specimens are required. The use of bronchoscopes with an outer diameter of 4.0 mm allows us to select fourth- and fifth-generation bronchi; these are two or three generations more peripheral than can be reached with a standard bronchoscope of around 6 mm in outer diameter.

How to Identify the Drainage Bronchus Leading to the Target Lesion

Identification of the Bronchial Branch Using Computed Tomography Imaging

See Chapter 7.

Identification of the Bronchial Branch Using a Navigation System

In recent years, two methods of navigation for PPLs have been developed. The electromagnetic navigation system is a localization device that assists with positioning endobronchial equipment in the desired area of the lung. It uses low-frequency electromagnetic waves emitted from an electromagnetic board placed under the bronchoscopy table mattress [13]. In a technical note, Harms et al. [14] introduced a new approach to the treatment of inoperable peripheral lung tumors, which combined an electromagnetic navigation system and EBUS with endobronchial brachytherapy planned in three dimensions. Asano et al. [15–17] have developed a bronchoscope insertion guidance system that produces virtual images by extracting the bronchi using automatic threshold adjustment and then searching for the bronchial route to the determined target. They used this system in combination with a thin bronchoscope and EBUS-GS. The system automatically produced virtual images to fifth-generation bronchi, on average. EBUS visualized 93.8% of the cases successfully, providing tissue diagnoses for 84.4%. This bronchoscope insertion guidance system readily produces virtual images for successfully guiding the bronchoscope to the target. The method shows promise for becoming a routine part of PPL biopsy techniques.

Signal Attenuation Caused by the Guide Sheath

The signal attenuation caused by the guide sheath can be used for accurately positioning the sheath within a PPL. The PPL should first be delineated using EBUS and the guide sheath positioned at the point where the lesion appears at its largest and clearest. Then, without disturbing the guide sheath, the assistant should withdraw the ultrasonic probe slowly until the probe transducer enters the guide sheath. As soon as the transducer has completely entered the guide sheath, the sheath will reflect the ultrasonic pulse and the ultrasound image will suddenly become darker. If the site of this phenomenon is within the lesion, the guide sheath will be placed precisely within the PPL.

Moving the Probe within the Lesion

Using Fluoroscopy to Select Another Bronchial Branch When a Lesion Cannot Be Delineated Using EBUS

When a lesion cannot be delineated using EBUS, bend the bronchoscope tip with the up–down angle lever and try to move the probe and guide sheath (probe/GS) close to the lesion using fluoroscopy (Figure 9.2). For example, while moving the probe/GS close to the lesion under fluoroscopy using the down angle lever, the probe/GS should be pulled back and then advanced to the lesion. If a bronchus enters the lesion from the bronchi in which the probe/GS is currently positioned, it may be possible to insert the probe/GS within the lesion.

Using the EBUS Image to Select Another Bronchial Branch

When the probe is adjacent to the lesion, bend the bronchoscope tip with the up–down angle

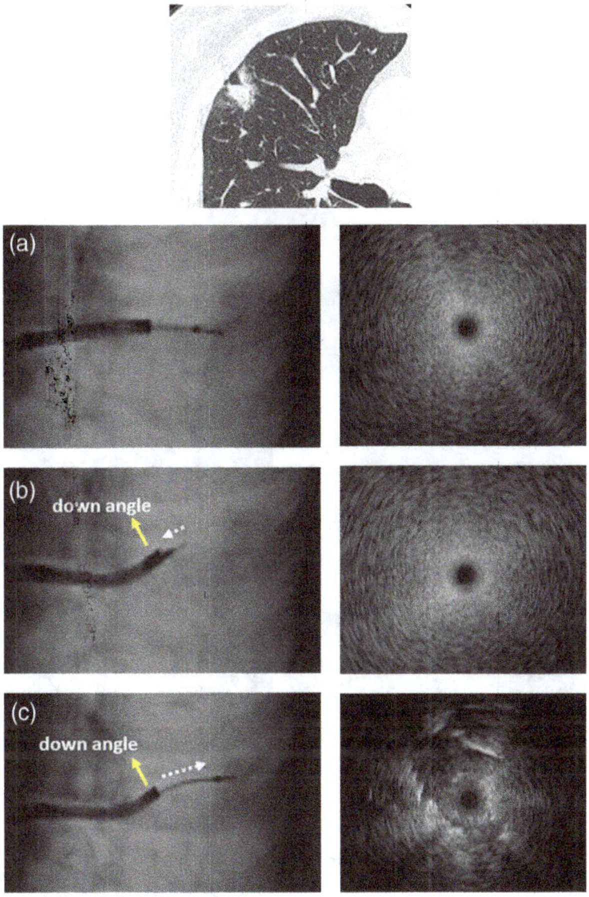

Figure 9.2 Selecting another bronchial branch using fluoroscopy when the lesion cannot be delineated using endobronchial ultrasonography (EBUS). (a) The lesion cannot be delineated using EBUS. (b) The probe and guide sheath are moved close to the lesion under fluoroscopy using the down angle lever. (c) The probe and guide sheath are pulled back and advanced to the lesion, ending up within the lesion.

lever and see whether the probe approaches the lesion on the EBUS image (Figure 9.3). For example, while moving close to the lesion on the EBUS image using the up lever, the probe/GS should be pulled back and then advanced to the lesion. If a bronchus enters the lesion from the bronchi in which the probe/GS is currently positioned, it may be possible to place the probe/GS within the lesion.

Using the EBUS Image with the Rotated Bronchoscope to Select Another Bronchial Branch

When the probe is adjacent to the lesion, bend the bronchoscope tip up and down with the angle lever and observe whether the probe approaches the lesion on the EBUS image (Figure 9.4). However, when the bronchoscope tip is bent by applying an up or down angle, the probe may move tangentially to the direction of the lesion border. If that happens, the bronchoscope should be linearized and rotated around its long axis. The bronchoscope tip should then be bent up or down again with the angle lever, checking whether the probe moves close to the lesion on the EBUS image. For example, while moving close to the lesion on the EBUS image using the up lever with the rotated bronchoscope, the probe/GS is pulled back and then advanced to the lesion. If a bronchus enters the lesion from the bronchi in

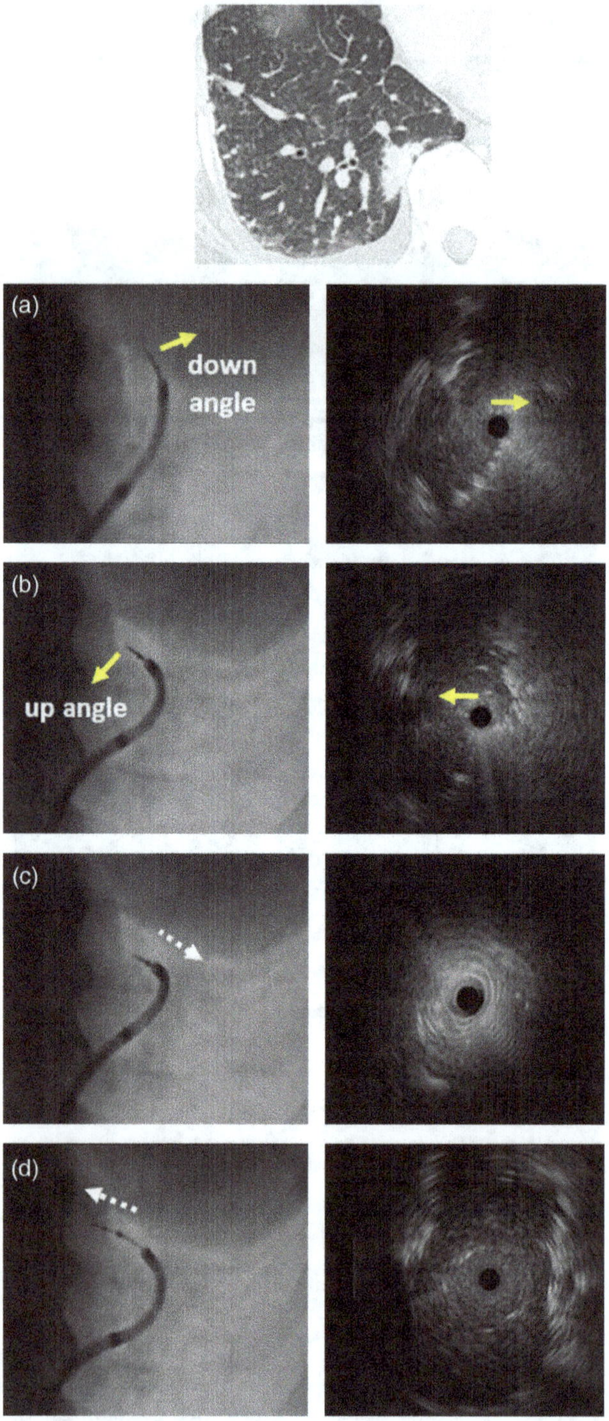

Figure 9.3 Selecting another bronchial branch using the endobronchial ultrasonography image when the probe is adjacent to the lesion. (a) With the probe adjacent to the lesion, the bronchoscope tip is bent with the down angle lever and the probe moved away from the lesion. (b) Bending the bronchoscope tip with the up angle lever, the probe is moved close to the lesion. (c) The probe and guide sheath are pulled back. (d) The probe and guide sheath are advanced into the lesion, ending up within it.

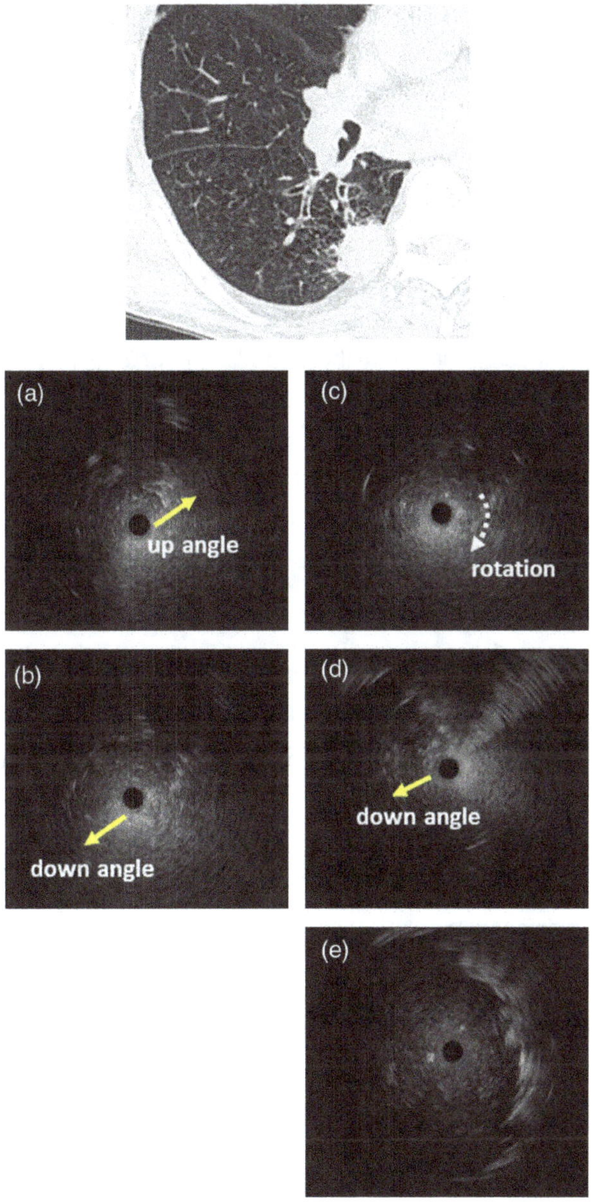

Figure 9.4 Selecting another bronchial branch with the rotated bronchoscope using the endobronchial sonography (EBUS) image when the probe is adjacent to the lesion. (a) With the probe adjacent to the lesion, the bronchoscope tip is bent with the up angle lever. The probe moves in a direction tangential to the border of the lesion. (b) The bronchoscope tip is bent with the down angle lever. The probe moves in a direction tangential to the border of the lesion. (c) The bronchoscope itself is linearized and rotated around its long axis. (d) The bronchoscope tip is then bent again by applying the down angle lever, and the probe is moved close to the lesion. (e) The bronchoscope is rotated and the bronchoscope tip moved to approach the lesion on the EBUS image using the down angle lever. The probe and guide sheath are pulled back and reinserted, and it may be possible to insert them within the lesion.

which the probe/GS is currently positioned, it may be possible to place the probe/GS within the lesion.

Management of Post-Biopsy Hemorrhaging

When hemorrhaging occurs following brushing or biopsy via the guide sheath, the blood usually passes into the guide sheath rather than into the airway. This is because the outer surface of the guide sheath is snug against the bronchial lumen. Wait about two minutes before withdrawing the guide sheath and in almost all cases it can be withdrawn without any further hemorrhage. We experienced one case in which a large intrapulmonary hemorrhage occurred, but the presence of the guide sheath meant that no further treatment was necessary; only a small amount of blood escaped into the airway.

Conclusion

EBUS-GS permits more accurate collection of samples from PPLs than other methods, as well as facilitating multiple biopsies from the same site and protecting against bleeding into the proximal bronchus from the biopsy site.

References

1. Kurimoto, N., Murayama, M., Yoshioka, S. et al. (2002). Analysis of the internal structure of peripheral pulmonary lesions using endobronchial ultrasonography. *Chest* 122: 1877–1894.
2. Kurimoto, N., Miyazawa, T., Okimasa, S. et al. (2004). Endobronchial ultrasonography using a guide sheath increases the ability to diagnose peripheral pulmonary lesions endoscopically. *Chest* 126: 959–965.
3. Mori, K., Yanase, N., Kaneko, M. et al. (1989). Diagnosis of peripheral lung cancer in cases of tumors 2 cm or less in size. *Chest* 95: 304–308.
4. Popvich, J. Jr., Kvale, P.A., Eichenhorn, M.S. et al. (1982). Diagnostic accuracy of multiple biopsies from flexible fiberoptic bronchoscopy—a comparison of central versus peripheral carcinoma. *American Review of Respiratory Diseases* 125: 521–523.
5. Radke, J.R., Conway, W.A., Eyler, W.R. et al. (1976). Diagnostic accuracy in peripheral lung lesions: factors predicting success with flexible fiberoptic bronchoscopy. *Chest* 76: 176–179.
6. Stringfield, J.T., Mrkowitz, D.J., Bentz, R.R. et al. (1977). The effect of tumor size and location on diagnosis by fiberoptic bronchoscopy. *Chest* 72: 474–476.
7. Fletcher, E.C. and Levin, D.C. (1982). Flexible fiberoptic bronchoscopy and fluoroscopically guided transbronchial biopsy in management of solitary pulmonary nodules. *Western Journal of Medicine* 135: 477–483.
8. Wallace, J.M. and Deutch, A.L. (1982). Flexible fiberoptic bronchoscopy and percutaneous lung aspiration for evaluating the solitary pulmonary nodule. *Chest* 81: 665–671.
9. Hadson, R.R., Zavala, D.C., Rhodes, M.L. et al. (1976). Transbronchial biopsy via flexible fiberoptic bronchoscope; results in 164 patients. *American Review of Respiratory Diseases* 114: 67–72.
10. Kvale, P.A., Bode, F.R., and Kini, S. (1976). Diagnostic accuracy in lung cancer; comparison of techniques used in association with flexible fiberoptic bronchoscopy. *Chest* 69: 752–757.
11. Shiner, R.J., Rosenman, J., Katz, I. et al. (1988). Bronchoscopic evaluation of peripheral lung tumors. *Thorax* 43: 887–889.
12. Yoshikawa, M., Sukoh, N., Yamazaki, K. et al. (2007). Diagnostic value of endobronchial ultrasonography with a guide sheath for peripheral pulmonary lesions

without X-ray fluoroscopy. *Chest* 131 (6): 1788–1793.

13 Schwarz, Y., Mehta, A.C., Ernst, A. et al. (2003). Electromagnetic navigation during flexible bronchoscopy. *Respiration* 70: 516–522.

14 Harms, W., Krempien, R., Grehn, C. et al. (2006). Electromagnetically navigated brachytherapy as a new treatment option for peripheral pulmonary tumors. *Strahlentherapie und Onkologie* 182: 108–111.

15 Asano, F., Matsuno, Y., Matsushita, T. et al. (2002). Transbronchial diagnosis of a pulmonary peripheral small lesion using an ultrathin bronchoscope with virtual bronchoscopic navigation. *Journal of Bronchology* 9: 108–111.

16 Asano, F., Matsuno, Y., Shinagawa, N. et al. (2006). A virtual bronchoscopic navigation system for pulmonary peripheral lesions. *Chest* 130: 559–566.

17 Asano, F., Matsuno, Y., Tsuzuku, A. et al. (2008). Diagnosis of pulmonary peripheral lesions using a bronchoscope insertion guidance system combined with endobronchial ultrasonography with a guide sheath. *Lung Cancer* 60: 366–373.

10

Endobronchial Ultrasonography with a Guide Sheath: Up to Date

David I.K. Fielding

Royal Brisbane and Women's Hospital, Herston, Queensland, Australia

Introduction

The endobronchial ultrasound (EBUS) guide sheath (GS) became available in the early 2000s and since that time has held its place as a safe and elegant way to sample peripheral nodules (Figures 10.1 and 10.2) [1]. Prior to that lesions could only be accessed by conventional transbronchial lung biopsy with fluoroscopy guidance and the yields were poor [2]. Traditional bronchoscopic biopsy of peripheral nodules had diagnostic yields of only 14–34% for nodules less than 2 cm, and has been found to be as low as 14% [3, 4].

Literature Review Including Meta-analyses

Kurimoto et al.'s study of 150 patients from 2004 at once showed the safety as well as the great diagnostic potential of the EBUS GS [5]. Importantly, most lesions less than 20 mm in diameter could not be visualized on simultaneous fluoroscopy, so EBUS was offering a unique and vital means of confirming lesion location prior to biopsy. The diagnostic yield of 21 lesions <10 mm was 76%, of lesions 10–15 mm was 76%, of 35 lesions 15–20 mm was 66%, and of 43 lesions 20–30 mm was 77%. An important concept was defined, namely whether the probe was located within the lesion (circumferentially surrounded by pathology) or adjacent to it, implying that no airway directly led into the lesion and effectively having the brush and forceps approaching the lesion from a less advantageous position. Cases within the lesion had a significantly higher diagnostic yield (105/121 cases, 87%) than cases with probe was adjacent to the lesion (8/19 cases, 42%). No pneumothoraces were observed.

This safety profile has remained; recently a review of almost 1000 cases from the National Cancer Centre Hospital done over two years reported an overall complication rate of 1.3% (13/965) [6]. Pneumothorax incidence was 0.8% (8/965) and 0.5% (5/965) for pulmonary infection. There was nil significant hemorrhage, air embolism, tumor seeding, or procedure-related death.

A number of studies have directly compared EBUS GS and computed tomography fine-needle aspiration (CT-FNA), due to higher rates of diagnostic success of CT-FNA. Recently Zhan et al. reported a systematic review and meta-analysis of EBUS-guided transbronchial lung biopsy (TBLB) and CT-guided transthoracic lung biopsy for the diagnosis of peripheral

Endobronchial Ultrasonography, Second Edition. Noriaki Kurimoto, David I.K. Fielding, Ali I. Musani, Christopher Kniese, and Katsuhiko Morita.

Companion website: www.wiley.com/go/kurimoto2e

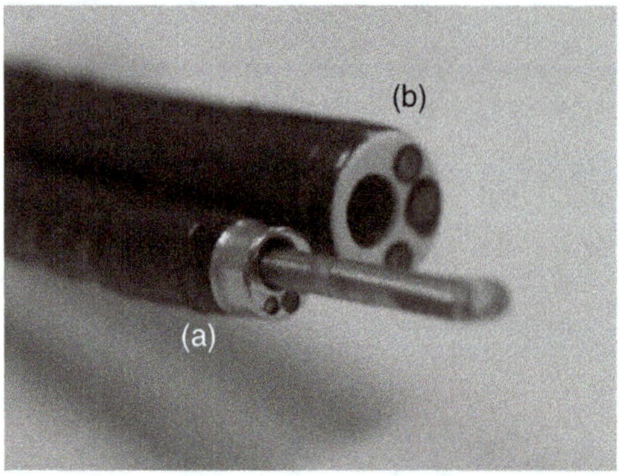

Figure 10.1 A comparison of bronchoscopes. (a) Thin bronchoscope (XBF-3B260Y1, 3.4-mm distal end diameter, Olympus, Tokyo, Japan) and thin ultrasonic probe (XUM-S20-17R, Olympus). (b) Standard bronchoscope (BF-1T260, 5.9-mm distal end diameter; Olympus).

lung cancer (PLC) [7]. This review had 31 publications dealing with EBUS-TBLB and 14 of CT-PTNB (percutaneous transthoracic needle biopsy). EBUS-TBLB had sensitivity of 0.69 (95% confidence interval [CI]: 0.67–0.71), which was less than CT-PTNB (0.94, 95% CI: 0.94–0.95). However, complications with EBUS-TBLB were lower than those reported for CT-PTNB. This meta-analysis showed that EBUS-TBLB is a safe and relatively accurate tool in the investigation of PLC. Although the yield remains lower than that of CT-PTNB, the procedural risks are lower. CT-PTNB had a pooled incidence of 0.32% (36/11 234) for severe bleeding and 1.09% (127/11 697) for pneumothorax that needed chest tube drainage. The pooled rate for EBUS GS across all included studies was 0.087% (2/2284) for severe bleeding and 0.48% (11/2284) for pneumothorax that needed chest tube drainage.

A persistent theme in analyses of yield is the importance of a positive bronchus sign on pre-procedure CT scans. Minezawa et al. recently reported results of 149 patients who had undergone thin section (0.5 mm slices) CT [8]; from EBUS GS the total diagnostic yield was 72.5%. In a multivariate analysis the only significant factor for diagnostic success was the presence of a CT bronchus sign; compared to

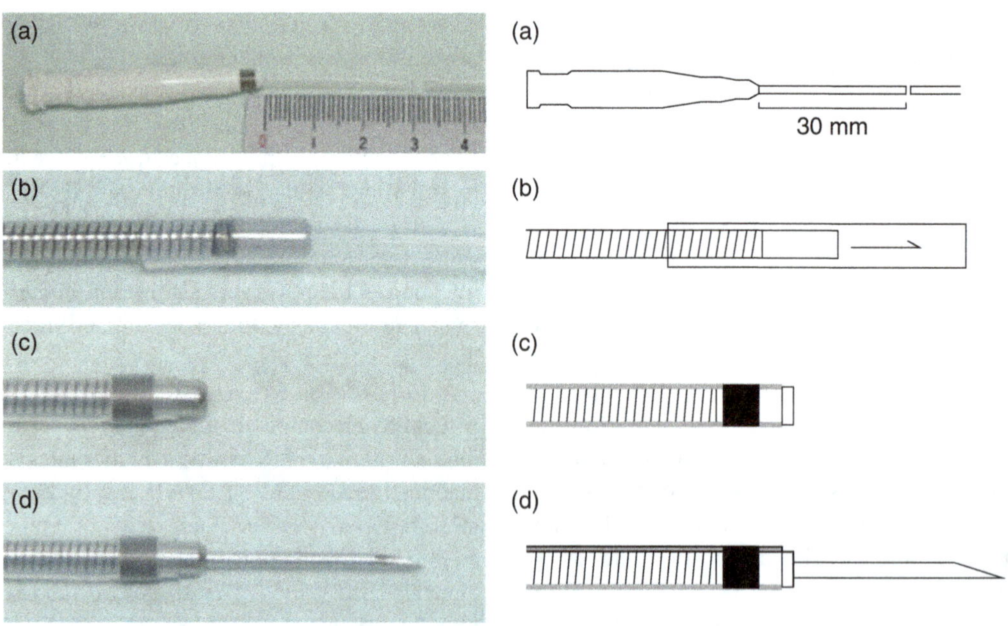

Figure 10.2 Preparation of guide sheath (GS) for transbronchial needle aspiration (TBNA). (a) Cut 30 mm from the proximal end. (b, c) When the TBNA sheath is inserted into the GS, note that the tip of the metallic sheath will coincide with the distal tip of the GS. (d) This way, the needle will not damage the GS during aspiration.

reference lesions which clearly did not have a bronchus sign, in cases with a clear bronchus visible within the lesion there was a hazard ratio of successful biopsy of 11.1 (2.99–41.2, p<0.001). Figure 1 from that paper demonstrates the classification of bronchus signs.

Asano has recently reviewed the associated technologies and adaptations that have followed and combined with EBUS GS, advancing the place of bronchoscopic sampling of peripheral nodules [1]. These included virtual bronchoscopic assistance in navigation, electromagnetic bronchoscopy, and ultrathin bronchoscopy. Each of these addresses difficulties of the biopsy and can be regarded as adjunctive approaches, almost as team work in the ultimate goal of obtaining tissue diagnosis. Most importantly, EBUS GS remains central to the final biopsy site selection, even when other tools including virtual bronchoscopy (VB) and electromagnetic navigation (EMN) are utilized.

With VB, after inserting the starting position and the peripheral target lesion, the software gives a fly-through of the most ideal route to the target lesion during the bronchoscopy. This can either be manually tracked by an assistant, or linked to the bronchoscopic image with side-by-side displays of the virtual path and real image. Two well-known VB platforms are Bf-NAVI® (Olympus Corporation, Tokyo, Japan) and LungPoint® (Broncus Medical, San Jose, CA, USA) [9, 10]. Ishida reported a randomized study of VB navigation-assisted (VBNA) EBUS versus non-VBNA EBUS. The VBNA group had higher diagnostic yield than the non-VBNA group (80.4% vs. 67.0%; p = 0.03) [10]. The overall procedure duration and the time elapsed until the start of sample collection were reduced in the VBNA compared with the non-VBNA group: median 24.0 minutes (range 8.7–47.0) versus 26.2 minutes (range 11.6–58.6) = 0.016 and 8.1 minutes (2.8–39.2) versus 9.8 minutes (2.3–42.3), p = 0.045, respectively. Eberhardt et al. first reported LungPoint in a small series of 25 cases and showed in 25 lesions of mean size 28 mm that the planned route was correct in all cases, and that the bronchoscope could be advanced all the way to the lesion bronchus in 54% of cases [9]. The median planning time was 5 minutes, and definitive diagnosis was possible in 20 cases (80%).

Others have shown that VBN can shorten the time needed to determine the biopsy position [11]. In a comparative study of 112 cases, Oshige et al. reported diagnostic yield of 84.2% for the VBN/EBUS GS group and 80.0% for the EBUS GS group [11]. The time to reach the biopsy position was significantly less in the VBN/EBUS GS group (5.5 ± 0.6 minutes in the VBN/EBUS GS group vs. 9.3 ± 0.9 minutes in the EBUS GS group, p < 0.01).

Matsumoto et al. have reported a more readily available VBN approach utilizing a widely available radiological workstation [12]. They used EBUS with a GS after planning on a CT workstation (Ziostation, Ziosoft, Tokyo, Japan) for small peripheral pulmonary lesions. Of 112 cases planned with the Ziostation group, there was significantly higher diagnostic yield than for the 113 cases in the non-Ziostation group (77.7% vs. 64.6%, p = 0.030). Also the EBUS detection rate was significantly higher in the Ziostation group (94.2% vs. 75.2%, p < 0.001). Procedure time was significantly shorter in the Aiostation group (24.0 ± 7.4 minutes vs. 26.9 ± 7.9 minutes, p = 0.005).

Ultrathin and thin bronchoscopes are ideally suited to the EBUS GS methods because of the need for better access to the periphery of the lung through the small branching airways. Oki et al. reported the use of a 3.4 mm thin bronchoscope and a 1.4 mm ultrasonic probe for peripheral pulmonary lesions without a GS, as the sheath would not fit the smaller 1.7 mm channel [13]. A total of 71 lesions (mean size 31.2 ±12.7 mm) were studied. The mean bronchus level reached with the thin bronchoscope was 4.6 generations (range 2nd to 7th generations). Diagnostic pathology was obtained in 49 of 71 patients (69%: 80% for malignant lesions and 52% for benign lesions). A definitive diagnosis of malignancy for lesions less than 20 mm and lesions greater than 20 mm was made in 82% (31/38) and 67% (4/6), respectively.

This study is important because this bronchoscope has a sufficient channel size to permit miniprobe deployment. Previous ultrathin scope studies used channel sizes of 1.2 mm, limiting lesion confirmation and size of instruments. Typically the thin bronchoscope can be inserted as far as the 6th-generation airway, and if necessary the ultrasound probe is then inserted under vision into the opening of the 7th-order bronchus.

EMN has been described in detail elsewhere [14]. It allows the bronchoscopist to steer endoscopic tools to peripheral pulmonary lesions. The diagnostic yield of EMN-guided bronchoscopy (ENB) has been as high as 74.1%. EMN utilizes EBUS miniprobes at the end of navigation to confirm lesion localization. One example study showed that diagnostic yield of the combined procedure (EBUS plus ENB; 88%) was greater than EBUS (69%) or ENB alone (59%; p = 0.02) [15]. The combined procedure's yield was independent of lesion size or lobar distribution. Another study showed that utilizing EMN with EBUS at completion of navigation, the diagnostic yield was 93% when EBUS verified the lesion location after navigation and only 48% when lesion location was not confirmed [9].

Wang Memoli has recently reported a meta-analysis of studies utilizing these complementary technologies (ENB, VB, radial (R)-EBUS, ultrathin bronchoscope, and/or GS) in the diagnosis of peripheral nodules [2]. A total of 3052 lesions from 39 studies were included. The overall (inverse variance weighted) diagnostic yield was 70.0% (95% CI: 67.1–72.9%). It establishes that the weighted diagnostic yield is significantly better than that reported for traditional flexible bronchoscopy, but the yield remains lower than that of transthoracic needle aspiration (TTNA) [7]. The range of yields across studies was 46.0–86.2% and the Q statistic indicated that there was significant ($p<0.0001$) variation in the diagnostic yield estimates. That paper's Table 2 lists the pooled diagnostic yield estimates for groups of studies that used various technologies. As reported, three modalities had a higher diagnostic yield than the overall yield: VB, R-EBUS, and the use of a GS. The diagnostic yield appeared to be highest (73.2%) when a GS was used, although there was significant variation across studies (Q statistic = 63.8, $P<0.0001$). The yields for VB (72.0%) and R-EBUS (71.1%) were also higher than the overall weighted diagnostic yield. The GS acts as an extended working channel to maintain the location of the forceps and brushes during biopsy, with that position having been found by the miniprobe within that sheath. Hence, these two "technologies" (the sheath is simply a plastic catheter) may help ensure better biopsy positivity. The finding of a higher weighted diagnostic yield for VB than ENB was of interest to these authors. It may simply be, as per the Eberhardt study, that ENB requires EBUS to confirm the final lesion location and that without this the yield is less.

Diagnostic yield of lesions of less than (629 lesions) or more than 20 mm (767 lesions) were reported from 20 studies. They were 60.9% (95% CI: 54.0–67.7%) and 82.5% (95% CI: 78.6–86.4%) for lesions less than and more than 20 mm, respectively. This had a weighted difference in diagnostic yield of 19.6% (95% CI: 11.7–27.6%; $p<0.001$) for the two groups based on size.

In terms of adverse events rate, there was 1.5% pneumothorax and 0.6% chest tube rates (an absolute number of 10 intercostal catheter insertions across the full range of studies) and only 0.7% of all cases required intervention. This compares with up to an overall 5% chest tube rate with TTNA in some series. The only other adverse event was a single instance of an aspiration event, which was presumably related to the anesthetic.

Regarding current guidelines for the use of these technologies, in 2013 the American Thoracic Society (ATS) gave the following recommendations as they apply to the use of EBUS GS [3]:

3.3.2.1. In patients suspected of having lung cancer, who have a peripheral lung nodule, and a tissue diagnosis is required due to uncertainty of diagnosis or poor surgical candidacy, radial EBUS is recommended as an adjunct imaging modality (Grade 1C). Remark: Radial EBUS can confirm in real time the ideal location of bronchoscopic sampling and increase the diagnostic yield over conventional bronchoscopy for peripheral nodules.

3.4.2.1. In patients with peripheral lung lesions difficult to reach with conventional bronchoscopy, electromagnetic navigation guidance is recommended if the equipment and the expertise are available (Grade 1C). Remark: The procedure can be performed with or without fluoroscopic guidance and it has been found complementary to radial probe ultrasound. Remark: If electromagnetic navigation is not available, TTNA is recommended.

3.5.2.1. In patients suspected of having lung cancer who have a peripheral lesion, and who require tissue diagnosis before further management can be planned, TTNA is a diagnostic option. However, it is recommended that further testing be performed if TTNA results are nondiagnostic and suspicion of lung cancer remains (Grade 1B).

Up-to-Date Advances in EBUS-Guided Peripheral Nodule Biopsy

Adding a TBNA Needle Sample

This is a simple addition to the sampling part of the EBUS GS procedure, whereby a TBNA needle is added to biopsies and brushes. Ostensibly this is to overcome difficulties posed when EBUS shows that a lesion is "eccentric" rather than centrally placed around the probe. Takai reported 37 cases using the following equipment (all Olympus, Tokyo, Japan): 1T-260 or LF-TP bronchoscope, K203 GS kit, and NA-1C-1 needle apparatus, customized by cutting the GS 30 mm from the proximal end to fit well with the needle [16]. There were 21 cases when the EBUS probe was located within the lesion (56.8%) and it was outside in 16 cases (43.2%). There was no significant difference in diagnostic rate for the two groups: 90% in "within" cases compared to 81% in "outside" cases ($p = 0.42$). The authors comments that GS-TBNA is effective not solely by itself, but in combination with other devices. They postulated that transbronchial forceps may cut a hole in the bronchus, thereby enabling the needle to more easily penetrate the lesion when it is eccentric to the bronchus.

Hayama et al. have also reported on this technique [6]. They retrospectively reviewed 67 cases where the lesion could not be visualized by EBUS: 22 cases had TBNA and the remainder had standard EBUS GS samples. The addition of GS-TBNA samples significantly improved the diagnostic yield: 55% versus 18%, $p < 0.01$.

Adding a Suction Catheter

A catheter suction device (Olympus Cannula PR-2B-1, 2.0 mm in diameter) can be added to diagnostic EBUS GS samples. Zaric et al. in 2016 reported 168 patients comparing the yield of the device to transbronchial biopsy in the same case [17]. Overall there was no difference in the yield of the samples (both more than 90%, in a series of mean lesion diameter of approximately 4 cm). These authors regarded the catheter as being complementary to other samples.

Eberhardt et al. used the same catheter in a series of EMN (and EBUS) cases [18], in which 53 lesions of less than 3 cm were analyzed; 40 samples (75.5%) were diagnostic. Compared to forceps biopsy, catheter aspiration was more likely to give positive tissue diagnosis with a higher success rate (36/40 vs. 22/40; $p = 0.035$).

The diagnostic yield was 93% when EBUS verified the lesion location after navigation and only 48% when lesion location was not confirmed. Therefore these authors considered that the suction catheter was particularly useful when the EBUS did not confirm the position of the lesion.

EBUS without GS

Zhang et al. reported the use of the EBUS miniprobe without the GS as a potentially cost-saving measure [19]. They termed this "EBUS with distance," meaning that the site of the lesion as carefully shown by EBUS was measured as to how distant it was from the tip of the bronchoscope – samples were taken at that distance. In a prospective study, 47 lesions with mean diameter 30.2 mm ± 13.5 mm were analyzed. Two interesting findings were firstly that using the "distance" method it took approximately 2 minutes longer on average to take biopsies (7.4 minutes vs. 5.2 minutes for GS). Also there were five cases in the "distance" method where there was more than 50 ml of airway bleeding after biopsy. Despite these findings there was equivalence in sample positivity (both more than 70%), although the authors commented that yield was less for smaller, more peripheral subpleural lesions. They commented that larger biopsy samples could be obtained when the GS was not used, which is consistent with clinical experience and was relevant in this series for the diagnosis of a mucosa-associated lymphoid lymphoma by the "distance" method.

Cryobiopsy

Adding a peripheral cryobiopsy also theoretically could overcome the problem of the lesion which is localized by EBUS but is "eccentric" to the probe. Presently the cryoprobe size means that the largest sheath needs to be used, hence there is some limitation potentially in terms of accessing more difficult upper-lobe airways with the necessary larger bronchoscope. Schuhmann et al. reported on 39 cases, in which the lesion was reached by EBUS in 31 cases [20]. Each case had 3 standard and 3 cryo transbronchial biopsies in random order. Importantly, as expected the biopsy size was larger than with conventional forceps (11.17 vs. 4.69 mm^2, $p = 0.001$). Secondly, there were 19 cases where the diagnosis was made by both conventional and cryobiopsies, but 4 cases where the diagnosis was only made by cryobiopsy. Importantly, also there was only 1 case of moderate bleeding. The technique does require the whole sheath to be removed, as the biopsy cannot fit back into the sheath to be removed, hence there is a difference to the usual situation of the sheath tamponading the bronchus where the biopsy was performed.

Franke et al. have reported the use of cryobiopsies through a 21 gauge EBUS-TBNA needle in pre-clinical experiments, demonstrating much larger biopsy sizes of lymph node tissue [21]. The way forward with this method is likely to be adaptation of the instrumentation, possibly with a smaller-size cryoprobe which will allow better access to smaller lesions, still giving the benefits of larger biopsies.

References

1 Asano, F. (2016). Advanced bronchoscopy for the diagnosis of peripheral pulmonary lesions. *Respiratory Investigation* 54 (4): 224–229.

2 Wang Memoli, J.S., Nietert, P.J., and Silvestri, G.A. (2012). Meta-analysis of guided bronchoscopy for the evaluation of the pulmonary nodule. *Chest* 142 (2): 385–393.

3 Rivera, M.P., Mehta, A.C., and Wahidi, M.M. (2013). Establishing the diagnosis of lung cancer: Diagnosis and management of lung cancer, 3rd ed: American College of Chest

Physicians evidence-based clinical practice guidelines. *Chest* 143 (5 Suppl): e142S–e165S.

4 Baaklini, W.A., Reinoso, M.A., Gorin, A.B. et al. (2000). Diagnostic yield of fiberoptic bronchoscopy in evaluating solitary pulmonary nodules. *Chest* 117 (4): 1049–1054.

5 Kurimoto, N., Miyazawa, T., Okimasa, S. et al. (2004). Endobronchial ultrasonography using a guide sheath increases the ability to diagnose peripheral pulmonary lesions endoscopically. *Chest* 126 (3): 959–965.

6 Hayama, M., Izumo, T., Chavez, C. et al. (2017). Additional transbronchial needle aspiration through a guide sheath for peripheral pulmonary lesions that cannot be detected by radial EBUS. *Clinical Respiratory Journal* 11 (6): 757–764.

7 Zhan, P., Zhu, Q.-Q., Miu, Y.-Y. et al. (2017). Comparison between endobronchial ultrasound-guided transbronchial biopsy and CT-guided transthoracic lung biopsy for the diagnosis of peripheral lung cancer: a systematic review and meta-analysis. *Translational Lung Cancer Research* 6 (1): 23–34.

8 Minezawa, T., Okamura, T., Yatsuya, H. et al. (2015). Bronchus sign on thin-section computed tomography is a powerful predictive factor for successful transbronchial biopsy using endobronchial ultrasound with a guide sheath for small peripheral lung lesions: a retrospective observational study. *BMC Medical Imaging* 15: 21.

9 Eberhardt, R., Kahn, N., Gompelmann, D. et al. (2010). LungPoint—a new approach to peripheral lesions. *Journal of Thoracic Oncology* 5 (10): 1559–1563.

10 Ishida, T., Asano, F., Yamazaki, K. et al. (2011). Virtual bronchoscopic navigation combined with endobronchial ultrasound to diagnose small peripheral pulmonary lesions: a randomised trial. *Thorax* 66 (12): 1072–1077.

11 Oshige, M., Shirakawa, T., Nakamura, M. et al. (2011). Clinical application of virtual bronchoscopic navigation system for peripheral lung lesions. *Journal of Bronchology & Interventional Pulmonology* 18 (2): 196–202.

12 Matsumoto, Y., Izumo, T., Sasada, A. et al. (2017). Diagnostic utility of endobronchial ultrasound with a guide sheath under the computed tomography workstation (ziostation) for small peripheral pulmonary lesions. *Clinical Respiratory Journal* 11: 185–192.

13 Oki, M., Saka, H., Kitagawa, C. et al. (2012). Randomized study of endobronchial ultrasound-guided transbronchial biopsy: thin bronchoscopic method versus guide sheath method. *Journal of Thoracic Oncology* 7: 535–541.

14 Herth, F.J. and Eberhardt, R. (2008). Endobronchial ultrasound and electromagnetic navigation bronchoscopy in the diagnosis of peripheral lung lesions. *Expert Opinion on Medical Diagnostics.* 2 (5): 461–466.

15 Eberhardt, R., Anantham, D., Ernst, A. et al. (2007). Multimodality bronchoscopic diagnosis of peripheral lung lesions: a randomized controlled trial. *American Journal of Respiratory and Critical Care Medicine* 176 (1): 36–41.

16 Takai, M., Izumo, T., Chavez, C. et al. (2014). Transbronchial needle aspiration through a guide sheath with endobronchial ultrasonography (GS-TBNA) for peripheral pulmonary lesions. *Annals of Thoracic and Cardiovascular Surgery* 20 (1): 19–25.

17 Zaric, B., Stojsic, V., Carapic, V. et al. (2016). Radial Endobronchial Ultrasound (EBUS) Guided Suction Catheter-Biopsy in Histological Diagnosis of Peripheral Pulmonary Lesions. *Journal of Cancer* 7 (1): 7–13.

18 Eberhardt, R., Morgan, R.K., Ernst, A. et al. (2010). Comparison of suction catheter

versus forceps biopsy for sampling of solitary pulmonary nodules guided by electromagnetic navigational bronchoscopy. *Respiration; International Review of Thoracic Diseases* 79 (1): 54–60.

19 Zhang, S.-J., Zhang, M., Zhou, J. et al. (2016). Comparison of radial endobronchial ultrasound with a guide sheath and with distance by thin bronchoscopy for the diagnosis of peripheral pulmonary lesions: a prospective randomized crossover trial. *Journal of Thoracic Disease* 8 (11): 3112–3118.

20 Schuhmann, M., Bostanci, K., Bugalho, A. et al. (2014). Endobronchial ultrasound-guided cryobiopsies in peripheral pulmonary lesions: a feasibility study. *European Respiratory Journal* 43 (1): 233–239.

21 Franke, K.-J., Nilius, G., Ruehle, K.-H. et al. (2013). The cryo-needle: a new tool for histological biopsies. A feasibility study. *Lung* 191 (6): 611–617.

11

Endobronchial Ultrasonography for Ground-Glass Opacity Lesions

David I.K. Fielding

Royal Brisbane and Women's Hospital, Herston, Queensland, Australia

Ground-glass lesions present particular difficulties in endobronchial ultrasonography sampling with a guide sheath (EBUS-GS). Firstly, the ultrasound features are subtle and can be missed if the probe is not withdrawn very slowly through the suspected location region. Secondly, the lesions are not invasive and sit extrinsic to the bronchus, and biopsy forceps often cannot catch the lesions.

Chavez et al. reported a case defining the "blizzard" appearance of ground-glass opacities (GGOs) on EBUS, commonly due to well-differentiated adenocarcinomas [1]. The difference to the normal snowstorm of the lung was the distance the coarser shadows extended radially from the probe: more than 1 cm for blizzard and less than 1 cm for snowstorm (Figure 11.1). A cytology specimen was collected by brushings and five standard forceps samples were taken for histology (the forceps had a 1.9 mm maximum outer diameter). Cytology samples were negative. Regarding the biopsies, the first and second specimens were negative, the third showed a few atypical cells, and the fourth and fifth specimens showed adenocarcinoma with lepidic growth pattern. The lesion was surgically confirmed as minimally invasive adenocarcinoma. The case demonstrates the subtle EBUS appearance and also how difficult it can be to make the tissue diagnosis. Izumo et al. further illustrated this finding [2].

In another case report, Sasada et al. commented on the need for seven biopsies and the difficulty in sampling these completely radiologically (by fluoroscopy) invisible lesions (Figure 11.1) [3]. In this case, definitive diagnosis was successfully obtained from seven transbronchial biopsy (TBB) specimens by using the usual 1.8 mm biopsy forceps included in the larger K-203 Guide Sheath Kit (Olympus Corporation, Tokyo, Japan). The authors recommended this larger forceps compare to the often-used smaller forceps in the small GS kit (K201) because of the often subtle nature of the pathology, particularly in the in situ or minimally invasive cases.

Izumo et al. have reported the results of EBUS GS on 116 patients with GGO to further classify and define the EBUS appearances [2]. All had been previously confirmed as having adenocarcinoma by the procedure and their findings were compared to computed tomography (CT). Also, in 103 patients the EBUS images

Endobronchial Ultrasonography, Second Edition. Noriaki Kurimoto, David I.K. Fielding, Ali I. Musani, Christopher Kniese, and Katsuhiko Morita.

Companion website: www.wiley.com/go/kurimoto2e

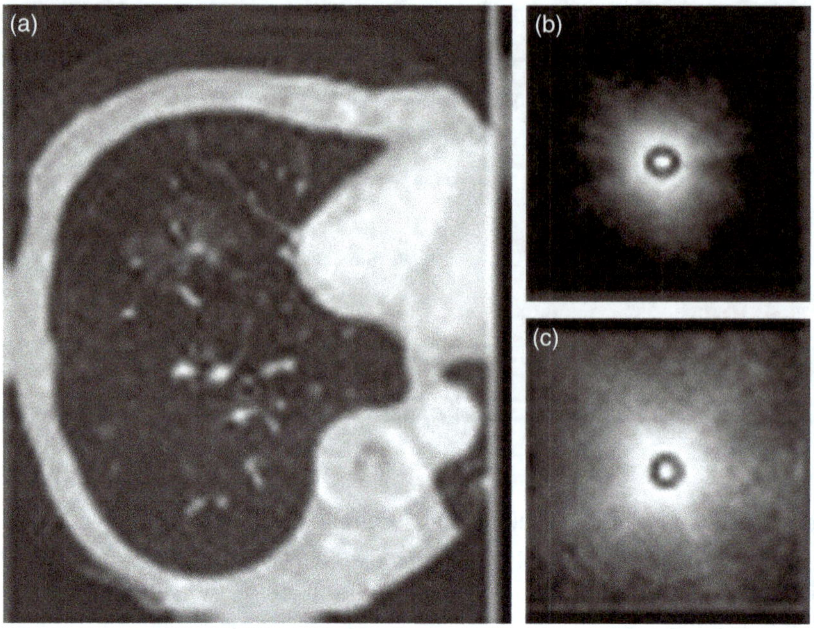

Figure 11.1 Images from a case showing (a) Ground glass opacity (GGO) lesion which could be approached due to a patent bronchus using virtual bronchoscopy. (b) Initial endobronchial ultrasound scanning through the right B8bi showed a whitish acoustic shadow that represented normal air-filled alveoli. EBUS image shown is on a 2 mm scale. (c) The Blizzard Sign. When the endobronchial ultrasound probe was inserted further and more distally, there was a subtle but noticeable increase in the intensity and radius of the whitish acoustic shadow more than 1 cm from the center of the EBUS image. *Source:* Sasada et al. [3]. Reprinted with permission from Elsevier.

were correlated with the histologic surgical specimens. The EBUS appearance was characterized as either "blizzard" type (an enlarged, diffuse, hyperintense acoustic shadow) or a "mixed blizzard" (a combination of blizzard and some diffuse heterogeneity with several hyperechoic dots and vessels). The latter have previously been shown to represent partially compressed parenchymal airways. All of the nine pure GGO lesions had the pure blizzard appearance on radial (R)-EBUS. For part-solid GGOs, the percentage of mixed blizzard was inversely related to the amount of the GGO component. Histologic findings from surgery revealed that all blizzard lesions were on the spectrum of adenocarcinoma in situ to well-differentiated adenocarcinoma, while the majority (33/64) of mixed blizzard lesions were moderately to poorly differentiated adenocarcinoma.

Nakai et al. reported predictive factors for obtaining a positive tissue diagnosis after EBUS GS for GGOs [4]. From 254 cases, 167 were diagnosed using EBUS-GS (65.7% diagnostic yield). The key finding was that a positive bronchus sign was a significant factor for higher diagnostic yield (72.9% vs. 34.0%; $p < 0.001$) by univariate analysis. Multivariate analysis indicated that both a bronchus sign and the use of virtual bronchoscopy planning were significantly associated with higher diagnostic yield ($p < 0.001$, odds ratio [OR] 5.35; $p < 0.001$, OR 1.97, respectively). These authors demonstrated the utility of a positive bronchus sign within the GGO on CT.

References

1 Chavez, C., Sasada, S., Izumo, T. et al. (2014). Image-guided bronchoscopy for histopathologic diagnosis of pure ground glass opacity: a case report. *Journal of Thoracic Disease* 6: E81–E84.

2 Izumo, T., Sasada, S., Chavez, C. et al. (2015). Radial endobronchial ultrasound images for ground-glass opacity pulmonary lesions. *European Respiratory Journal* 45: 1661–1668.

3 Sasada, S., Izumo, T., Chavez, C., and Tsuchida, T. (2014). Blizzard sign as a specific endobronchial ultrasound image for ground glass opacity: A case report. *Respiratory Medicine Case Reports* 12: 19–21.

4 Nakai, T., Matsumoto, Y., Suzuk, F. et al. (2017). Predictive factors for a successful diagnostic bronchoscopy of ground-glass nodules. *Annals of Thoracic Medicine* 12: 171–176.

12

Techniques for Comparing Endobronchial Ultrasonography Images of Peripheral Pulmonary Lesions with Macroscopy and Histopathology Findings

Katsuhiko Morita[1,2]

[1] *Department of Thoracic Surgery, Japan Community Health Care Organization (JCHO), Shimonoseki Medical Center, Shimonoseki City, Yamaguchi Prefecture, Japan*
[2] *Shimane University, Izumo City, Shimane Prefecture, Japan*

Introduction

Peripheral pulmonary lesions (PPLs) include those in small bronchi. Since it is difficult to observe the involved bronchi directly by bronchoscopy, many clinicians use endobronchial ultrasonography (EBUS) to confirm the presence of PPLs. However, the endobronchial ultrasonography with guide sheath (EBUS-GS) method is inadequate for diagnosis of lesions that cannot be seen with EBUS. Diagnosis using this method would require introduction of the guide sheath with probe (probe/GS) beyond the margin of the lesion in order to raise the diagnostic rate. Although computed tomography (CT) images are also used for the diagnosis of pulmonary pathologies, in the case of solid lesions EBUS images are considered to provide more detailed information about the internal structure of the lesion, including its vascularity, than CT images. Diagnosis could be further aided by contrasting pathologic images of the excised specimens with EBUS images. However, comparison of the EBUS images of PPLs with macroscopic evaluation of the resected specimen and microscopic images of the biopsied specimen is not always easy, for the following reasons.

- The bronchi involved in PPLs are so small that it is difficult for even versatile bronchoscopes appropriate for use with the EBUS-GS method to reach the bronchi. Moreover, it is impossible to observe the entire surface of the lesion from within the bronchial lumen, unlike what can be done for gastrointestinal lesions, since it is like looking at only the tip of the iceberg that is the entire PPL (Figure 12.1).
- It is unclear from which part of the lesion the ultrasound image was obtained.
- It is difficult to identify the exact site on the resected specimen that was biopsied. Direct invasion by tumor, as indicated by the pleural indentation sign, makes identification of the lesion in the excised lung easy. However, if a solid tumor does not extend to the visceral pleura of the excised lung, as evidenced by contact, invasion, pleural indentation, or any other involvement, the lesion can only be found by palpation after collapse of the excised lung. The lesion in the excised specimen becomes even more obscure after fixation with formalin. Therefore, it is difficult to accurately dissect the tissue to be histopathologically evaluated from the excised specimen.

Endobronchial Ultrasonography, Second Edition. Noriaki Kurimoto, David I.K. Fielding, Ali I. Musani, Christopher Kniese, and Katsuhiko Morita.

Companion website: www.wiley.com/go/kurimoto2e

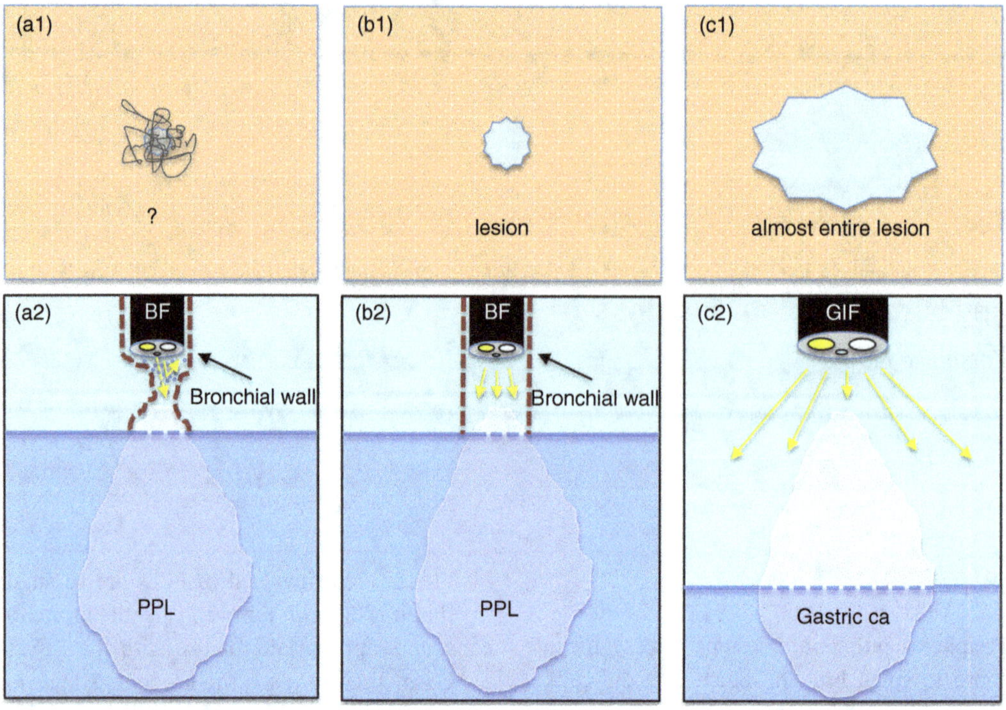

Figure 12.1 Direct bronchoscopic observation of the peripheral pulmonary lesion (PPL). The part of the PPL seen with the bronchoscope can be considered as being only the tip of the iceberg that is the entire PPL even in the best condition (b1 and b2). (a1, a2) Even when approaching the PPL with the bronchoscope, the collapsed bronchus containing mucous substance obscures visualization of the PPL. (b1, b2) Part of the PPL can be observed via the bronchoscope inside the open bronchus. (c1, c2) The large lumen-like stomach or colon permits visualization of the entire surface of the lesion with the endoscope. BF, bronchoscope; ca, cancer; GIF, gastrointestinal fiber scope.

For these reasons, we judged that it is necessary to directly observe peripheral lesions endoscopically in order to accurately compare EBUS images and pathologic findings. To achieve this goal, a thin bronchoscope should be positioned as close as possible to the target area of the lung, and factors hindering direct observation of the lesion should be eliminated. An example of an ultrathin bronchoscope that can be used to reach peripheral lesions is shown in Figure 12.2a. Ultrathin bronchoscopes can be inserted up to just beneath the pleura compared with thin bronchoscopes, as shown in Figure 12.2b. However, with insertion of the ultrathin bronchoscope, the peripheral airways tend to collapse easily because their walls are not stiff, unlike those of central airways. In addition, even if mucus secretions that obscure the visual field are reduced to some extent by suction, the mucus remaining in the working channel is pushed out of the channel when inserting the GS probe, again interfering with visualization of the lesion.

In such cases, even if the peripheral bronchus is in a state of collapse, it is possible to prevent airway collapse or reopen the collapsed airway by injecting a small amount of physiological saline into the airway, simultaneously eliminating any obstructing mucus (Figure 12.3a). Further, although injection of physiological saline into the respiratory tract may allow direct visualization of only a very small part of the lesion, it allows accurate visualization and record-keeping of the particular bronchial branch leading up to the

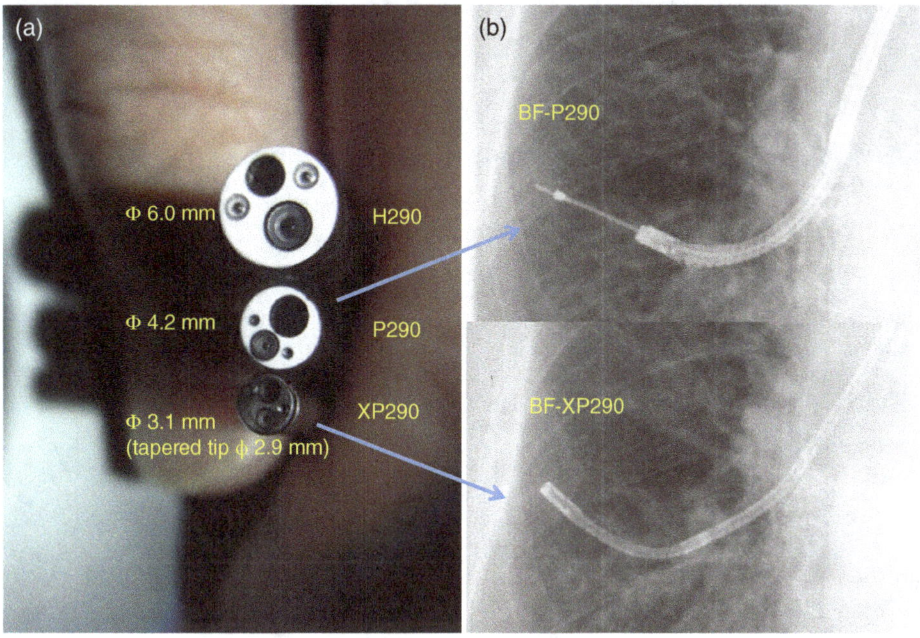

Figure 12.2 (a) The tips of three kinds of bronchoscopes with different thicknesses that are commonly used: conventional bronchoscope (BF-H290), thin bronchoscope (BF-P290), and ultrathin bronchoscope (BF-XP290). (b) The ultrathin bronchoscope (BF-XP290), which is not designed for use with a guide sheath kit, can be inserted up to just beneath the pleura, compared to the thin bronchoscope (BF-P290).

lesion, allowing accurate localization of the biopsy site with respect to the bronchial tree. The part directly observable by the bronchoscope was clarified, and we decided to leave the record-keeping track of which part of the lesion was observed from which peripheral airway (Figure 12.3b). Even when direct observation of the lesion is not possible by bronchoscopy, knowledge of the peripheral airway through which the probe/GS is inserted and related observations provide useful information.

In order to accurately locate the lesion and identify the peripheral airway via which it is observed endoscopically and scanned by EBUS, it is necessary to accurately assess the bronchi involved in the lesion using CT scans before the examination. If the lesion to be biopsied is relatively close to the center of the lung, that is a lesion that is likely to be reached by a thin bronchoscope (BF-P290, Olympus Corporation, Tokyo, Japan) with a tip diameter of 4.2 mm, approximately 5 cc of physiological saline is injected into the working channel of the scope just before inserting the probe/GS into the target bronchus, so as to prevent the involved bronchus from collapsing, and the probe/GS is guided under direct vision for scanning of the bronchus. For more peripheral lesions, an ultrathin bronchoscope (BF-XP290, Olympus) with a tip diameter of 3.1 mm (tapering to 2.9 mm) is used for direct observation (Figure 12.2a). When the ultrathin bronchoscope is used to identify the bronchus that is assumed to be the involved bronchus, a smaller volume of about 3 cc of physiological saline (due to the smaller volume of the working channel of the XP290) is injected to obtain a good field of vision.

Using this technique and an ultrathin bronchoscope, we were able to directly observe lesions such as stenosis in about 50% of cases in which CT indicated that the lesion might be present in a more peripheral bronchus than the fourth-generation bronchus, corresponding to the sub-subsegmental area branch. Next,

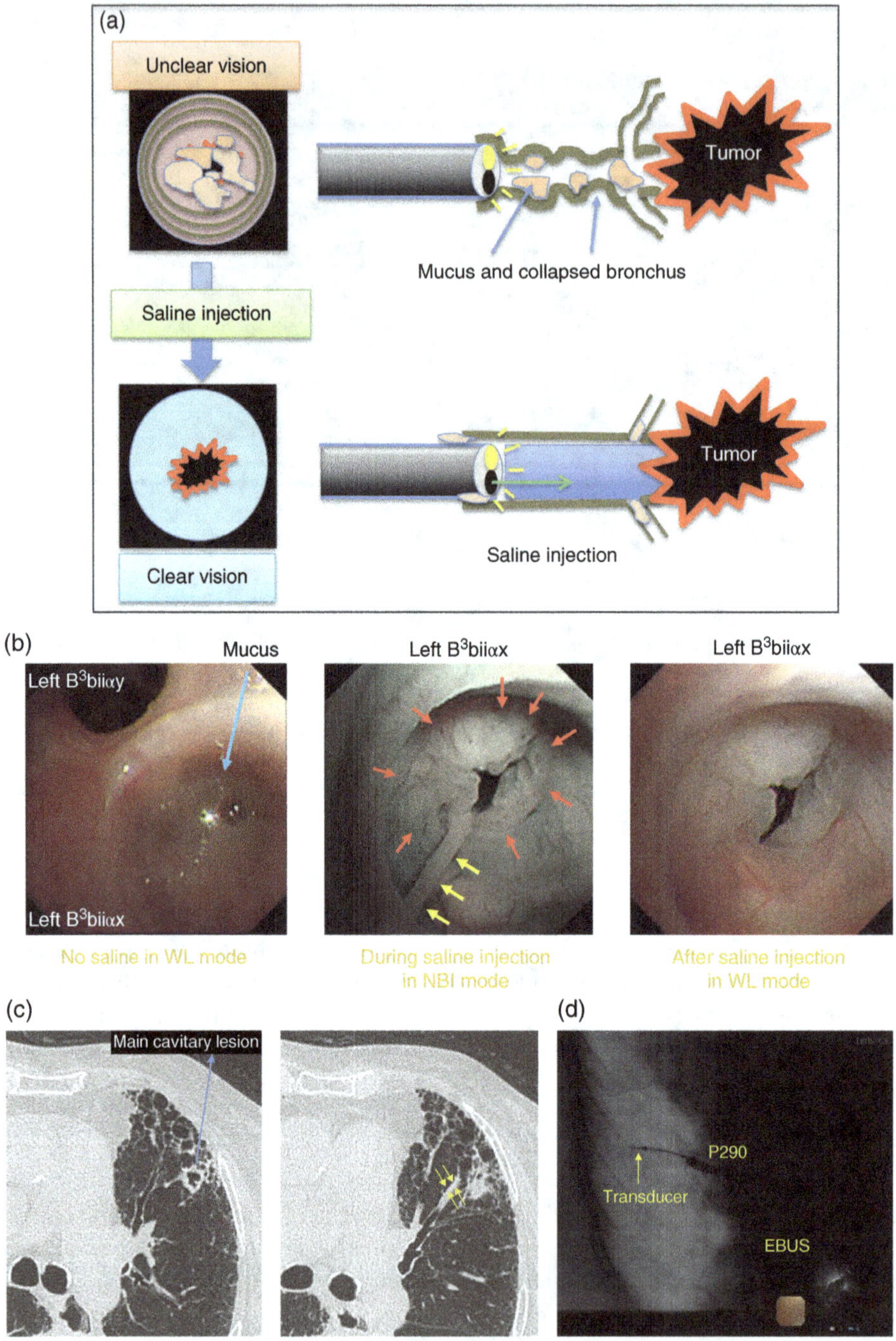

Figure 12.3 Injection of physiological saline into the peripheral airway to facilitate clear bronchoscopic visualization of peripheral pulmonary lesions. (a) The effect of saline injection into the airway. It is possible to prevent airway collapse or reopen a collapsed airway by filling the airway with a small amount of physiological saline, which simultaneously eliminates mucus. (b) Bronchoscopic image before, during, and after saline injection into the left B^3biiαx bronchus, showing that the BF-XP290 can reach and visualize peripheral lesions. The red arrow in the middle narrow band imaging (NBI) image indicates the main lesion and the yellow arrow indicates the mucus material like a pillar in the saline. WL, white light. (c) The arrow in the right computed tomography image indicates the involved bronchus (left B^3biiαx). (d) Fluoroscopic image during endobronchial ultrasound (EBUS) scanning using the BF-P290 is synchronized with an EBUS image in the right lower small window. Note: The case shown in Figures 12.3, 12.4, and 12.5 is different from the case in Figures 12.9–12.14.

in order to perform transbronchial biopsy (TBB) by the EBUS-GS method, the ultrathin bronchoscope (BF-XP290) is replaced by a thin bronchoscope (BF-P290), the probe/GS is inserted into the involved bronchus identified by the BF-XP290 ultrathin bronchoscope after injecting physiological saline into the airway, and the lesion is scanned. In our previous study, the BF-P290 could reach one branch in the bronchial tree before that accessible by the BF-XP290, and there was a significant possibility of the lesion identified by BF-XP290 being directly observable by the BF-P290 by injecting an appropriate amount of physiological saline via its working channel. The effect of physiological saline instillation into the airway in allowing direct observation of the PPL is explained in Figure 12.3.

Once the lesion and the involved bronchi have been localized by detailed bronchoscopic evaluation and CT images, they are surgically resected. After removal of the diseased lung, the next step is to re-examine the bronchial tree of the resected specimen for a complete understanding of the branching pattern of the route to the lesion. This can also be done bronchoscopically immediately after surgery. Although, unlike in vivo, it is impossible to control the airway diameter of the resected bronchus by inspiration and expiration, a surprisingly beautiful bronchoscopic image can be obtained by continuously injecting physiological saline through the working channel of the bronchoscope to prevent airway collapse and to ensure a good field of view. Once the ex vivo specimen has been bronchoscopically evaluated, pre-operative in vivo and post-operative ex vivo bronchoscopy images are compared. For this, it is necessary to arrange the images obtained by pre-operative bronchoscopy from the center toward the periphery of the bronchial tree in order, and to clarify the position of each branch leading to the lesion. The method we usually follow to compare the in vivo bronchoscopic findings of peripheral lesions with those of the excised specimen is described in what follows.

"Branch Reading": Identification of Involved Bronchi Leading to Target Lesion Using CT Images

1) Identify which bronchi are involved in lesions from pre-operative CT images (hereinafter called "branch reading") and hand draw the assumed bronchoscopic image (hereinafter called "branch reading image"). In addition to the axial image, we also refer to coronal and sagittal images to acquire an image of the bronchial tree. Oblique images are also useful in cases where optimal branches are difficult to distinguish by axial, coronal, and sagittal images (Figure 12.4).
2) A virtual bronchoscopic image (hereinafter referred to as "navigation image") is created by a doctor using a virtual bronchoscope navigation device (DirectPath, Olympus; Figure 12.5a). Meanwhile, virtual bronchoscope images are also created by a radiology technician using special software for the creation of virtual bronchoscopic images (Vincent bronchoscope software, Fujifilm Medical, Tokyo, Japan; Figure 12.5b). We compare the branch reading image obtained by hand and the navigation images obtained digitally and finally create a more accurate branch reading image (Figure 12.4).
3) This branch reading image serves as a guide to the lesion during the subsequent diagnostic bronchoscopy.

Diagnostic Bronchoscopy

1) After sufficient pharyngeal anesthesia, the patient is asked to lie supine on the examination bed, and a single chest X-ray image in the anterior–posterior direction is obtained (Figure 12.6a and b). When the lesion can be seen with X-rays, the positional relationship between the lesion and the ribs in the background, the diaphragm, and so on is assessed and the lesion is

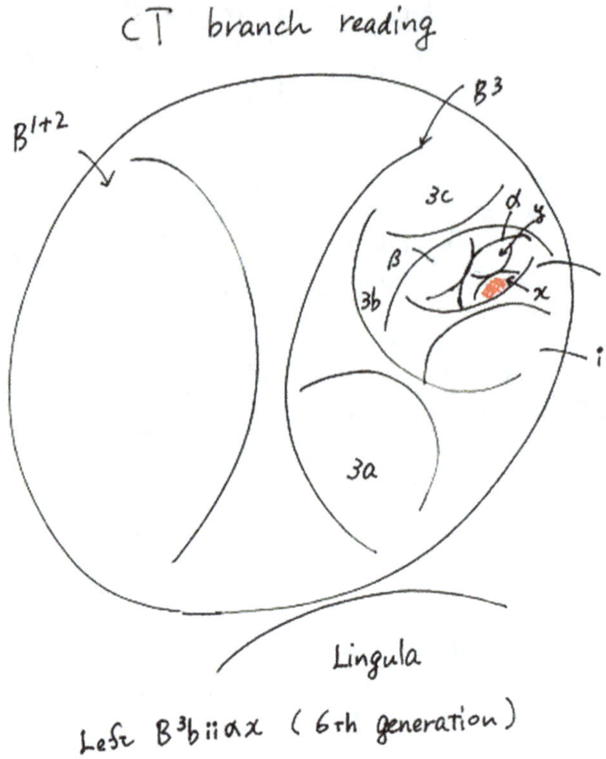

Figure 12.4 Hand-drawn "branch reading" image. CT, computed tomography.

marked on the X-ray. Since the chest X-ray is taken in the anterior–posterior direction with the patient in the supine position, the image is quite similar to the scout image of CT, allowing marking of the X-ray to be done with considerable ease and accuracy. It is recommended to use a small paper tag (Post-it®, 3M, St. Paul, MN, USA) to put a mark directly on the chest X-ray film or the screen monitor, if available, and to use editing software such as DirectPath or Vincent to mark the position of the lesion. With DirectPath virtual navigation software, the target is automatically displayed on the virtual chest X-ray picture, although the lesion is always displayed as a circle or an ellipse (Figure 12.5a). On the other hand, with Vincent software, the automatic tumor extraction function identifies the location and extent of the tumor in a single CT section, meaning the shape and location of the target can be accurately marked on the virtual chest X-ray (Figure 12.5b). A virtual chest X-ray picture created with these types of image editing software is convenient because the orientation of the virtual chest X-ray picture can be changed to match the patient's position. The three images of coronal CT, the virtual bronchial tree with target fused on the virtual X-ray, and the real X-ray image in the anterior–posterior direction are then displayed side by side on the monitor by a radiology technician to compare them (Figure 12.6c and d). The bronchoscopist can confirm their correlation on a monitor mounted on the wall of the examination room (Figure 12.6e). The radiology technician replaces the real X-ray image in the anterior–posterior direction with the real X-ray image taken at EBUS scanning or biopsy for correlation after bronchoscopy (Figure 12.6f).

2) Since the bronchoscope is usually inserted nasally, after confirming that the patient has

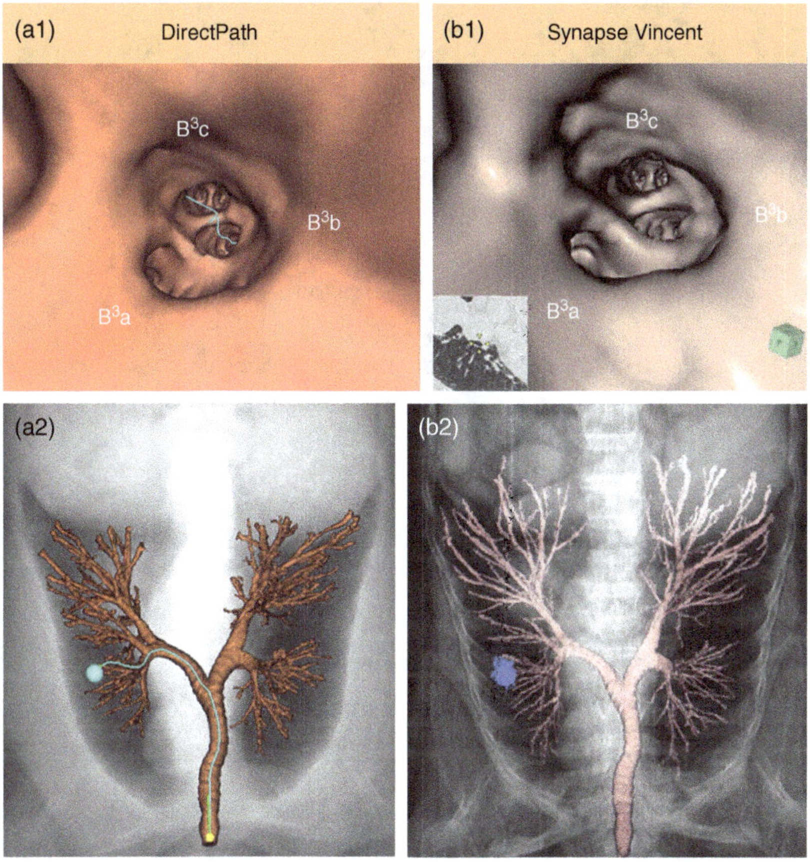

Figure 12.5 Representative virtual bronchoscopic navigation images by DirectPath and Synapse Vincent software (left B^3 orifice). (a1, a2) Virtual bronchoscopic image and virtual bronchial tree created by DirectPath software showing the target lesion. (b1, b2) Virtual bronchoscopic image and virtual bronchial tree created by Vincent software showing the target lesion. DirectPath is operated by the doctor, while Vincent is operated by the radiology technician.

no history of allergy, we inject a small amount of xylocaine jelly into the nostril through which the bronchoscope is to be inserted. A silicon protector, called a nose clip, is inserted into the nostril to protect it (Figure 12.7). Then, the ultrathin bronchoscope (BF-XP290) is inserted nasally and the bronchial tree up to the left and right subsegmental bronchial level are examined. Next, the bronchoscope is withdrawn to the level of the tracheal bifurcation and, under the advice of the supervising doctor, it is guided back into the bronchial tree in the direction of the target lesion, using the branch reading image and navigation image as a guide. Once the lesion is visualized by bronchoscopy, or even if no lesion can be visualized, the location of the bronchoscope tip near the lesion is confirmed by fluoroscopy at this time. In principle, when visualization is poor, a small amount of physiological saline is injected via the working channel into the peripheral airway. By doing so, airway branching and direct findings can be more accurately observed. However, this step is limited only to cases where the biopsy target is not a pure ground-glass opacity (GGO) on CT, since, unlike solid lesions, pure GGOs are more likely to be difficult to identify with EBUS after injecting saline. EBUS findings of pure GGO can only be identified with subtle

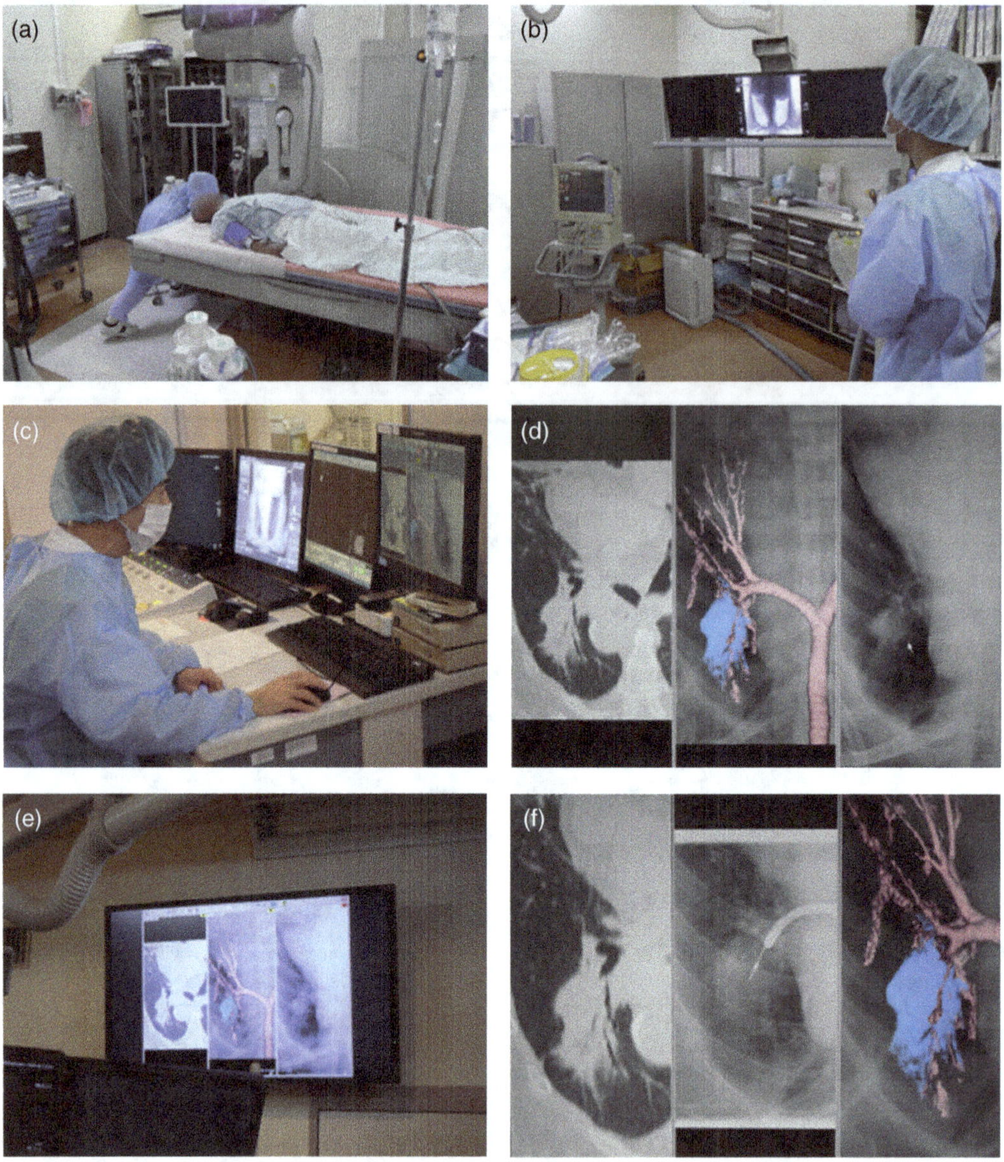

Figure 12.6 (a) Position of the patient on the X-ray bed. (b) Chest X-ray image in the anterior–posterior direction. (c) Radiology technician manipulating the image software on site. (d) Correlation between coronal computed tomography (CT) images, the virtual bronchial tree on virtual chest X-ray, and an antero-posterior chest X-ray image. (e) TV monitor mounted on the wall of the X-ray fluoroscopy room to display the correlation image. (f) Correlation between chest X-ray, scan of the lesion by the probe/guide sheath, and coronal CT image and virtual image.

echogenic enhancement. At this time, only one or two brushings are obtained for cytologic evaluation.

3) Next, the ultrathin bronchoscope (BF-XP290) is replaced with a thin bronchoscope (BF-P290) and, referring to the branch reading image and navigation image, the bronchoscope is introduced as deep as possible from the tracheal carina to the lesion, with a small amount of physiological saline, usually about 5 cc and up to a maximum of 10 cc, being injected from the

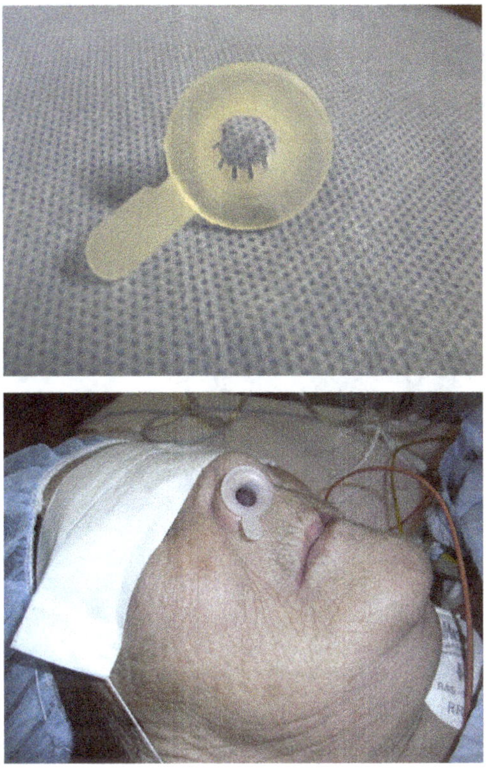

Figure 12.7 The nose clip used to protect the nostril during bronchoscopy and a picture of it fitted to the nostril.

working channel into the respiratory tract to improve visibility. Subsequently, a radial type ultrasonic probe covered with a guide sheath (hereinafter referred to as the probe/GS) is inserted into the bronchus assumed to lead to the lesion (Figure 12.3d). Then, under fluoroscopic visualization to confirm accurate positioning of the probe/GS in the vicinity of the lesion, ultrasonography is used to scan the lesion and confirm its presence. The probe/GS is moved in and out of the working channel of the bronchoscope, while adjusting the angle of the tip of the bronchoscope so that the transducer in the ultrasound probe tip extends beyond the border of the lesion.

4) Once the probe/GS seems to be optimally positioned, it should be confirmed that the ultrasound image darkens or brightens when the ultrasonic probe is slightly withdrawn and reintroduced while maintaining the guide sheath in the same position under fluoroscopy (hereinafter referred to as dark phenomenon; Figure 12.8). The reasons for the occurrence of this dark phenomenon on the ultrasound screen are attenuation and blockage of the ultrasound beam by withdrawing the transducer near the tip of the ultrasound probe into the guide sheath and to the level of the metal marker installed in the tip of the guide sheath, respectively. The original ultrasound image can be obtained by reintroducing the transducer beyond the guide sheath. When the lesion is visualized and the guide sheath positioned accurately, observation of the dark phenomenon by slightly withdrawing and reintroducing the transducer can help to confirm that the lesion exists immediately in front of the guide sheath.
5) In addition to repeated brushing and biopsy, bronchial washing, as well as flushing and collection of the cells adhering to the internal lumen of the guide sheath, is also performed. With rapid on-site evaluation (hereinafter referred to as ROSE) of stamp cytology, the number of brushes and biopsies can be reduced.

Bronchoscopy of the Excised Specimen

1) It is necessary to arrange the images obtained by pre-operative bronchoscopy in the order of larger to smaller bronchi – that is, from the center to the periphery – and to clarify the position of each branch leading to the lesion (Figure 12.9).
2) The resected specimen is typically a lung lobe in cases with primary lung cancer because lobectomy is usually performed in such cases. We try to perform ex vivo bronchoscopy as soon as possible after specimen removal. First, we start with observing the bronchial stump and identifying the correct segmental bronchus. In order to position

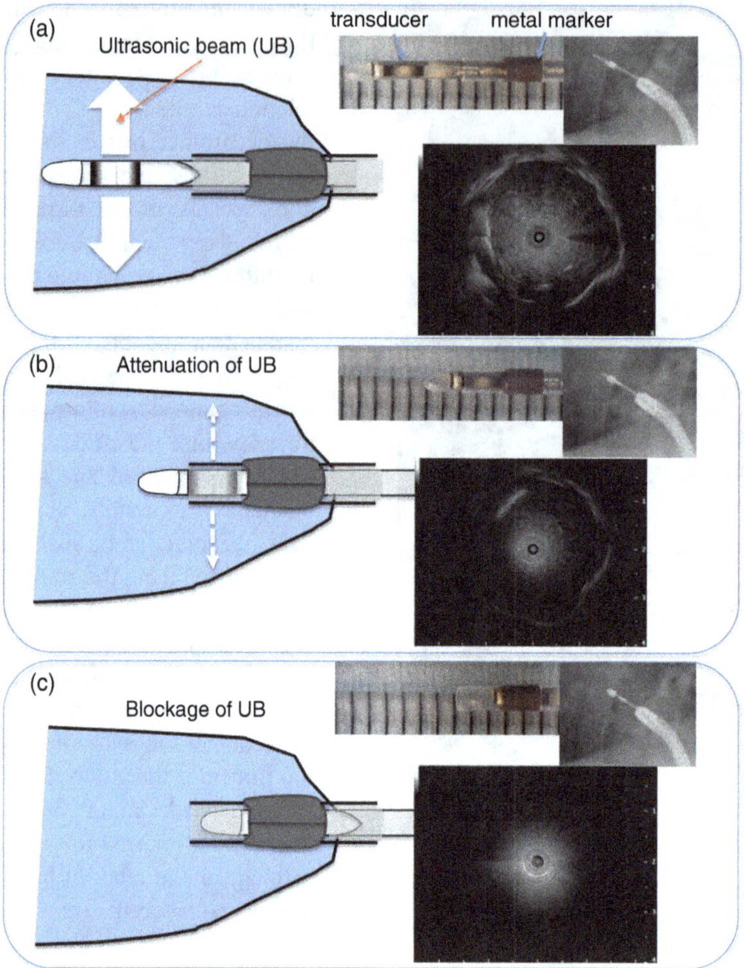

Figure 12.8 (a–c) Images of the dark phenomenon during ultrasonography and the corresponding positional relationship between the transducer installed in the tip of the probe and the metal marker installed in the tip of the guide sheath.

and support the resected specimen for ex vivo bronchoscopy, approximately 5 to 10 1-0 silk stitches are sutured onto the bronchial stump of the resected specimen and each end of the thread is gripped with Kocher's forceps. The resected lobe is put in a bucket for holding the specimen, and the tips of the Kocher's forceps are hooked onto the edge of the bucket to pull the silk threads upward, so that the bronchial stump of the specimen faces upward. Since the tip of the Kocher's forceps gets hooked onto the protruding rim of the bucket, when grasping the thread it is preferable to avoid using the tip of the Kocher's forceps, and instead to use the part just proximal to the tip. The length of the thread is adjusted so that the specimen is well lifted. The lobe is positioned in the bucket so that its bronchial stump faces upward (Figure 12.10).

3) In order to continuously inject physiological saline into the bronchi of the resected specimen when observing it with the BF-XP290 bronchoscope, we use an infusion tube to create a conduit for infusion from the physiological saline bag to the working channel

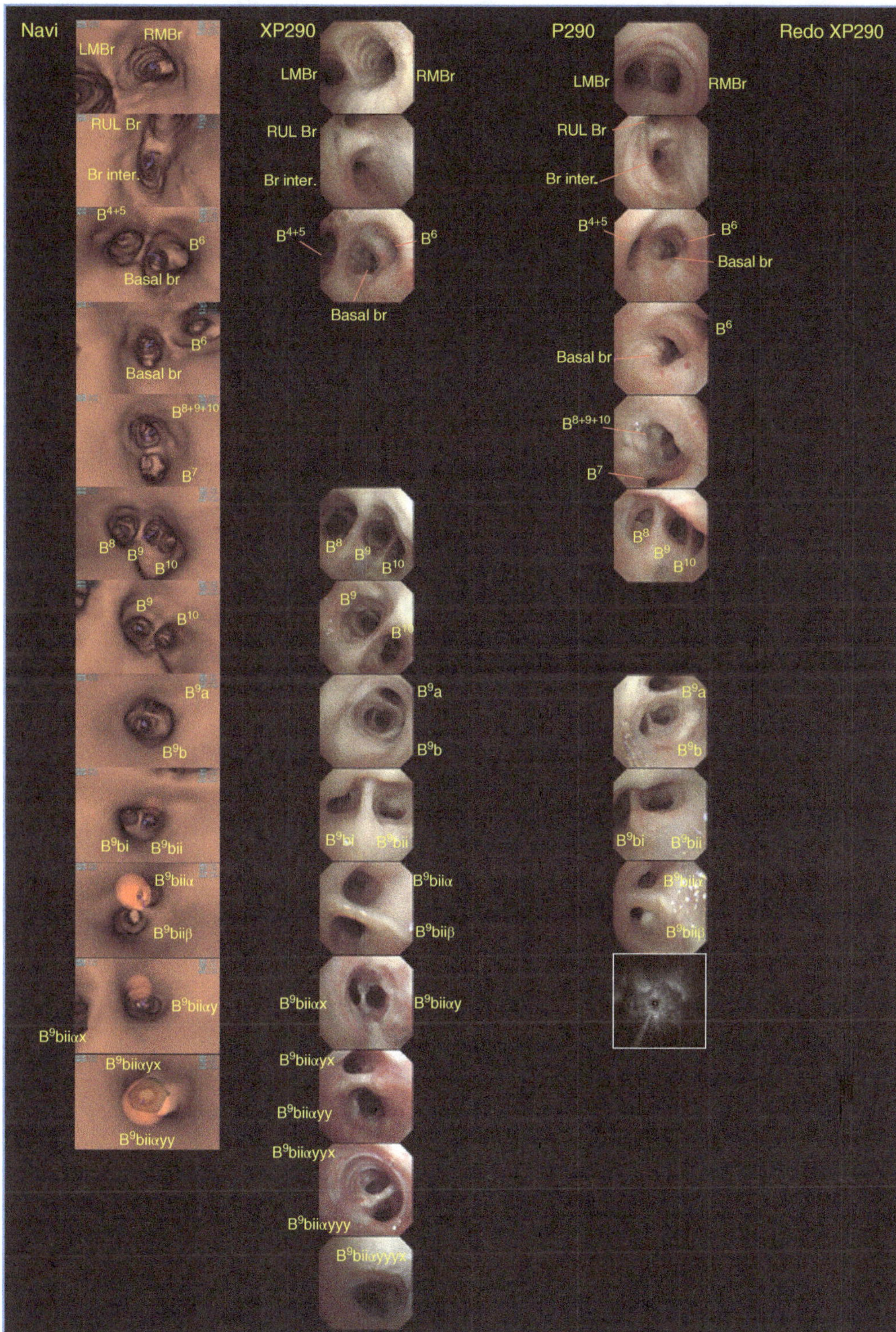

Figure 12.9 Rearrangement of bronchoscopic images obtained with different scopes.

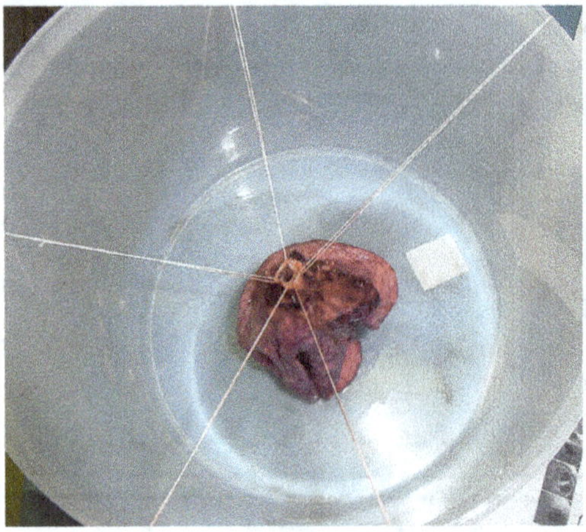

Figure 12.10 Positioning the resected lung lobe in a bucket so that the bronchial stump faces upward.

of the bronchoscope (Figure 12.11). During bronchoscopy of the resected specimen, as far as possible, we first observe the bronchial lumen without infusing physiological saline. If the field of view cannot be secured due to collapse of the bronchus or secretions, physiological saline is infused. Figure 12.12 shows representative bronchoscopic images with and without physiological saline injection into the bronchus of the resected specimen. The drip speed is adjusted with a clamp on the middle of the tube and by adjusting the height of the stand from which the saline bag is suspended. When the height of the stand is low and the speed of the drip is slow, it is convenient to

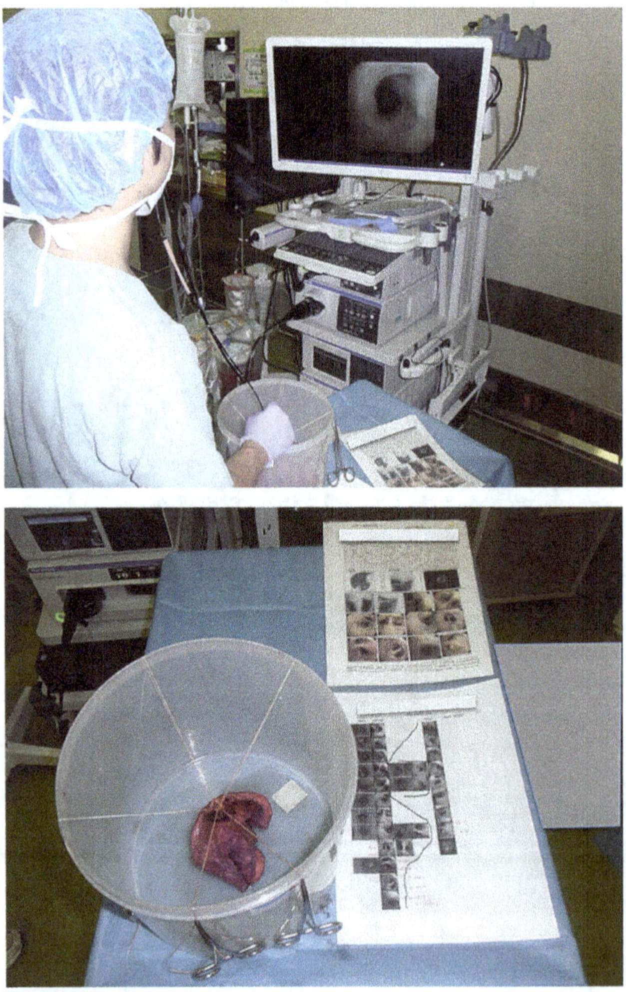

Figure 12.11 The setting in the operating room following excision of the lung specimen and its setup for subsequent bronchoscopy.

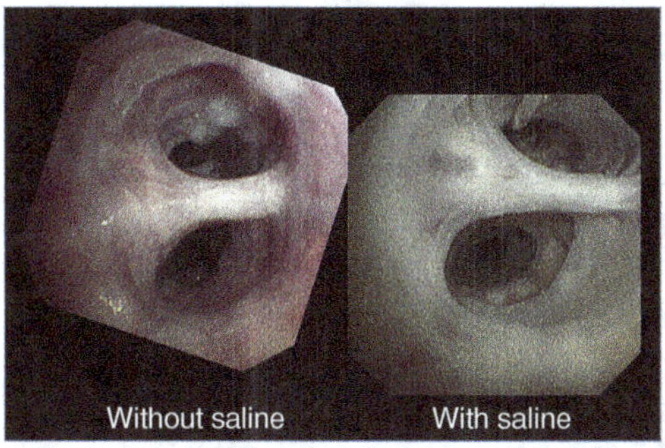

Figure 12.12 Representative bronchoscopic images with and without physiological saline injection into the bronchus of the resected specimen.

use a pressure bag. The drip speed should be the lowest possible that allows a clear field of vision, otherwise the specimen will get immediately filled with physiological saline, causing blood components and bubbles to flow backward. If too much physiological saline is injected, the findings of the EBUS to be performed subsequently may be significantly different from in vivo EBUS observations. If bubbles persist in front of the lens of the bronchoscope and interfere with the visual field, physiological saline infusion should be interrupted and suction should be applied to remove the bubbles. However, despite thorough suctioning, the bubbles remain in the working channel of the bronchoscope and are likely to re-obstruct the field of vision once saline is reinjected. Hence, flooding the specimen with saline should be avoided by maintaining the drip speed at a slow rate.

4) Bifurcation images are taken sequentially while comparing them with bronchoscopic images obtained before surgery, since there may be small bronchial branches that were not noticed in vivo (Figure 12.13).
5) Since the currently available ultrasound probe cannot be inserted into the working channel of the BF-XP290 bronchoscope, we withdraw the BF-XP290 a little and directly insert the ultrasound probe in the direction of the involved bronchus. With a clear visual field obtained by saline injection, it is often possible to guide the probe tip to the correct branch alongside the bronchoscope tip. While guiding the probe is easy if the lesion can be confirmed directly by endoscopy, scanning the area near the suspected location of the lesion with the probe is recommended in cases where direct confirmation of the lesion is not possible. Representative bronchoscopic and ultrasound images of radial probe scanning during infusion of saline into the resected specimen are shown in Figure 12.14. As already mentioned, when there is a lot of saline infused around the tumor, the resultant EBUS image might be quite different from the pre-operative EBUS image. Therefore, it is necessary to perform the evaluation as quickly as possible after resection of the specimen and with infusion of the minimum amount of saline required to ensure clear visualization.

Endobronchial Ultrasonography: Case Presentation

A 60-year-old woman was found to have a nodule in her right lower lung field on chest radiography during routine medical checkup for hypertension. CT revealed a well-defined round nodule measuring 13 × 12 × 14 mm and with a smooth margin in segment S^6 of the lower right lung lobe (Figure 12.15). Thin-slice CT before the bronchoscopy and bronchial branch reading showed that the right B^6biβxy bronchus was involved (Figure 12.16a). Using DirectPath virtual navigation software, it was possible to identify up to the B^6biβ bronchus by automatic bronchial extraction, after which the branch of B^6biβ was extended to the target by manual extraction (Figure 12.16b). Bronchial branches further peripherally from B^6biβ to the target could not be identified using DirectPath. With bronchial branch reading, it was possible to identify the sixth- and seventh-order branches

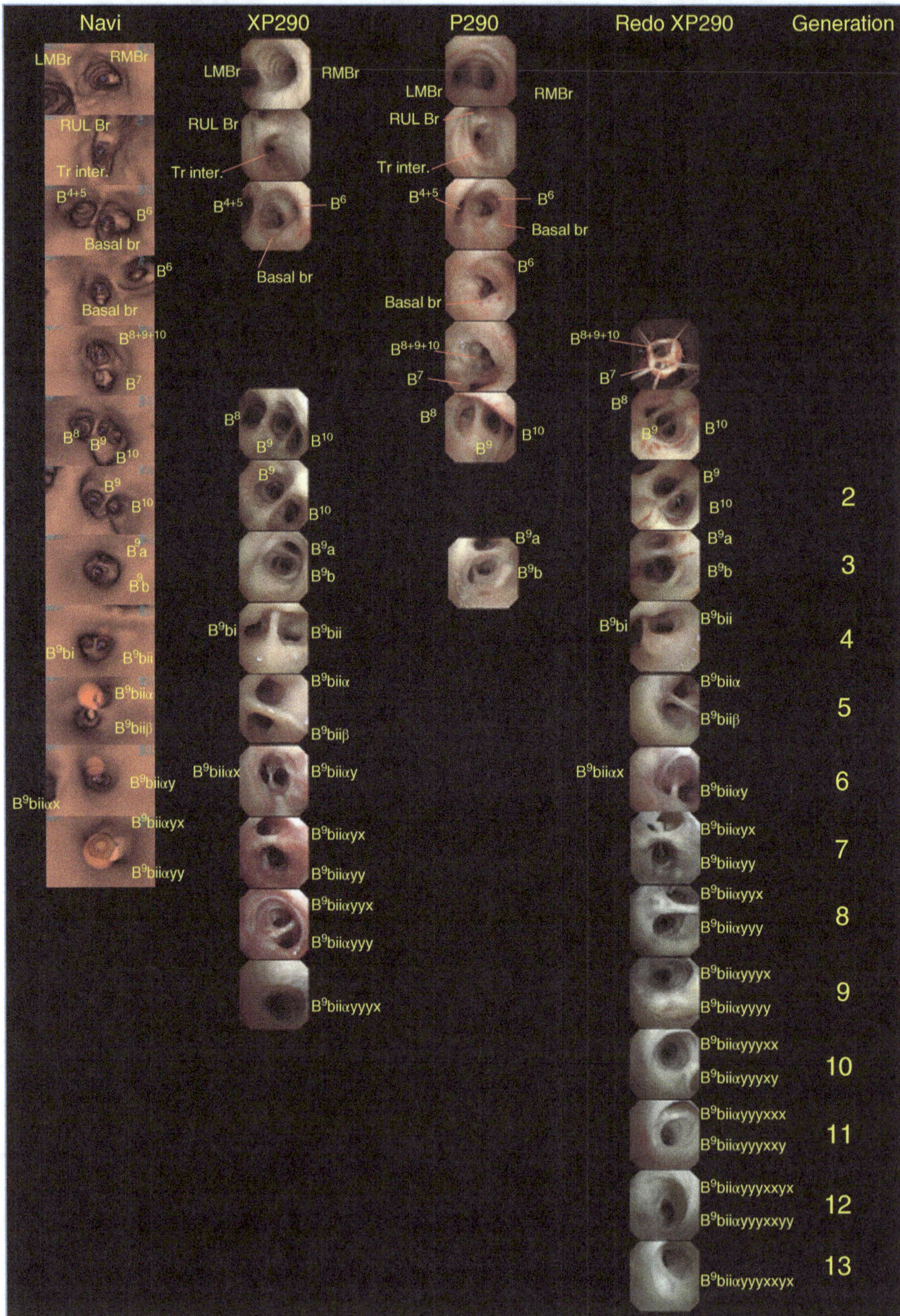

Figure 12.13 Representative bronchoscopic images of both the in vivo and ex vivo (redo XP290) lung.

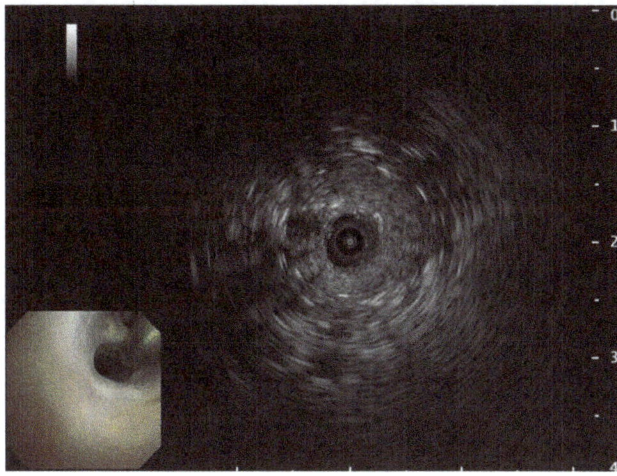

Figure 12.14 Representative bronchoscopic and ultrasound images of the resected specimen with radial probe scanning during physiological saline infusion.

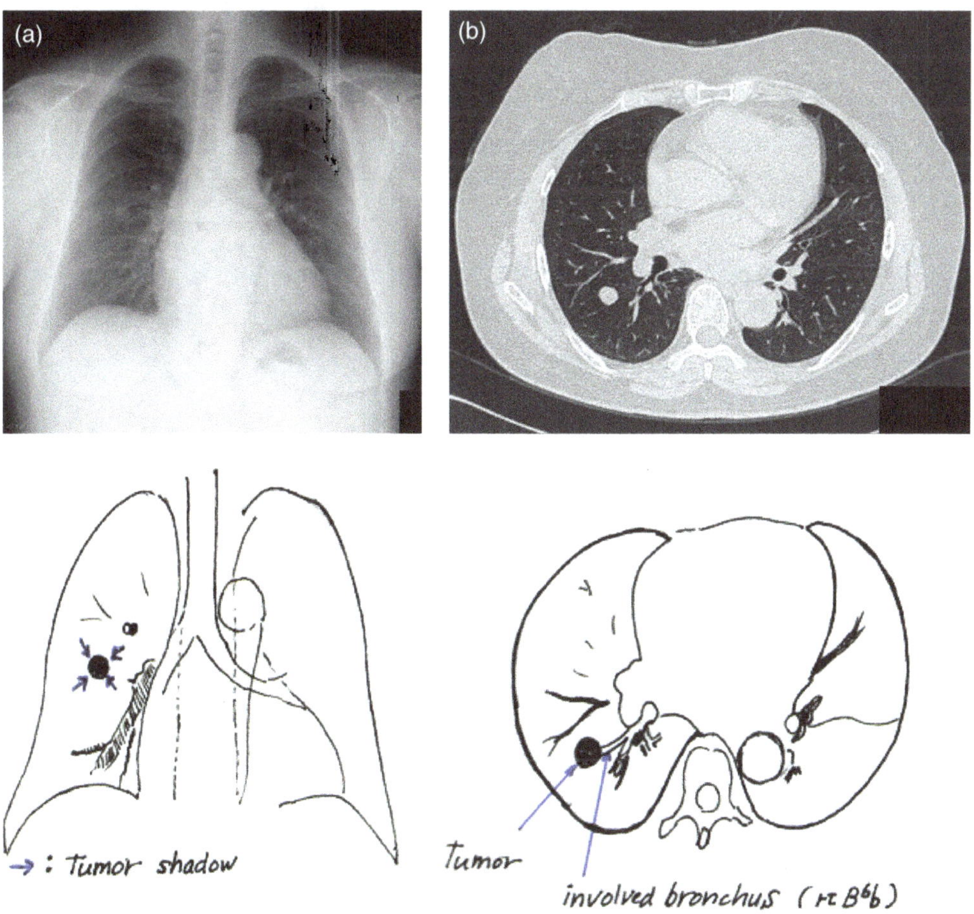

Figure 12.15 Chest X-ray (a) and computed tomography findings (b).

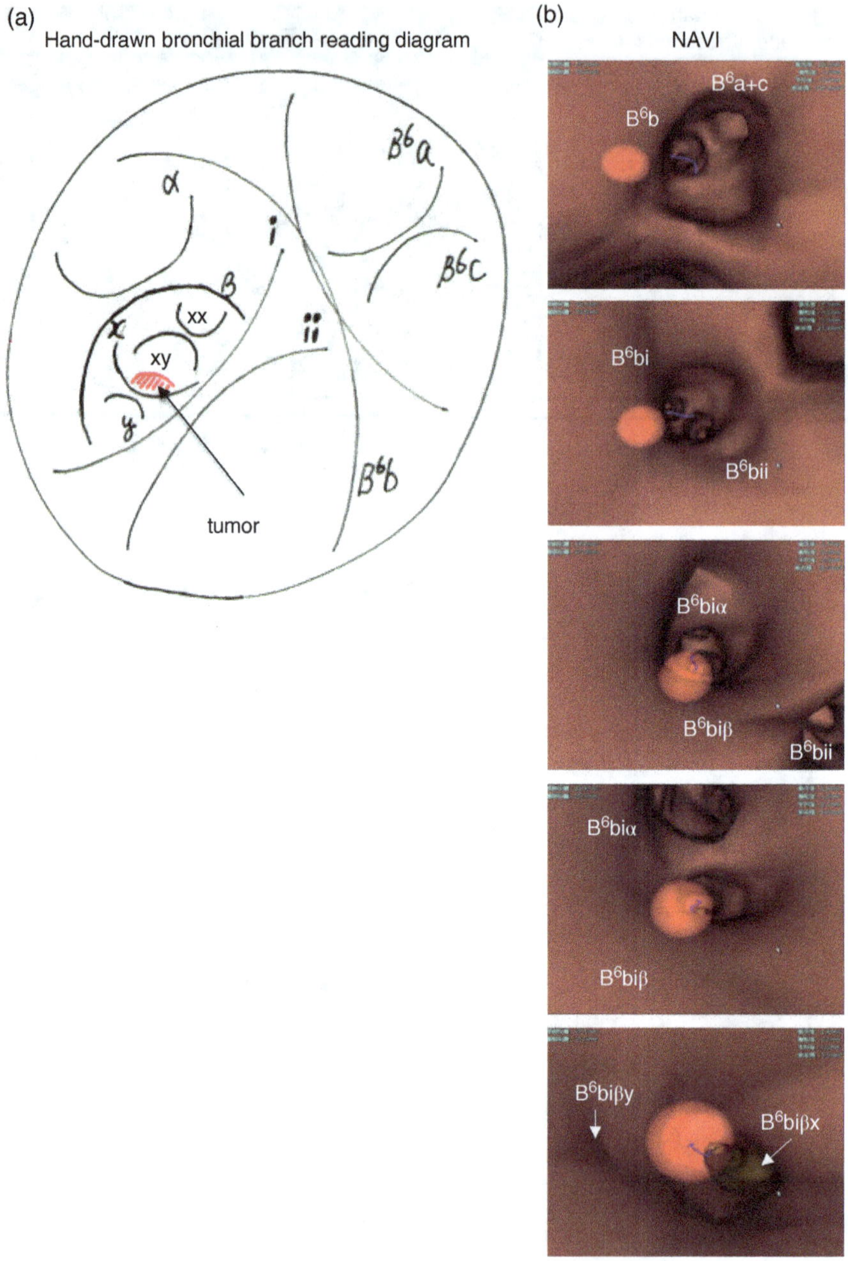

Figure 12.16 Bronchial branch reading diagram (a) and navigation image created using DirectPath virtual navigation software (b).

after B^{6}biβ using coronal CT sections; that is, up to B^{6}biβxy (Figure 12.16).

Actual bronchoscopy was first performed using the ultrathin bronchoscope, BF-XP290. During bronchoscope insertion according to the navigation image, the scope entered the B^{6}biβ bronchus (the B^{6}biβy bronchus corresponds to the part that can be seen as a slight indentation on the navigation screen; Figure 12.17: diagram at the bottom of the Navi row), and it could be inserted up to B^{6}biβx. With deeper advancement of the bronchoscope, B^{6}biβxx could be

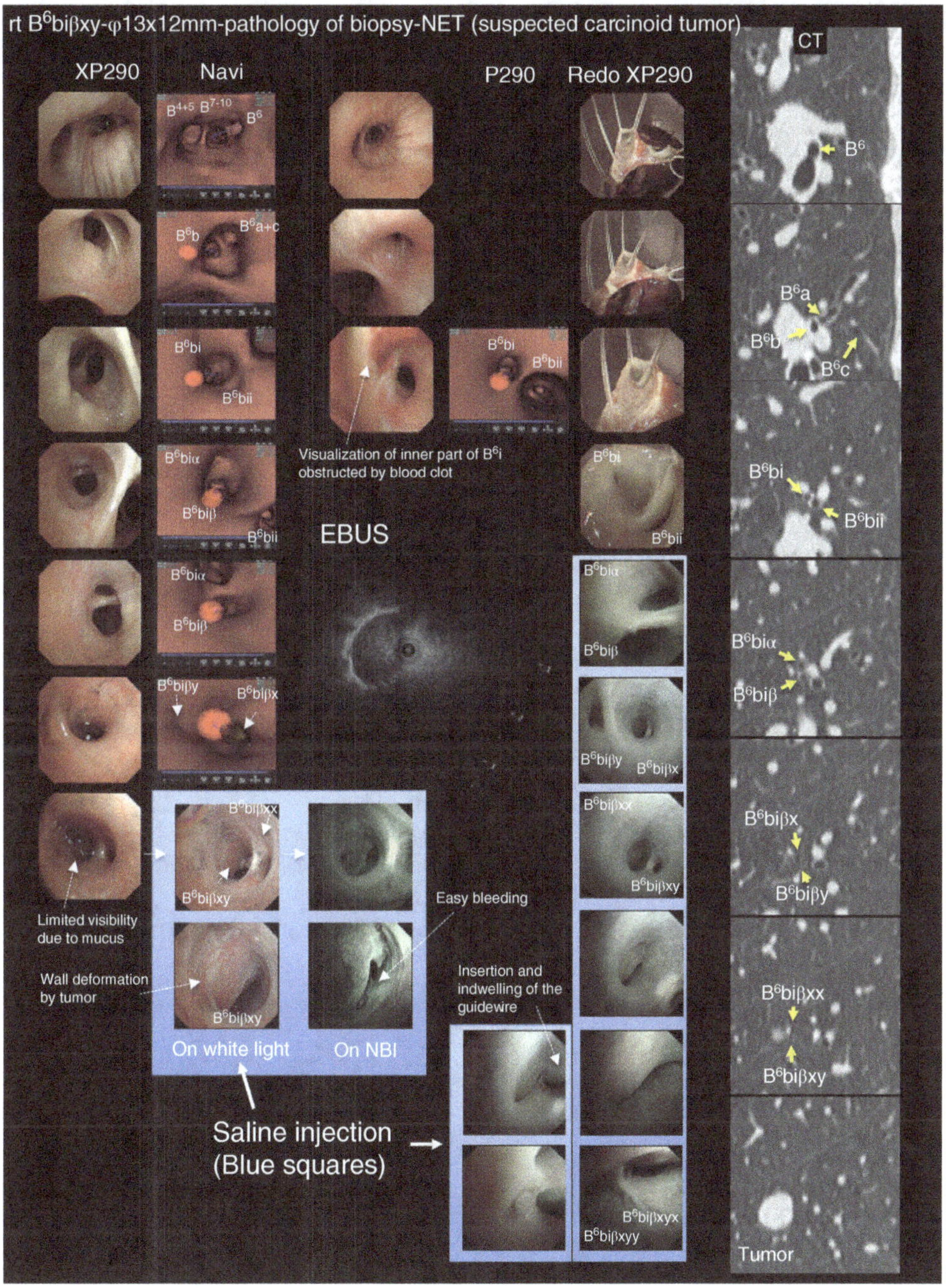

Figure 12.17 Correlation between bronchoscopy, endobronchial ultrasound, and computed tomography findings.

visualized, while the deeper part of B^{6}biβxy could not be visualized due to an abundance of mucus (Figure 12.17: diagram at the bottom of the XP290 row). Since there was slight resistance to further insertion of the scope, approximately 3 cc of physiological saline was injected into the respiratory tract from the working channel, in order to open the airway and to obtain a clear field of vision (Figure 12.17: upper pictures in the blue squares were obtained under saline injection). The scope was further advanced one branch deeper and revealed the bronchial wall of B^{6}biβxy to be deformed semi-circumferentially. Although a central depression was identified, it was unclear whether this was triggered by the slight water pressure; however, slight bleeding was observed in the central depression (Figure 12.17: lower pictures in the blue squares were obtained under saline injection). While evaluating the angle and distance of this branching pattern, the BF-XP290 bronchoscope was gradually withdrawn and it was replaced with the BF-P290 bronchoscope. The entrance of B^{6}bi was seen to be filled with blood due to bleeding (Figure 12.17: bottom picture of the P290 row). From the bronchial branch reading diagram and the branch pattern of the peripheral airway observed with the BF-XP290, it was supposed that after B^{6}bi, advancing the probe/GS to the left sub-branch (y) of the right branch (x) of the lower bronchus (β) would lead to the lesion.

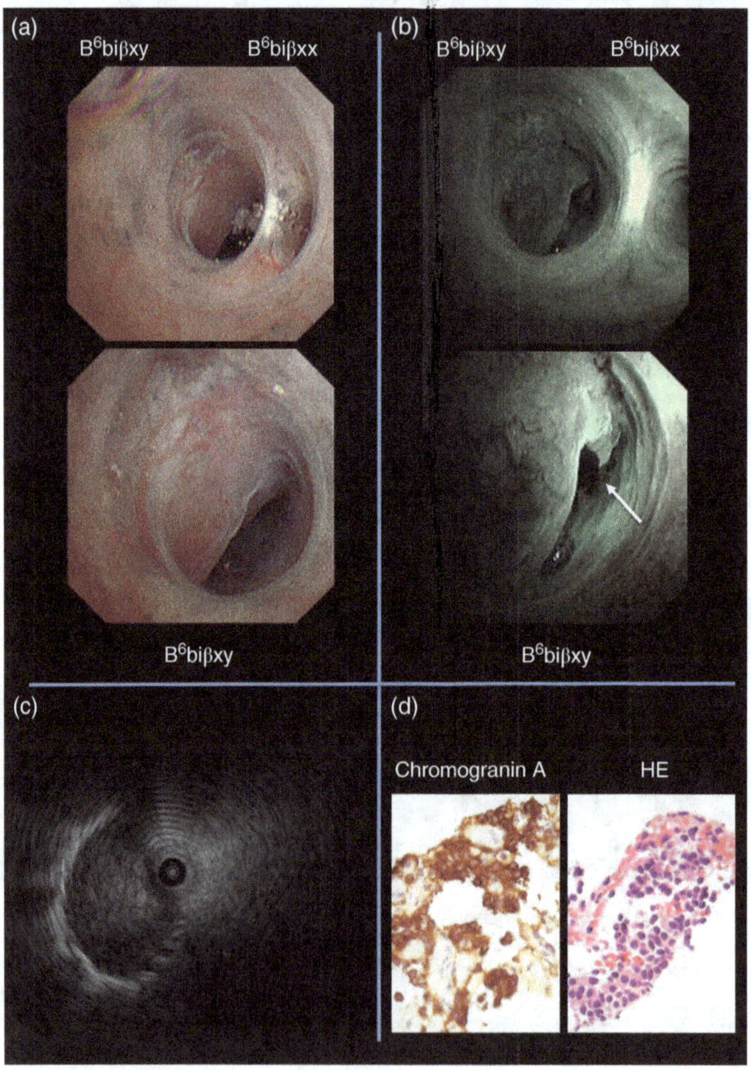

Figure 12.18 Direct endoscopic observation of protrusion of the left wall of the B^{6}biβxy bronchus: (a) white light image, b) narrow band imaging, (c) endobronchial ultrasound, (d) histopathology of preoperative biopsy specimen. Arrow: bleeding from the central indentation of the lesion.

The lesion was subsequently identified as an area of unevenness on the left wall of B^6biβxy (Figure 12.18a and b). When a small amount of physiological saline was injected from the working channel of BF-P290 and the probe/GS was inserted, the lesion was visualized from adjacent to the lesion on the EBUS monitor (Figure 12.18c). We tried brushing and biopsy of the lesion three times while angling the tip of the bronchoscope so that the forceps could approach the lesion. Histopathologic diagnosis of the biopsy specimen indicated carcinoid tumor (Figure 12.18d).

Whole body positron-emission tomography (PET)-CT scan and brain magnetic resonance imaging (MRI) were performed to rule out other tumors, and the patient was ultimately diagnosed with primary pulmonary carcinoid tumor without metastasis to the hilar mediastinal lymph nodes or distant organs; hence, right lower lobe resection was performed. The surgically resected right lower lobe was once again examined bronchoscopically using the BF-XP290 scope immediately after resection. Continuous injection of physiological saline into the respiratory tract helped to expand the airway, such that we could observe all the bronchial branches without interruption. In this case, it was possible to identify the next branch beyond the lesion; that is, the spur of B^6biβxyx and B^6biβxyy (Figure 12.17: redo XP290 bronchoscopy of the resected specimen after surgery). To enable complete excision along the long axis of the involved bronchus, a guidewire had been inserted intraoperatively below B^6biβxyy under bronchoscopic observation and, following resection of the lung lobe, the resected specimen was fixed with 10%

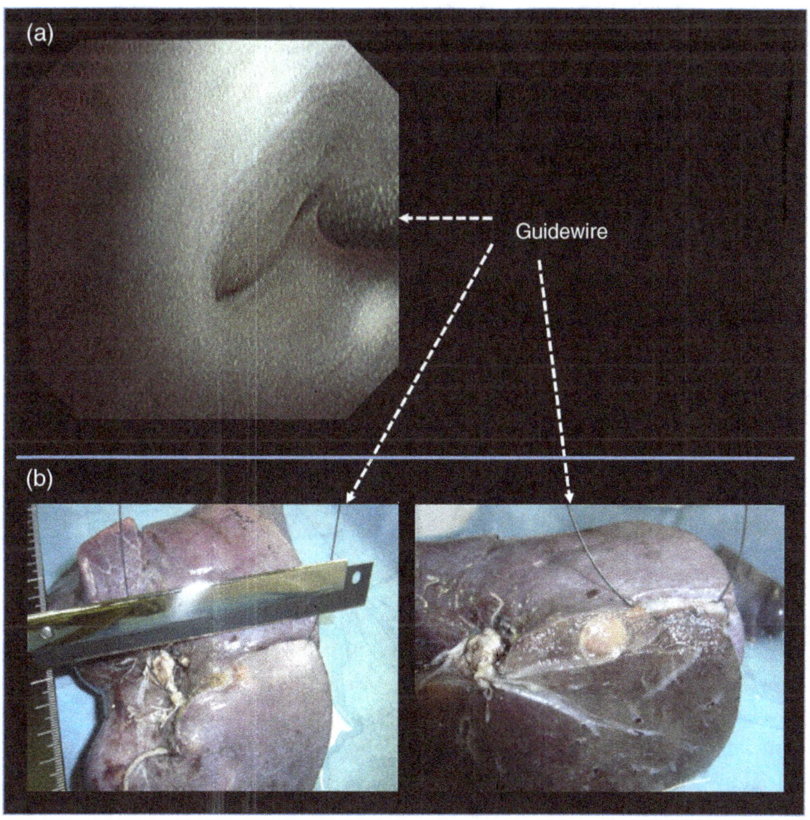

Figure 12.19 Method of cutting along the bronchus leading to the lesion: (a) guidewire insertion, (b) cutting along the guidewire.

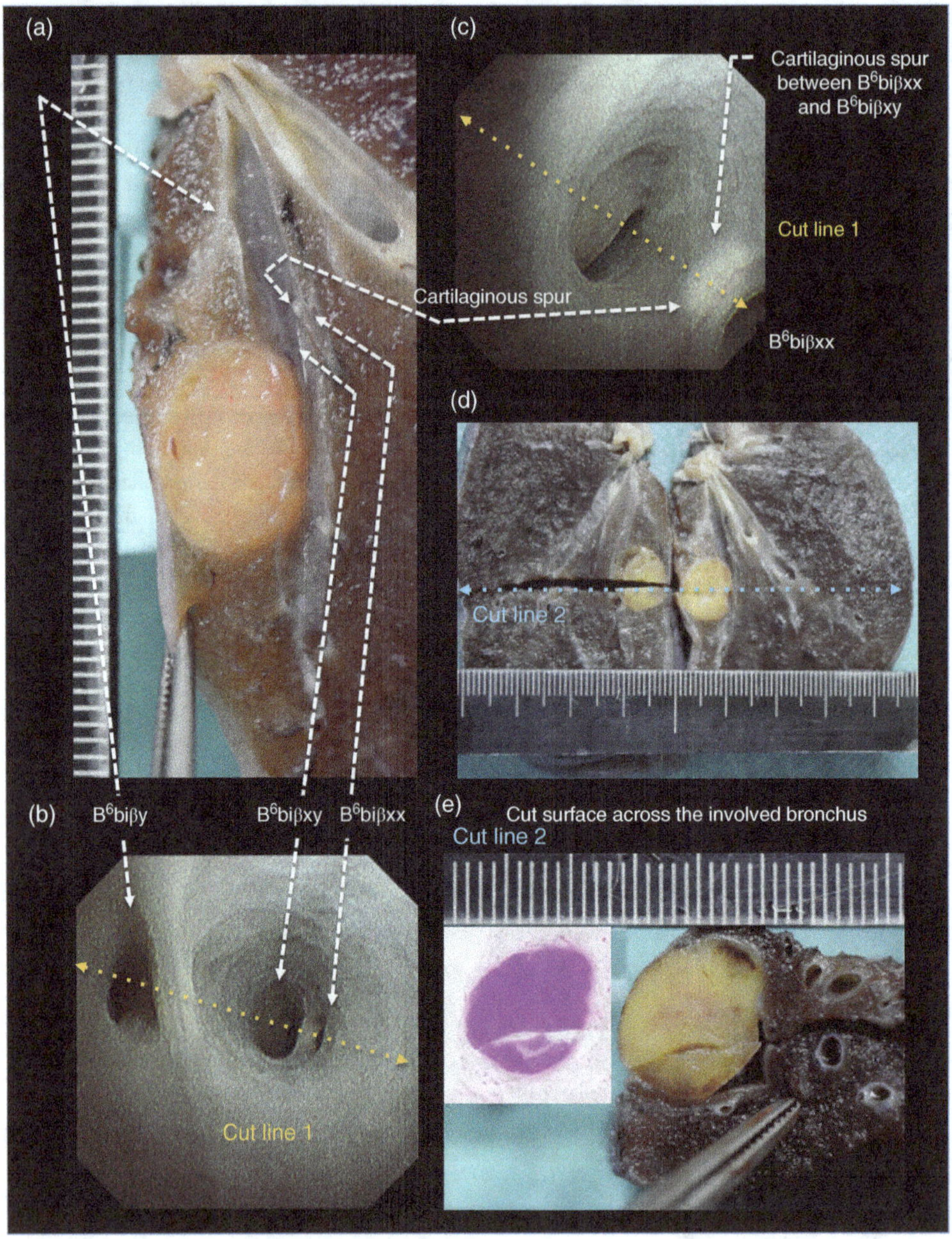

Figure 12.20 Cut surface of the specimen and its correlation with bronchoscopy.

buffered formalin with the guidewire in situ (Figure 12.19a). During post-operative evaluation of the excised specimen, by cutting along this guidewire we were able to accurately split the specimen along the plane of the involved bronchus and obtain a clear cross-section of the lesion and the bronchus (Figure 12.19b). In this case, the cartilage forming the spur of B^6biβxx and B^6biβxy and branches of B^6biβy on its central side were clearly resected. This indicated that the specimen was resected along cut line 1 shown in Figure 12.20a–c. The specimen was also resected along cut line 2 shown Figure 12.20d, in order to correlate the excised specimen with the EBUS findings (Figure 12.18d).

13

Endobronchial Ultrasonography of Airway Integrity and Tumor Involvement

David I.K. Fielding

Royal Brisbane and Women's Hospital, Herston, Queensland, Australia

Introduction

Since the first papers on this topic by Kurimoto and Herth [1, 2], the endobronchial ultrasound (EBUS) radial balloon (RB) method has remained the mainstay of assessment of the depth of penetration of endoluminal tumors through bronchus wall [3]. The depth of invasion determines staging and treatment choice. Superficial lesions can be treated by argon plasma coagulation, whereas deeper lesions will require diathermy, cryotherapy, or photodynamic therapy (PDT). Lesions suspected to go through the outside layers of the bronchus may be suitable for brachytherapy with curative intent in highly selected cases.

Kurimoto et al.'s elegant 1999 study established the utility of EBUS for superficial versus deep penetration of the bronchial wall [1]. It was an ex vivo experiment on 45 normal resection specimens and 24 lung cancer resected specimens. The findings were as follows. The cartilaginous portions of the extrapulmonary bronchi and the intrapulmonary bronchi exhibited a five-layer structure. Starting on the luminal side, the first layer (hyperechoic) was a marginal echo, the second layer (hypoechoic) was the submucosal tissue, the third layer (hyperechoic) was the marginal echo on the inner side of the bronchial cartilage, the fourth layer (hypoechoic) was bronchial cartilage, and the fifth layer (hyperechoic) was the marginal echo on the outer side of the cartilage. In the membranous portions, the first layer (hyperechoic) was a marginal echo, the second layer (hypoechoic) was smooth muscle, and the third layer (hyperechoic) corresponded to the adventitia (Figure 13.1). EBUS was able to accurately determine the depth of diagnosis of 23 of the 24 lung cancer specimens; in one case which overinterpreted the depth of invasion, this was due to lymphocyte infiltration (Figures 13.2–13.4).

These findings were tested in another elegant study determining how the EBUS RB method changed management in superficial endobronchial squamous cell carcinomas (Figures 13.5 and 13.6) [4]. Prior to PDT treatment in 18 superficial carcinomas, with no invasion by fine-cut chest computed tomography (CT), RB was performed to assess the depth of penetration; the findings were that nine lesions were diagnosed as intracartilaginous by EBUS. Long-term complete remission has been achieved in these patients with a median followup term after PDT of 32 months, confirming the EBUS interpretation. The remaining nine lesions were diagnosed as extracartilaginous by EBUS and were considered candidates for other therapies such as surgical

Endobronchial Ultrasonography, Second Edition. Noriaki Kurimoto, David I.K. Fielding, Ali I. Musani, Christopher Kniese, and Katsuhiko Morita.

Companion website: www.wiley.com/go/kurimoto2e

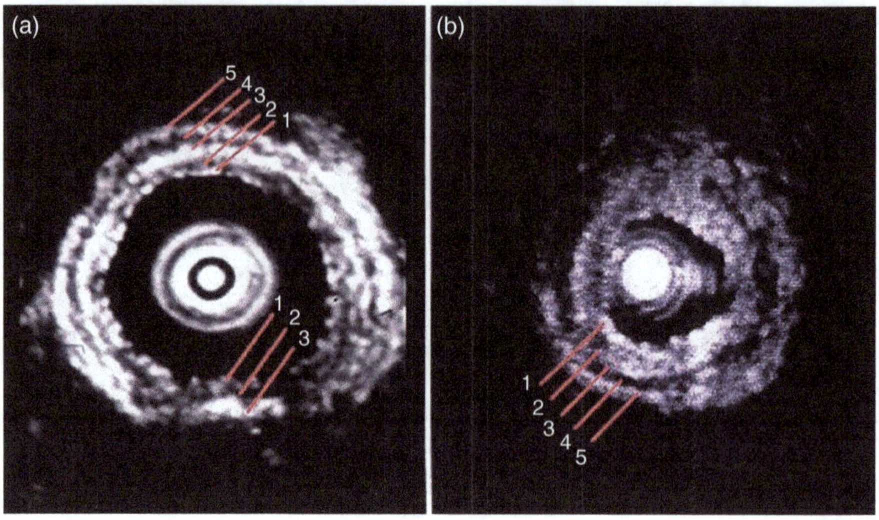

Figure 13.1 Layers of the bronchial wall by endobronchial ultrasound. The cartilaginous portion of the trachea and the extrapulmonary bronchi is visualized as five layers, and the membranous portion is visualized as three layers (a). The first layer (hyperechoic) is a marginal echo, the second layer (hyperechoic) is smooth muscle, the third layer (hyperechoic) is the marginal echo on the inner side of the bronchial cartilage, the fourth layer (hypoechoic) is cartilage, and the fifth layer (hyperechoic) is the marginal echo on the outer side of the cartilage. In the membranous portion of the extrapulmonary bronchi, the first layer (hyperechoic) is a marginal echo, the second layer (hypoechoic) is smooth muscle, and the third layer (hyperechoic) is the adventitia. The intrapulmonary bronchi are visualized as five layers (b). The first layer (hyperechoic) is a marginal echo, the second layer (hypoechoic) is submucosal tissue, the third layer (hyperechoic) is the marginal echo on the inner side of the bronchial cartilage, the fourth layer (hypoechoic) is cartilage, and the fifth layer (hyperechoic) is the marginal echo on the outer side of the cartilage. *Source:* Kurimoto et al. [1].

resection, chemotherapy, and radiotherapy, although two were invisible by high-resolution (HR)-CT, three were superficial, and five were 1 cm in diameter on observation by bronchoscopy. The depth of tumor invasion estimated by EBUS was proven to be accurate by histopathologic findings in six specimens after surgical resection. EBUS RB was therefore shown to be an indispensable addition to the endoluminal staging of these uncommon kinds of cases.

Radial probe (RP)-EBUS is also used with centrally located tumors adjacent to the trachea (Figures 13.5 and 13.6) to determine if there is tracheal invasion (clinical T4 stage) or if the tumor is just adjacent and not invading the trachea (clinical T1a–3 depending on lesion size; Figures 13.7–13.9). Herth et al. reported 131 cases with central thoracic malignancies potentially involving the central airways [2]. The bronchoscopists were blinded to the radiologist's interpretation of the chest CT before doing the EBUS. The ability of chest CT and EBUS to distinguish between compression and infiltration was measured against the histologic results.

All patients underwent chest CT followed by white-light bronchoscopy (WLB) and RP-EBUS, with subsequent surgical evaluation and radiology results blinded from the bronchoscopist. In 81 patients (77%), the CT scan was read by the radiologist as consistent with tumor invasion. EBUS only showed invasion in 49 cases (47%). Histology after surgery revealed a specificity of 100%, a sensitivity of 89%, and an accuracy of 94% for EBUS. Chest CT was far inferior, with a specificity of 28%, a sensitivity of 75%, and an accuracy of 51%. EBUS RB remains a key tool in this type of assessment.

Kita et al. have reported the utility of EBUS RB in assessing the layers of the airway in

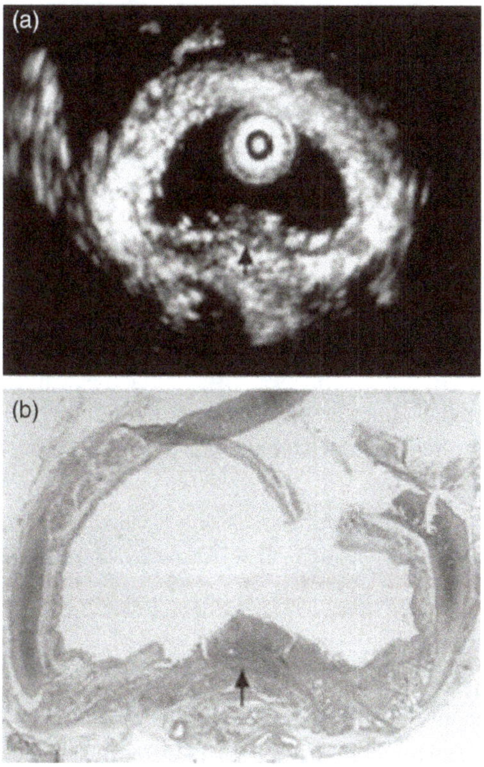

Figure 13.2 Comparison of ultrasonogram (a) and histopathologic findings (b) of a representative example of invasion above the smooth muscle of the membranous portion. A lesion was on the luminal side in contact with the hypoechoic second layer, which corresponds to smooth muscle (black arrow), and this was confirmed on the histopathologic specimen (b: hematoxylin-eosin, original ×5). *Source:* Kurimoto et al. [1].

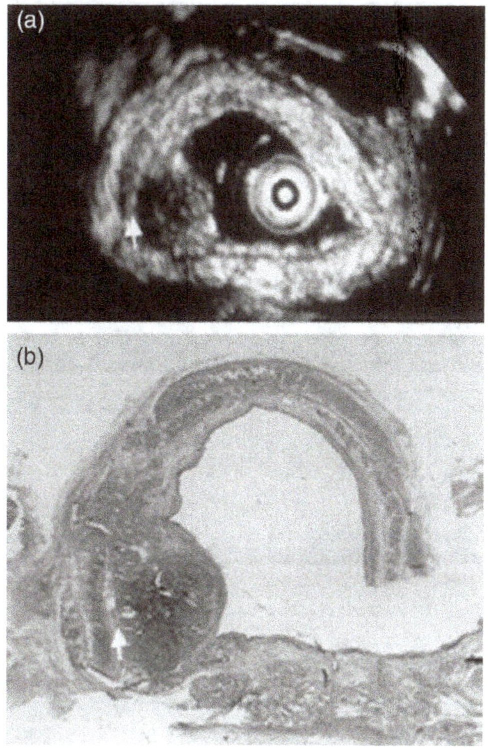

Figure 13.3 Comparison of ultrasonogram (a) and histopathologic findings (b) of a representative example of invasion at submucosal tissue. A lesion was on the luminal side in contact with the hyperechoic third layer (inner marginal echo of cartilage; white arrow), and a tumor in contact with the inner surface (white arrow) of the cartilage was observed histopathologically. Histopathologic findings confirmed this ultrasound determination of the depth of tumor invasion (b: hematoxylin-eosin, original ×5). *Source:* Kurimoto et al. [1].

asthma patients specifically as they relate to bronchial hyper-responsiveness [5]. These authors studied 24 asthmatic patients and placed the 20 MHz balloon EBUS probe in the bronchus intermedius. The percentage of airway wall thickness was determined by EBUS and was defined as outer diameter minus lumenal diameter divided by outer diameter times 100. Bronchial hyper-responsiveness to methacholine was measured with a standard PC_{20} protocol. As expected, the percentage wall thickness measured by EBUS was significantly greater in patients with asthma than that in non-asthma control subjects ($p<0.01$). The mean (standard deviation) wall thickness percentage measured by EBUS images was 27.2% (± 3.9%) in the patients with asthma and 18.9% (± 2.6%) in subjects without asthma. The evaluation of the laminar structure using EBUS indicated that the thickness of the second layer in patients with asthma was greater than that in subjects without asthma ($p<0.05$). PC_{20} was negatively correlated with the thickness of the second layer ($r = 0.52$, $p<0.01$), but was not significantly correlated with other layers in patients with asthma. It was assumed that the observed EBUS thickening resulted from the cellular changes of asthma (edema and inflammatory cell infiltration), and from structural

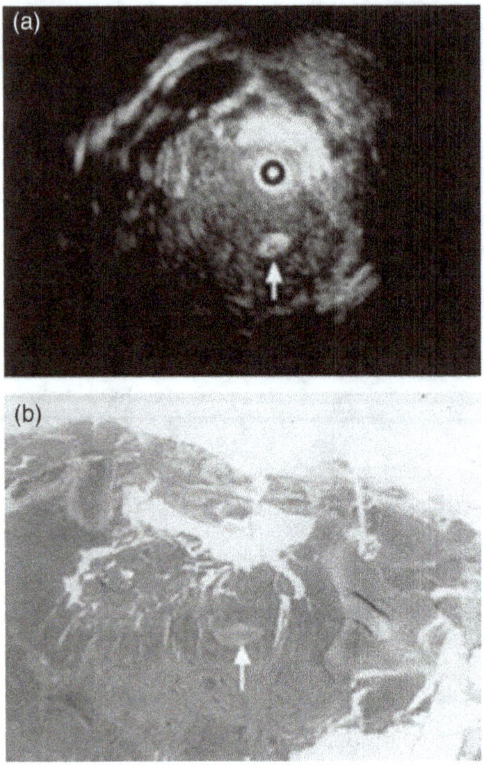

Figure 13.4 Comparison of ultrasonogram (a) and histopathologic findings (b) of a representative example of invasion beyond the bronchial wall. An island-like area (white arrow) was thought to be cartilage within the tumor on the basis of the ultrasonographic findings. Cartilage having exactly the same shape was observed at the same location (white arrow) in the histopathologic specimen (b: hematoxylin-eosin, original ×5).
Source: Kurimoto et al. [1].

changes, such as mucous gland hyperplasia, reticular basement membrane thickening, vascular proliferation, and airway smooth muscle hypertrophy and hyperplasia. In particular, the authors inferred that the EBUS technique was showing differences in the thickness of the submucosal tissue containing smooth muscle in patients with asthma which were greater than that in non-asthmatic subjects, as the second layer predominantly comprises smooth muscle. It remains to be seen whether these encouraging findings are used in asthma medication studies, but certainly they are being tested in the response of airways to bronchial thermoplasty [6].

Optical Coherence Tomography

The main competition for the RP-EBUS technique in airway assessment is optical coherence tomography (OCT) [9]. Recent studies have compared the accuracy of OCT to that of CT chest, because the spatial resolution of CT does not allow small airways to be visualized and there are still concerns about the sensitivity of the measurements obtained from these airways. Bronchoscopic OCT by contrast has exceptional spatial resolution; due to the use of low-coherence light, OCT can produce images

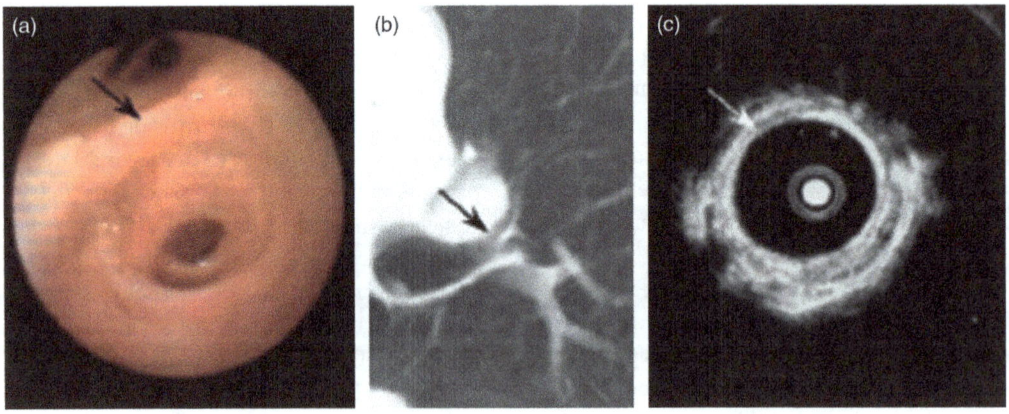

Figure 13.5 A case of carcinoma in situ. (a) Bronchoscopic view shows an irregular thickness at the spur between superior and lingual bronchi of the left upper lobe (arrow). (b) The lesion is invisible on high-resolution computed tomography scan. (c) Endobronchial ultrasound shows a normal layered structure of the bronchial wall and the tumor is not observed. *Source:* Miyazu et al. [4]. Reprinted with permission from American Thoracic Society.

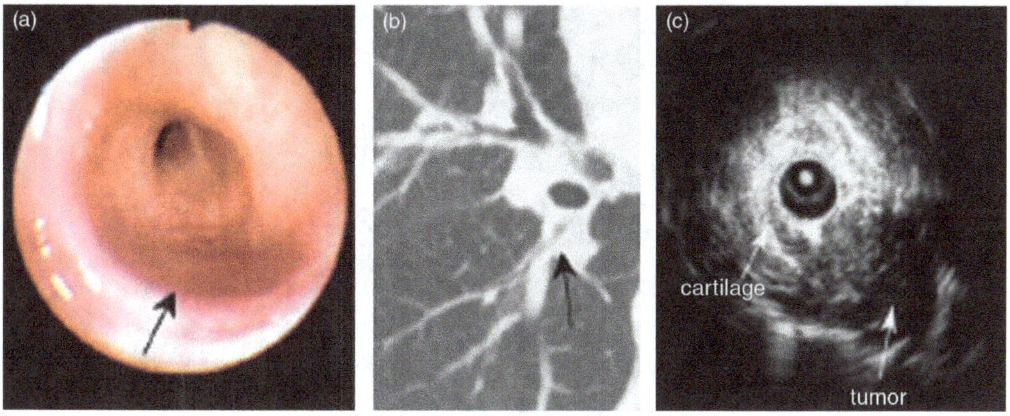

Figure 13.6 A case of squamous cell carcinoma at the orifice of the right B6. (a) The bronchoscopic view showed a reddish superficial tumor at the orifice of B6 (arrow). The tumor appeared superficial and was 0.5–1.0 cm in diameter. (b) High-resolution computed tomography showed an obscure lesion at the site. Because there was little contrast between it and surrounding mediastinal connective tissue, we diagnosed it as invisible. (c) Endobronchial ultrasound can delineate the tumor (arrow) and shows that the cartilage layer is involved and interrupted around the tumor. Accordingly, it was diagnosed as extracartilaginous. *Source:* Miyazu et al. [4]. Reprinted with permission from American Thoracic Society.

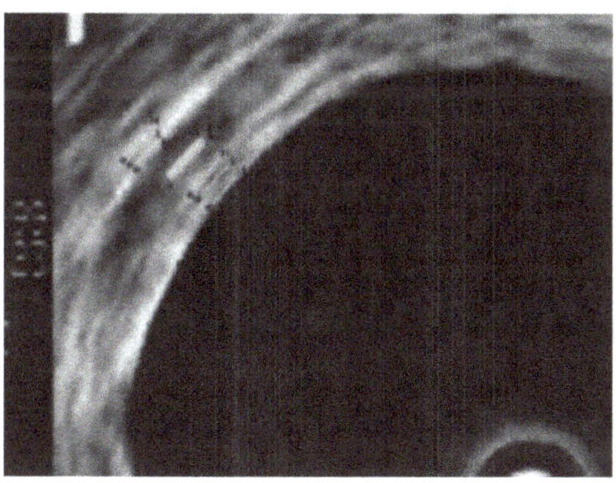

Figure 13.7 Example of a normal airway wall as shown by endobronchial ultrasound (magnified). Shown is the seven-layer structure as visualized with a 20 MHz probe. Identifiable structures from the inside out are mucosa (H), submucosa (L), endochondrium (H), cartilage (L), perichondrial layer (H), connective tissue (L), adventitia (H). L, low-density layer; H, high-density layer. *Source:* Herth et al. [2]. Reprinted with permission from American College of Chest Physicians.

with resolution in the range of 5–15 mm [7, 8]. Such methods may allow chronic obstructive pulmonary disease (COPD) phenotype to be better defined on the basis of small airway phenotype and hence allow tailoring of therapy.

One study correlated OCT measurements of airway dimensions with measurements assessed using CT scans and lung function in 44 current and former smokers [9]. Lumen and wall area as measured by CT and OCT were strongly correlated (r = 50.84, p = 0.001, and r = 50.89, p = 0.001, respectively; Figure 13.10). Compared with CT, OCT measurements were lower for both lumen and wall area by 31% and 66%, respectively. The correlation between forced expiratory volume (FEV1%) predicted and CT and OCT measured wall area (as a percentage of the total area) of fifth-generation airways was very strong (r = 520.79, r = 520.75), but the slope of the relationship was much steeper using OCT than using CT (y = 520.33, x = 182, y = 520.1, x = 178), indicating greater sensitivity of OCT in detecting changes in wall measurements that relate to FEV1 (Figure 13.10). These findings were consistent with OCT being more sensitive to changes in small airway dimensions than CT.

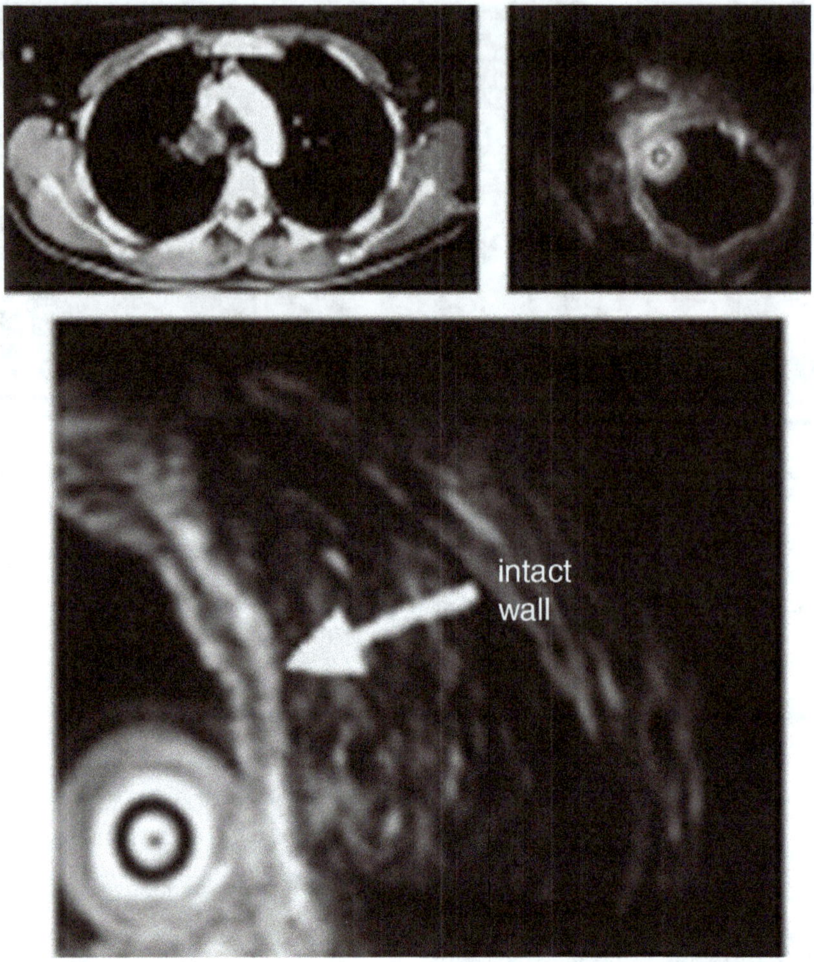

Figure 13.8 Top left: example of a chest computed tomograph with central mass abutting the airway. This mass was classified as infiltrating the airway, as no plane could be identified between tumor and airway; R, right. Top right: the corresponding endobronchial ultrasound (EBUS) examination demonstrates an intact outermost airway layer and as such no evidence of infiltration. The EBUS finding was confirmed at time of surgery. Bottom: magnified EBUS image demonstrating the intact bronchial wall. *Source:* Herth et al. [2]. Reprinted with permission from American College of Chest Physicians.

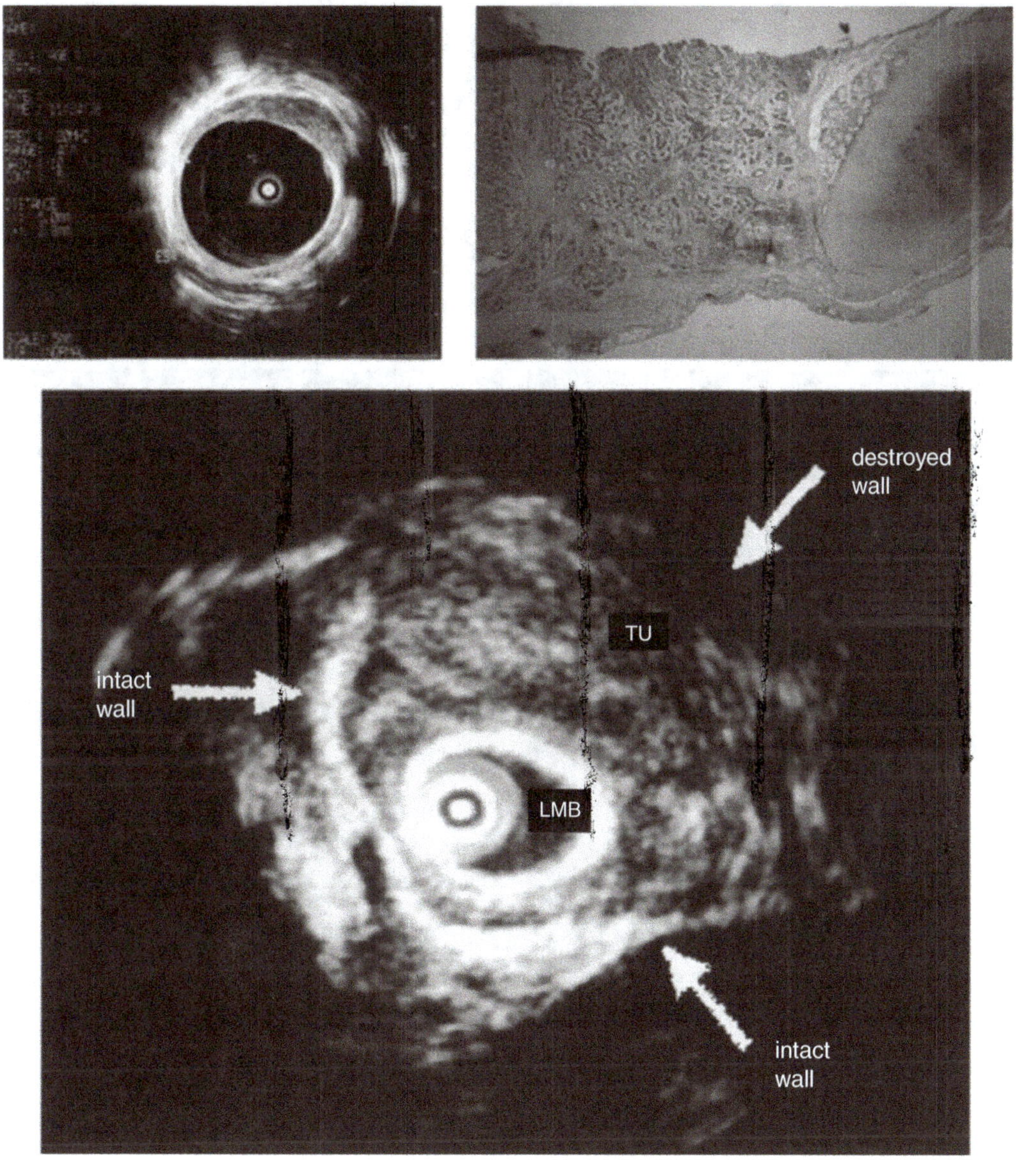

Figure 13.9 Top left: Endobronchial ultrasound (EBUS) image showing tumor infiltration (Tu) of a tracheal wall. Top right: the histologic correlate shows cartilage destruction by tumor (hematoxylin-eosin, original, 160). ES, esophagus; TR, trachea. Bottom: magnified image of a tumor infiltration of the bronchial wall of the left main bronchus. The difference between the intact wall and the destroyed area is clearly visible. LMB, left main bronchus; TU, tumor. *Source:* Herth et al. [2]. Reprinted with permission from American College of Chest Physicians.

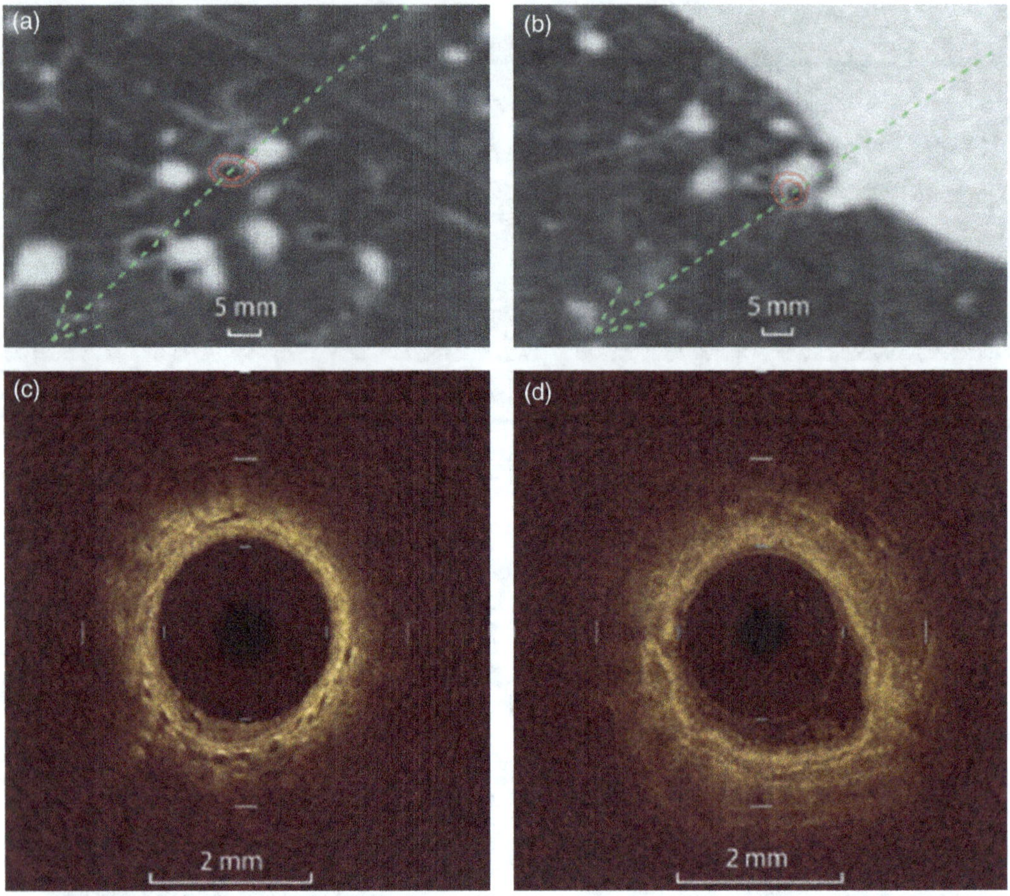

Figure 13.10 Images of fifth-generation airways obtained using computed tomography (CT) (a, b) and optical coherence tomography (OCT) (c, d). The airways in (a) and (c) were obtained from a subject with normal forced expiratory volume (FEV1; 118% predicted) and in (b) and (d) are obtained from a subject with an FEV1 of 52% predicted. The percentage of wall area measured using CT is only 5% different (69% vs. 74%), but 29% different (43% vs. 72%) using OCT. The green dotted arrow in the CT images (a and b) represents the orientation of the longitudinal plane of the reformatted airway path from which the cross-sectional image is obtained (see Figure 13.1). *Source:* Coxson et al. [9]. Reprinted with permission from American Thoracic Society.

References

1 Kurimoto, N., Murayama, M., Yoshioka, S. et al. (1999). Assessment of usefulness of endobronchial ultrasonography in determination of depth of tracheobronchial tumor invasion. *Chest* 115 (6): 1500–1506.

2 Herth, F., Ernst, A., Schulz, M., and Becker, H. (2003). Endobronchial ultrasound reliably differentiates between airway infiltration and compression by tumor. *Chest* 123 (2): 458–462.

3 Leong, S., Shaipanich, T., Lam, S., and Yasufuku, K. (2013). Diagnostic bronchoscopy—current and future perspectives. *Journal of Thoracic Disease* 5 (Suppl 5): S498–S510.

4 Miyazu, Y., Miyazawa, T., Kurimoto, N. et al. (2002). Endobronchial ultrasonography in the assessment of centrally located early-stage lung cancer before photodynamic therapy.

American Journal of Respiratory and Critical Care Medicine 165 (6): 832–837.

5 Kita, T., Fujimura, M., Kurimoto, N. et al. (2010). Airway wall structure assessed by endobronchial ultrasonography and bronchial hyperresponsiveness in patients with asthma. *Journal of Bronchology & Interventional Pulmonology* 17 (4): 301–306.

6 Kirby, M., Ohtani, K., Lopez Lisbona, R.M. et al. (2015). Bronchial thermoplasty in asthma: 2-year follow-up using optical coherence tomography. *European Respiratory Journal* 46 (3): 859–862.

7 Armstrong, J.J., Leigh, M.S., Sampson, D.D. et al. (2006). Quantitative upper airway imaging with anatomic optical coherence tomography. *American Journal of Respiratory and Critical Care Medicine* 173 (2): 226–233.

8 Huang, D., Swanson, E.A., Lin, C.P. et al. (1991). Optical coherence tomography. *Science* 254 (5035): 1178–1181.

9 Coxson, H.O., Quiney, B., Sin, D.D. et al. (2008). Airway wall thickness assessed using computed tomography and optical coherence tomography. *American Journal of Respiratory and Critical Care Medicine* 177 (11): 1201–1206.

14

Endobronchial Ultrasonography in Interventional Bronchoscopy

Christopher Kniese[1] and Ali I. Musani[2]

[1] *Indiana University School of Medicine, Indianapolis, IN, USA*
[2] *Division of Pulmonary Sciences & Critical Care Medicine, University of Colorado School of Medicine, Denver, CO, USA*

Introduction

Endobronchial ultrasound (EBUS) has gained widespread use in recent years. However, many of the earliest applications of this technology came during interventional bronchoscopy procedures [1]. These applications are still used today in selected centers, particularly in those that see a large volume of patients with large obstructive airway lesions. One of the largest series of EBUS applications was described by Becker and Herth in Heidelberg, Germany [2]. This series reflects the experience of these authors with rigid bronchoscopy and the management of central airway obstruction, as well as their pioneering role in the use of EBUS in different clinical situations. The early techniques predominantly used the 360° radial probe. In this setting, radial EBUS is used to evaluate and visualize the layers of the bronchial wall and determine whether tumor invasion has occurred, either from endobronchial lesions within the airway lumen or from external lesions. Conventional bronchoscopy, whether rigid or flexible, can only provide superficial inspection of the bronchial mucosa, with little insight into the underlying pathology. EBUS technology enhances the evaluation, allowing more accurate staging via direct assessment of tissue invasion in both early- and late-stage disease. EBUS can provide information not available via other imaging modalities, and various studies have shown superior sensitivity as a diagnostic modality when compared with conventional imaging techniques such as computed tomography (CT) or magnetic resonance imaging (MRI) [2].

Earlier chapters discussed the assessment of smaller endobronchial lesions, including assessing the depth of invasion. In this chapter additional techniques will be described, including distinguishing external airway compression from true invasion, which may have substantial treatment implications, including affecting decision-making regarding a patient's surgical candidacy. Large multicenter studies are largely lacking on these topics; however, discussing these techniques can provide a deeper understanding of the benefits of ultrasound in bronchoscopy.

Technique

In contrast to the miniature radial probe used to evaluate peripheral pulmonary lesions, ultrasound imaging of the central airways requires use of a saline-filled balloon (XMAJ-643R,

Endobronchial Ultrasonography, Second Edition. Noriaki Kurimoto, David I.K. Fielding, Ali I. Musani, Christopher Kniese, and Katsuhiko Morita.

Companion website: www.wiley.com/go/kurimoto2e

Olympus Corporation, Tokyo, Japan). The probe (XUM-BS20-26R) is passed through the working channel of the bronchoscope (channel diameter 2.8 mm or greater) and positioned adjacent to the wall at the desired evaluation site. The balloon is inflated under bronchoscopic visualization until it fills the airway lumen, in contact with the airway wall (see Figure 14.1). The most detailed EBUS images are obtained with approximately 1 cm of distance between the probe (inside the balloon) and the wall. However, it is possible to image structures up to 4 cm from the bronchial wall with this technique [3]. When assessing an airway over a given length, the preferred technique is to insert the probe and balloon at the distal end of the area of interest, inflate the balloon, then slowly retract the probe along the wall of the bronchus while viewing the ultrasound image. This ensures that the balloon is not inflated in a larger proximal airway and then forced into smaller airways, which can increase trauma and potentially damage the balloon. To inflate the balloon, the recommended procedure is to fill the balloon until it makes firm contact with the bronchial wall. Airway obstruction often occurs, including central airways that include the mainstem bronchi and trachea; however, this is generally tolerated well for short periods of time. Careful monitoring of oxygenation and ventilation parameters is paramount during this time. Prior literature has described tolerance of apnea for up to three or four minutes during evaluation of mediastinal lesions, although caution is recommended [4].

This method can also be employed with examining airways with external compression, in that the probe can be inserted past the narrowed airway with the balloon uninflated, then gently inflated to “open” the airway. Care should be taken to not overinflate the balloon to the point of causing airway injury. However, this technique will allow the operator to assess the structures external to the airway that are responsible for the compression.

To assess the ultrasound images, it is important to understand the appearance of various structures. The mucosa directly adjacent to the balloon will appear hyperechoic, with the underlying submucosal layer comparatively hypoechoic. The next two layers, the endochondrium and perichondrium, will again appear as hyperechoic layers, and at times may obscure visualization of soft tissue structures that are directly adjacent (this includes connective tissues of the mediastinum). Vascular structures such as blood vessels will appear hypoechoic

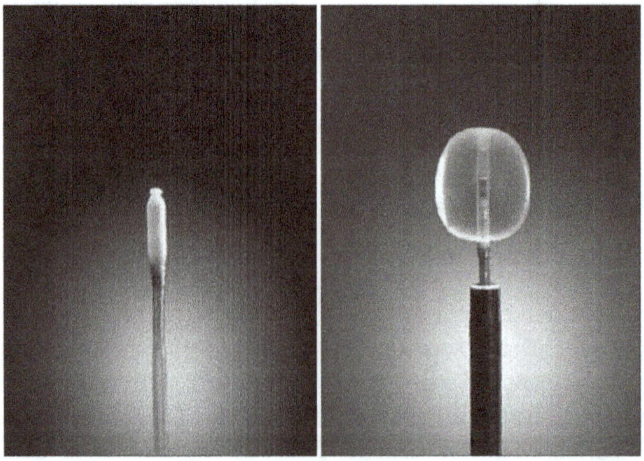

Figure 14.1 Radial probe with balloon deflated (left) and probe with balloon inflated (right) within working channel of bronchoscope. Source: Images obtained via Creative Commons license from https://openi.nlm.nih.gov/detailedresult.php?img=PMC2813108_LI-26-17-g001&query=radial+probe+ultrasound&it=xg&req=4&npos=15.

and are usually identifiable by pulsations that can be seen in real time. Detailed knowledge of the anatomic structures surrounding the airways is a necessity for the proceduralist, and comfort with identifying these structures is improved by repetition and experience. By comparison to blood vessels, lymph nodes will generally appear hyperechoic.

As a reference, important structures surrounding the right mainstem bronchus include the pulmonary trunk and the right main pulmonary artery. The left mainstem bronchus is surrounded by the pulmonary trunk, the right and (particularly) left main pulmonary artery, the ascending aorta, and the aortic arch. The distal trachea is bordered by the superior vena cava on the right, the aortic root on the left, and the azygous vein crossing at the level of the right tracheobronchial angle (see Figure 14.2).

Evaluating Tracheal Compression versus Tracheal Wall Invasion

Herth et al. reported in 2003 on the ability of EBUS to differentiate between external tumor compression and airway infiltration [5]. In this report, tumors were defined as masses adjacent to the trachea or within either tracheobronchial angle. The authors evaluated 131 patients, many of whom were believed not to be surgical candidates for a variety of reasons, including visible tumor in the trachea, contralateral disease, evidence of N3 nodal disease, and metastatic disease. In this series, 105 of these patients ultimately underwent surgery, with a majority of patients having either adenocarcinoma or squamous cell carcinoma of the lung. CT scans were performed prior to EBUS evaluation, and 81 of the 105 patients (77%) were believed to have tumor invasion, while 24 of 105 (23%) were believed to have extrinsic compression based on imaging interpretation. However, when the authors performed EBUS examination, only 49 of the 105 patients (47%) had evidence of invasion, while 56 of 105 (53%) only showed extrinsic compression. The authors then compared these results to the surgically resected specimens, considered the gold standard for evaluating airway invasion. The surgical specimens revealed that 55 of the 105 patients (53%) had airway invasion, whereas 50 patients (48%) had extrinsic compression. Therefore, radial EBUS was more accurate than CT at predicting airway invasion, with a calculated sensitivity of

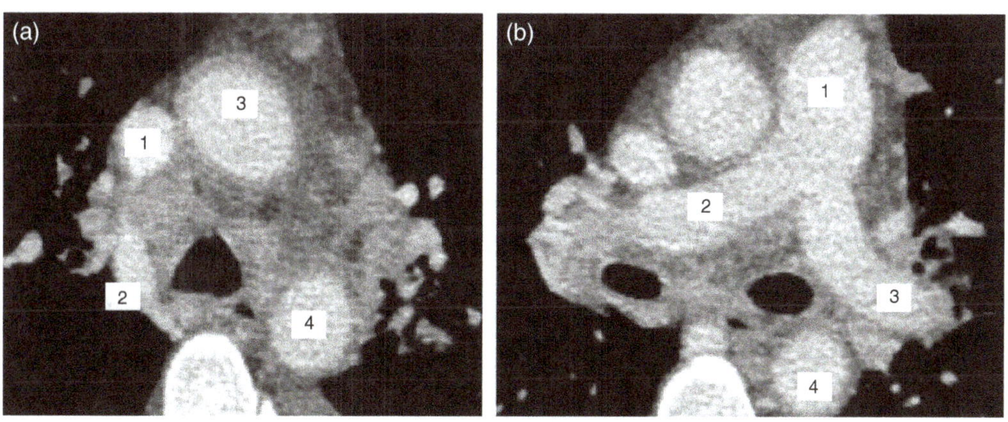

Figure 14.2 (a) Image of the distal trachea in a patient with mediastinal adenopathy. Note the following structures adjacent to the trachea: superior vena cava (1), azygous vein (2), ascending aorta (3), and descending aorta (4). (b) Computed tomography image of the left and right mainstem bronchi in the same patient. Note the following structures: main pulmonary artery (1), right pulmonary artery (2), left pulmonary artery (3), descending aorta (4).

89%, specificity of 100%, and accuracy of 94% (compared to CT with sensitivity, specificity, and accuracy of 75%, 28%, and 51%, respectively). In this series EBUS missed six cases of invasion, but overall showed a statistically significant correlation with surgical findings, whereas CT scan did not. The technique was safe, and took on average 3.5 minutes to perform, thus it represents an attractive option for staging patients with tumor adjacent to the airway. Another study reported in 2012 also assessed patients with central airway tumors with concern for invasion, and correlated EBUS imaging findings with surgical specimens [6]. In this study, radial EBUS again had a sensitivity of 89%, specificity of 100%, and accuracy of 90% for diagnosing invasion, which is quite similar to the prior results. However, this experience has not yet been validated in large, multicenter studies.

Wakamatsu et al. reported in 2006 on patients with primary thyroid and esophageal tumors [7]. They again compared EBUS to imaging modalities that included CT and MRI in the evaluation of airway invasion. However, an important difference in this study is that the EBUS findings were used to determine a patient's eligibility for surgical resection. If invasion was seen on EBUS, then patients were referred for chemotherapy and radiation. In this population, EBUS was found to have sensitivity and specificity of 92% and 83%, respectively, for detecting airway invasion. This again compared favorably to CT (sensitivity 59%, specificity 56%) and MRI (sensitivity 75%, specificity 73%). When evaluating the patients who ultimately underwent surgery, EBUS accurately diagnosed invasion in 91% of such patients, compared to approximately 50% and less that were identified on CT and MRI. This provides further support for the superiority of EBUS over these two imaging modalities for identifying airway invasion. One possible explanation for this is the superior ability of ultrasound to visualize the adventitial layer of the airway wall, which is often too small to visualize on imaging such as MRI. More recently, authors have described applying EBUS in a similar fashion to assess a patient with mucoepidermoid carcinoma in order to assess depth of invasion in the airway wall after initial endoscopic resection [8]. In this case, EBUS allowed for pre-operative assessment, and ultimately the patient was referred for curative therapy with surgical resection.

Shirakawa and others provided a nice summary of using EBUS to evaluate the various layers of the airway wall [9]. Not only did EBUS provide good resolution of the outer layers of the airway wall (unlike CT and MRI), but it also extended beyond the airway wall, providing visualization of adjacent lymphatic and vascular structures. The authors proposed a five-layered system for classifying the tracheal wall and used this system to help diagnose tracheobronchial tumor invasion. They also noted imaging patterns that seemed to point toward invasion. For example, when the outermost layer of the trachea could not be distinctly seen in the setting of an adjacent tumor, invasion was diagnosed. In addition, they noted that esophageal cancers tend to invade membranous portion of the trachea. On ultrasound, the outermost layer of this membranous portion is the adventitia; thus, interruption of this layer was used to diagnose invasion of the membranous trachea. Identification of the adventitial layer does require some experience and may be difficult for novice users initially. These authors also noted, similar to prior reports, that disruption of the tracheobronchial cartilage could be easily identified on ultrasound.

Nakamura et al. described the use of a 30 MHz probe (compared to a 20 MHz probe) in order to improve imaging resolution and better assess the layers of the airway wall [10]. In this same study they assessed a specialized software package designed to determine depth of tumor invasion in the wall of the trachea or bronchi. More importantly, they described five layers (or lamina) seen on ultrasound. These were, starting from the airway lumen, as follows: first layer, corresponding to balloon sheath and bronchial epithelium; second layer, corresponding to submucosa and smooth muscle; third layer, corresponding to luminal aspect of bronchial cartilage; fourth layer, corresponding to the bronchial cartilage; and fifth layer, corresponding to the outer edge of the cartilage and the outer bronchial wall [10]. The ultrasound images, coupled with the software program, were used to generate echo intensity curves. The authors found that the 30 MHz probe not only generated higher-resolution images, but also showed statistically significant superiority at identifying airway invasion when coupled with that particular software program. However, this software is not currently in routine use, and the most valuable conclusion is that the higher MHz probe generated higher-resolution images (albeit at the cost of lower depth of penetration).

Relapsing Polychondritis with Tracheobronchomalacia

Relapsing polychondritis (RP) is a condition that is well described in Japan and provides further insight into the broad applicability of radial probe EBUS. Miyazawa et al. first described their experience with using radial EBUS to guide stent placement in airway obstruction due to lung cancer [11]. Next, they described two patients with RP in whom EBUS played integral roles in management, one of who had previously undergone emergent tracheostomy and had developed new respiratory symptoms [12]. Bronchoscopy revealed significant tracheobronchomalacia with excessive dynamic airway collapse on expiration. Prior CT imaging had revealed significant thickening of the airway wall. EBUS performed at the time of bronchoscopy showed submucosal edema with disruption of the cartilaginous tissue in both the trachea and mainstem bronchi. Subsequent biopsies confirmed degeneration of the cartilage with inflammatory cell infiltrate consistent with RP. The second patient had EBUS evidence of cartilage degeneration demonstrated by ultrasound assessment of the airway walls, with subsequent biopsies confirming the diagnosis. In both cases the patients were treated with nitinol stents, with EBUS aiding in stent placement.

Some of these same authors again reported in 2013 on a patient who was ultimately diagnosed with RP who demonstrated cartilaginous degeneration on ultrasound imaging as well as submucosal edema [13]. Therefore, these three patients, all with RP, demonstrated two distinct ultrasound imaging patterns (fragmentation and edema); this was not previously described in the literature. Recognition of these patterns on ultrasound imaging may help differentiate RP from other forms of tracheobronchomalacia, in which the cartilaginous layers will appear intact on EBUS imaging.

Endobronchial Stenting

When placing stents to maintain airway patency, one must first determine the appropriate-sized stent. Proper sizing of the stent is essential to avoid complications such as stent migration (which primarily occurs when the stent is too small) or excessive radial force that can apply undue pressure on the airway wall (often occurring if the stent is too large). The dynamic changes in airway diameter in patients with malignant central airway obstruction can often make this size estimation difficult. The same is true in patients with tracheobronchomalacia and excessive dynamic airway collapse. These size estimations were often performed with static imaging modalities, including CT or MRI, which fail to account for the dynamic changes in airway diameter that occur with spontaneous respiration. In the same series of two patients with RP previously highlighted, the authors used radial EBUS to measure airway diameter in real time to get a better estimation of these dynamic changes [12]. This is accomplished by inflating the balloon until it is in close contact with the airway wall, and then measuring the diameter of the inflated balloon on the ultrasound image. This does require comfort on the part of the operator to determine the proper fit of the balloon in the airway, in order to prevent placement of an inappropriately sized stent. As with most applications of EBUS technology, this comfort level can be achieved with experience.

A separate series by Iwamoto et al. described patients with airway stenosis due to tuberculosis [14] who were referred for therapeutic bronchoscopy. They used EBUS in four such patients, and described the typical ultrasound findings, which included thickening of the bronchial wall and destruction of the cartilage. Those patients found to have cartilaginous destruction were again treated with endobronchial stenting.

In malignant central airway obstruction, EBUS can be used to assess the degree of airway invasion, as previously described in this chapter. In addition to the aforementioned study by Miyazawa et al., the same authors have also described using EBUS to assess the airway proximal to the tumor in order to identify areas of weakened cartilage [11, 15]. This information was clinically relevant, in that these patients were prone to proximal migration of stents due to pressure from the obstruction and proximal weakness of the cartilage; identification of these weakened points allowed for additional stenting of the weakened areas proximal to the obstruction, which improved airflow through the stented areas, supported the weakened walls, and protected against stent migration. Neither standard bronchoscopy nor CT scanning was able to provide identification of this weakened cartilage proximal to the tumors.

Herth et al. also described the ability of EBUS to aid in stent placement in a large series of patients [16]. They emphasized the ability of EBUS to identify mucosal involvement proximal to the area of obvious tumor invasion (similar to the prior description of proximal cartilaginous involvement), which led to the placement of longer airway stents to support these areas in addition to the primary tumor site. They also used EBUS to again identify sites of extrinsic compression, which also led to longer stent placement. Ultimately, in their series, EBUS aided in stent placement in 51% of patients (out of a total of 235 patients).

Brachytherapy

EBUS imaging has been applied to additional therapeutic modalities, including brachytherapy. The large series by Herth et al. in 2002 described their experience in using EBUS in prospective fashion for all patients referred for therapeutic bronchoscopy [16]. This included patients who had been referred for brachytherapy as definitive therapy. EBUS was performed prior to therapeutic interventions, and in 28% of the patients in whom brachytherapy was meant to be curative, EBUS revealed local disease extension or lymph node metastases that were previously undiagnosed, thus changing management in a substantial proportion of patients. Bronchoscopy without EBUS may underestimate the degree of airway invasion in small endobronchial lesions, thus this could falsely lead providers to perform local ablative therapies when more potent interventions such as surgical excision or external beam radiation are more appropriate. Similar findings were also published by Miyazu et al. in patients who were evaluated with EBUS prior to planned photodynamic therapy [17].

Thermal Applications

Using EBUS to aid the performance of thermal techniques, including laser and argon plasma coagulation in endobronchial tumors, was described by Herth et al. [16]. In this series, EBUS was reported to change management in 123 of the 346 patients included (36%). EBUS was used primarily to evaluate the area being treated, including the adjacent external structures such as additional tumor or large blood vessels. The operators stopped debridement when ultrasound imaging demonstrated close proximity to the large vessels. In this series, none of the patients experienced significant bleeding or fistula formation. The authors obtained images demonstrating tumor invading the airways in close proximity to the pulmonary arteries (on the anterior aspects of the bilateral mainstem bronchi). In addition, imaging was able to demonstrate tumor adjacent to the descending aorta. Importantly, to obtain ultrasound imaging in this method, only partial inflation of the balloon is required, given the reduced airway lumen due to the obstructing tumor.

Miscellaneous Applications

As the use of EBUS has rapidly expanded over the past decade, so have the numerous applications of this technology. One only need perform a quick literature search to find several publications on novel uses of this technology. A few such uses will be briefly discussed here.

Nakajima et al. reported on EBUS-guided transbronchial needle aspiration (TBNA) of a mediastinal cyst [18]. In this case, the patient had a prior thyroid goiter that was surgically resected, and now had an enlarging cyst that was compressing the membranous portion of the trachea and causing respiratory symptoms. The cyst was not amenable to percutaneous aspiration due to adjacent vasculature, and the patient was not a surgical candidate. Thus, under local anesthetic and mild conscious sedation, EBUS was used for real-time imaging of the cyst and TBNA was performed for drainage. Multiple aspirations were performed due to septations in the cyst and the patient had relief of respiratory symptoms.

Convex-probe EBUS has been reported to identify a pericardial recess that was mimicking paratracheal lymph nodes [19]. EBUS imaging showed hypodensity and the absence of vasculature in the right lower paratracheal station (station 4R). TBNA for cyst drainage could also be performed here. A separate but recent report described the use of EBUS and guide sheath to drain a lung abscess [20].

More recently, authors have described the use of EBUS to perform diagnostic biopsies of locations normally reserved for alternate procedures. Convex-probe EBUS has recently been used to perform ultrasound-guided biopsy of the thyroid gland [21]. In a separate case, operators used a convex-probe EBUS scope to visualize pleural nodules that were accessible via the esophagus and perform biopsy when traditional methods of pleural biopsy proved to be non-diagnostic [22]. In this case, a diagnosis of clear cell carcinoma was made. Placement of fiducial markers to guide stereotactic body radiation therapy (SBRT) using EBUS guidance concurrent with the patients' diagnostic and staging bronchoscopy was recently reported [23]. In addition, authors from China have recently reported on the use of EBUS elastography to evaluate mediastinal lymph nodes in an attempt to ascertain benign versus malignant adenopathy [24].

Shaw reported in 2006 on using EBUS to assess airway wall thickening, with the goal of demonstrating changes in airway wall thickness in patients treated for airway conditions such as asthma [25]. They first reported results from animal studies comparing EBUS to actual airway measurements, and subsequently human studies comparing measurements obtained on EBUS to those obtained on high-resolution CT scanning. They showed statistically significant agreement in both human and animal models. The significance of this would be to assess airway wall thickness in such patients without exposing them to unnecessary radiation.

Lastly, Irani et al. reported on the use of radial EBUS to assess the airways of lung transplant recipients [26]. The goal was to quantitatively assess the airway wall structures adjacent to the anastomosis sites and correlate these findings with outcomes such as graft rejection and infection. The authors performed 20 EBUS examinations on 10 transplant recipients, saved the images, and used software to quantitatively assess the findings. Importantly, for each patient they obtained images proximal to the anastomosis (autologous tissue) and distal to the anastomosis (allogeneic tissue). Although the overall sample size was small, they did obtain some interesting findings. They noted that the relative thickness of the second layer of tissue (the submucosa, which appears hyperechoic) was smaller in patients with graft rejection compared to those with no rejection; this finding was statistically significant. Conversely, they found that this layer was larger in patients with infection compared to those without, which was also statistically significant. A main limitation of this study was that imaging findings could not be correlated with macroscopic findings in vivo; however, the procedure was safe and could be easily performed in patients undergoing surveillance bronchoscopy post-transplant, which is a routine procedure at most institutions. These findings have not been validated by larger, multicenter studies.

References

1 Becker HD. Endobronchial ultrasound - expensive toy or useful tool? *Proceedings of the 8th World Congress for Bronchoesophagology*, Munich 1994, abstract no. 237.

2 Becker, H.D. and Herth, F. (2000). Endobronchial ultrasound of the airways and the mediastinum. In: Progress in Respiratory Research. Vol 30: Interventional Bronchoscopy (eds. C.T. Bolliger and P.N. Mathur), 80–93. Basel-Freiburg: S. Karger.

3 Becker, H.D. (2005). The role of endobronchial ultrasound (EBUS) in diagnosis and treatment of centrally located early lung cancer. In: Textbook of Prevention and Detection of Early Lung Cancer (eds. F.R. Hirsh, P.A. Bunn, H. Kato and J.L. Mulshine), 168–175. London: Taylor and Francis.

4 Frietsch, T., Becker, H.D., Bulzebruck, H., and Wiedemann, K. (2000). Capnometry for rigid bronchoscopy and high frequency jet ventilation compared to arterial pCO_2. *Acta Anesthesiologica Scandinavica* 44: 391–397.

5 Herth, F.J., Ernst, A., Schulz, M. et al. (2003). Endobronchial ultrasound reliably differentiates between airway infiltration and compression by tumor. *Chest* 123: 458–462.

6 Li, J., Chen, P.P., Huang, Y., and Chen, Z.X. (2012). Radial probe endobronchial ultrasound scanning assessing invasive depth of central lesion in the tracheobronchial wall. *Chinese Medical Journal* 125 (17): 3008–3014.

7 Wakamatsu, T., Tsushima, K., Yasuo, M. et al. (2006). Usefulness of preoperative endobronchial ultrasound for airway invasion around the trachea: oesphageal cancer and thyroid cancer. *Respiration* 73: 651–657.

8 Rehman, S., Lovvorn, H.N. 3rd, Rickman, O.B. et al. (2018). Unique application of awake tracheoscopy and endobronchial ultrasound in the management of tracheal mucoepidermoid carcinoma. *Head & Neck* 40 (6): E58–E61.

9 Shirakawa, T., Tanaka, F., and Becker, H.D. (2001). Layer structure of the central airways viewed using endobronchial ultrasonography (EBUS). In: Bronchology and Bronchoesophagology. State of the Art (eds. H. Yoshimura, A. Kida, T. Arai, et al.), 921–923. Amsterdam: Elsevier.

10 Nakamura, Y., Endo, C., Sato, M. et al. (2004). New technique for endobronchial ultrasonography and comparison of two ultrasonic probes: analysis with a plot profile of the image analysis software NIH image. *Chest* 126: 192–197.

11 Miyazawa, T., Miyazu, Y., Iwamoto, Y. et al. (2004). Stenting of the flow limiting segment in tracheobronchial stenosis in lung cancer. *American Journal of Respiratory Critical Care Medicine* 169: 1096–1102.

12 Miyazu, Y., Miyazawa, T., Kurimoto, N. et al. (2003). Endobronchial ultrasonography in the diagnosis and treatment of relapsing

polychondritis with tracheobronchial malacia. *Chest* 124: 2393–2395.
13 Eksombatchai, D., Boonsarngsuk, V., Amornputtisathaporn, N. et al. (2013). Tracheobronchial involvement in relapsing polychondritis diagnosed on endobronchial ultrasound. *Internal Medicine* 52: 801–805.
14 Iwamoto, Y., Miyazawa, T., Kurimoto, N. et al. (2004). Interventional bronchoscopy in the management of airway stenosis due to tracheobronchial tuberculosis. *Chest* 126: 1344–1352.
15 Miyazawa, T., Yamakido, M., Ikeda, S. et al. (2000). Implantation of Ultraflex nitinol stents in malignant tracheobronchial stenosis. *Chest* 118: 959–965.
16 Herth, F., Becker, H.D., LoCicero, J., and Ernst, A. (2002). Endobronchial ultrasound in therapeutic bronchoscopy. *European Respiratory Journal* 20: 118–121.
17 Miyazu, Y., Miyazawa, T., Kurimoto, N. et al. (2001). Endobronchial ultrasonography in the assessment of centrally located early-stage lung cancer before photodynamic therapy. *American Journal of Respiratory Critical Care Medicine* 165: 832–837.
18 Nakajima, T., Yasufuku, K., Shibuya, K., and Fujisawa, T. (2007). Endobronchial ultrasound guided transbronchial needle aspiration for the treatment of central airway stenosis caused by a mediastinal cyst. *European Journal of Cardiothoracic Surgery* 32: 538–540.
19 Fielding, D., Hundloe, J., Windsor, M. et al. (2008). High riding pericardial recess: findings on EBUS TBNA. *Journal of Bronchology* 15: 182–184.
20 Miki, M. (2019). Standard and novel additional (optional) therapy for lung abscess by drainage using bronchoscopic endobronchial ultrasonography with a guide sheath (EBUS-GS). *Internal Medicine* 58 (1): 1–2. https://doi.org/10.2169/internalmedicine.0968-18.
21 Sapalidis, K., Kosmidis, C., Laskou, S. et al. (2018). Convex-probe endobronchial ultrasound for thyroid biopsy: a new hybrid method. *Respiratory Medicine Case Reports* 23: 125–127.
22 Kassirer, M., Wiesen, J., Atlan, K., and Avriel, A. (2018). Sampling pleural nodules with an EBUS scope: a novel application. *Respiratory Medicine Case Reports* 25: 36–38.
23 Seides, B.J., Egan, J.P. 3rd, French, K.D. et al. (2018). Fiducial marker placement for stereotactic body radiation therapy via convex probe endobronchial ultrasound: a case series and review of literature. *Journal of Thoracic Diseases* 10 (3): 1972–1983.
24 Gu, Y., Shi, H., Su, C. et al. (2017). The role of endobronchial ultrasound elastrography in the diagnosis of mediastinal and hilar lymph nodes. *Oncotarget* 8 (51): 89194–89202.
25 Shaw, T.J., Wakely, S.L., Peebles, C.R. et al. (2004). Endobronchial ultrasound to assess airway wall thickening: validation in vitro and in vivo. *European Respiratory Journal* 23: 813–817.
26 Irani, S., Hess, T., Hofer, M. et al. (2006). Endobronchial ultrasonography for the quantitative assessment of bronchial mural structures in lung transplant recipients. *Chest* 129: 349–355.

15

Cytopathology in Endobronchial Ultrasound-Guided Transbronchial Needle Aspiration of Mediastinal and Hilar Lymph Nodes

Christopher Kniese[1] and Ali I. Musani[2]

[1] *Indiana University School of Medicine, Indianapolis, IN, USA*
[2] *Division of Pulmonary Sciences & Critical Care Medicine, University of Colorado School of Medicine, Denver, CO, USA*

Introduction

Cytopathology refers to that branch of pathology that specifically focuses on the examination of cells obtained during tissue sampling to evaluate for the presence or absence of disease [1]. Sporadic reports of cytologic analyses appeared in the medical literature in the nineteenth century, but it was the work of Dr. Papanicolaou that is credited with expanding the field [1]. Today, cytologic analysis is performed on tissue samples obtained from a wide range of diagnostic and therapeutic procedures. This chapter will focus specifically on cytopathology as it pertains to bronchoscopy, with a particular focus on rapid on-site evaluation (ROSE). We aim to provide a brief overview of this practice, with an emphasis on recent publications that highlight the utility of ROSE from the perspective of the bronchoscopist. For a detailed description of this field, we recommend the reader consult the pathology literature.

Technique

ROSE refers to the practice of preparing cytologic specimens during bronchoscopy (or an equivalent tissue sampling procedure) and evaluating them as the procedure is ongoing. The main goal is to provide preliminary information regarding sampling adequacy and diagnosis [2]. This is generally accomplished by having a trained technician and cytopathologist come to the procedure room, collect specimens directly from the operator, and prepare slides for immediate evaluation.

ROSE is most commonly performed on transbronchial needle aspiration (TBNA) specimens, but can also be applied to forceps biopsies and brush specimens. The technique for performing TBNA is discussed in stepwise fashion in Chapter 4. Once a specimen is obtained, the needle is then taken to the cytotechnologist, and aspirate material is placed on slides using a touch preparation technique [3]. This should be performed immediately to avoid coagulation of aspirate material within the needle. First, the stylet is passed through the needle to expel material onto the slide, followed by air or saline instillation if needed. Any material left in the needle after slide preparation is collected in either saline- or formalin-filled containers for preparation of cell block. Slides are most commonly prepared using the Diff-Quik stain. This is an alcohol-based protocol that is a modification of prior staining techniques such as Giemsa stains and was designed for rapid preparation

Endobronchial Ultrasonography, Second Edition. Noriaki Kurimoto, David I.K. Fielding, Ali I. Musani, Christopher Kniese, and Katsuhiko Morita.

Companion website: www.wiley.com/go/kurimoto2e

and evaluation [4]. The slides are air-dried, then passed through successive solutions in a protocol that takes less than five minutes to complete [5]. When completed, this protocol produces slides with excellent cytologic detail, comparable to that of the Papanicolaou stain, that allow the pathologist to provide initial evaluation of TBNA or fine-needle aspiration (FNA) specimens [6]. These slides are then reviewed using microscopy, often with the pathologist in the operating room or bronchoscopy suite, to allow direct communication with the bronchoscopist about preliminary findings. See Figures 15.1 and 15.2 for an illustration of slide sample handling and slide preparation. Several examples of touch preparation slides with corresponding cell block images from samples obtained during EBUS-TBNA are shown in Figures 15.3–15.6.

It is important to note that ROSE only examines portions of specimens obtained during TBNA or FNA sampling. Additional material that is not prepared on slides is placed directly into containers for further processing. Thus, it is highly possible that specimens initially labeled "negative" or "non-diagnostic" on ROSE could later yield a diagnosis once the final pathologic evaluation is complete.

Role of Rapid On-Site Evaluation in Endobronchial Ultrasonography

ROSE aims to provide the bronchoscopist with preliminary information on the adequacy of tissue sampling. In theory, when initial sampling is deemed adequate to confirm a diagnosis, this should obviate the need for additional tissue sampling. However, data regarding its true utility is mixed. A prospective, randomized controlled trial comparing endobronchial ultrasonography (EBUS) with and without ROSE showed that patients who underwent EBUS with ROSE had a significantly lower need for additional bronchoscopic procedures, as well as a lower number of needle punctures performed on target lesions [8]. This same study showed no difference in mean procedure time. A recent systematic review assessing the available randomized controlled trials reached a similar conclusion, that ROSE could reduce the number of needle passes required during procedures and reduce the need for additional bronchoscopies [9].

Data regarding the effect of ROSE on diagnostic yield is less promising. In multiple studies, ROSE has not been shown to improve the diagnostic accuracy of EBUS-TBNA [9, 10]. Another recent study assessing 170 patients who underwent EBUS for mediastinal staging showed that despite ROSE suggesting inadequate tissue in 30 patients, 22 of those ultimately received a diagnosis from final pathologic assessment [11]. Thus, the authors concluded that ROSE did not significantly impact clinical decision-making during the procedure. This finding conflicts with prior studies suggesting that ROSE may reduce the number of needle passes performed during procedures. A separate study recently assessed the concordance rate between initial assessment via ROSE and final pathologic diagnosis, with an overall concordance rate of 94% [12]. Therefore, data reported in the literature to date is variable.

Another key factor in evaluating the efficacy of ROSE is assessment of sample adequacy, which differs from diagnostic yield. Sample adequacy refers to whether or not the tissue samples obtained were sufficient to yield a diagnosis. Much like diagnostic accuracy, sample adequacy is a key performance metric in the assessment of EBUS-TBNA. A recent meta-analysis that synthesized data from 25 studies concluded that on average, ROSE improved sample adequacy by 12% when compared with cohorts that did not use ROSE [13]. Given the emerging role of EBUS-TBNA as the initial minimally invasive staging procedure of choice, this improvement is significant.

EBUS-TBNA with the application of ROSE can be used outside of suspected pulmonary malignancy as well. There is an increasing body of literature regarding the diagnosis of lymphoma using mediastinal TBNA, and ROSE can

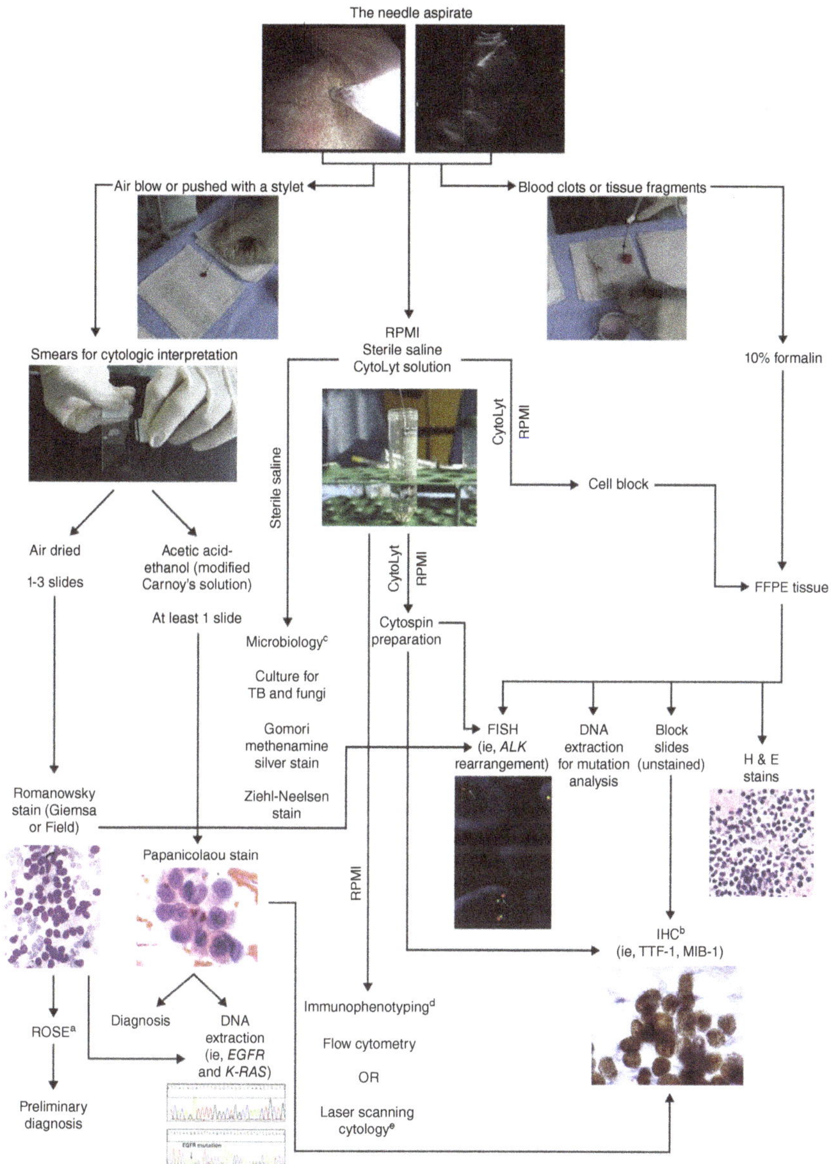

Figure 15.1 Handling of transbronchial needle aspiration specimens obtained during endobronchial ultrasonography-guided lymph node sampling. *Source:* Figure reprinted with permission from authors and Elsevier [7].

Diagram depicting a potential algorithm for sample preparation and handling of EBUS and conventional TBNA specimens in NSCLC, including recommendations for pathologic diagnosis and molecular testing.

Abbreviations: EBUS = endobronchial ultrasound; FFPE = formalin-fixed, paraffin-embedded; FISH = fluorescence in situ hybridization; H & E = hematoxylin and eosin stain; IHC = immuno-histochemistry; MIB-1 = monoclonal antibody against the Ki-67 antigen; NSCLC = non–small-cell lung cancer; ROSE = rapid on-site evaluation; RPMI = Roswell Park Memorial Institute (medium); TB = tuberculosis; TBNA = transbronchial needle aspiration; TTF-1 = thyroid transcription factor-1.

[a] ROSE is used to detect quantity and quality of the specimen for diagnosis and to allocate the specimen for cell block and IHC and molecular analysis.

[b] IHC is used if diagnosis needs to be confirmed but ideally 1 marker should be used (ie, TTF-1 for adenocarcinoma, p40 for squamous cell carcinoma).

[c] Microbiology studies are ordered based on clinical suspicion of infection and/or if ROSE showed granulomas with or without caseation; physicians should contact their local laboratories to determine the preferred medium for transport.

[d] Immunophenotyping is ordered when there is clinical suspicion of lymphoma and when ROSE shows "reactive lymphadenopathy."

[e] Laser scanning cytology requires 15,000 cells to run the full panel.

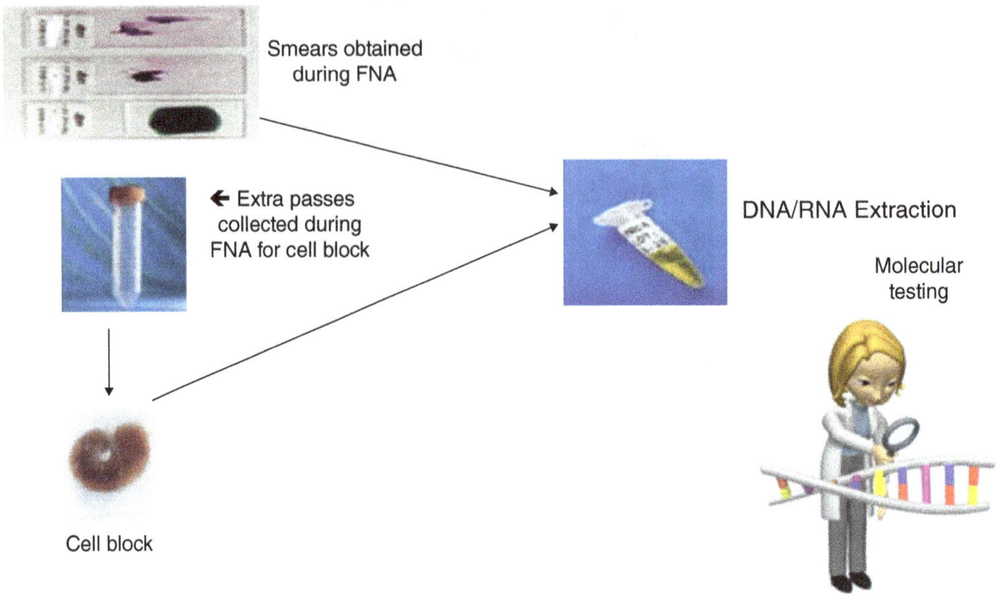

Figure 15.2 Further illustration of sample handling. FNA, fine-needle aspiration. *Source:* Figure reprinted with permission from authors and Elsevier [7].

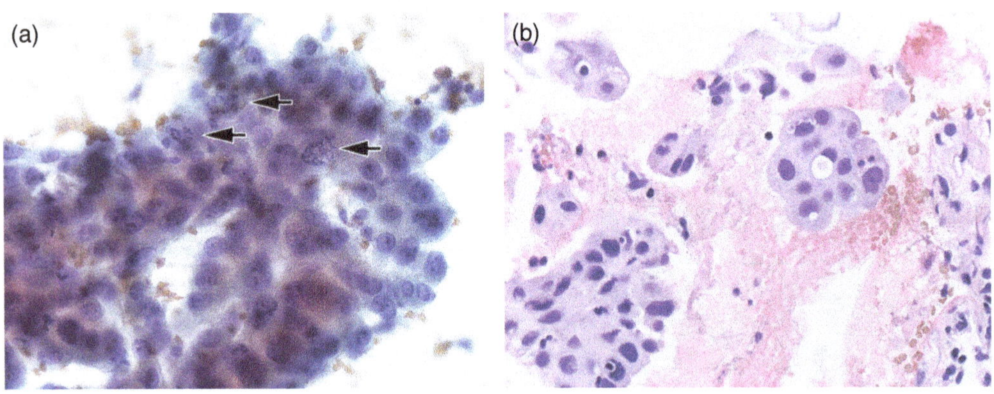

Figure 15.3 (a) Cytology slide using Papanicolaou stain at 400× magnification in a patient with adenocarcinoma. Arrows indicate mitotic figures. (b) Cell block material prepared from the same patient at 400× magnification. *Source:* Images courtesy of Sharon Sams, MD, and Lisa Litzenberger, Department of Pathology, University of Colorado Denver School of Medicine, USA.

assist in this regard. A recent prospective series demonstrated that TBNA, combined with ROSE, is reliable in not only diagnosing but also subtyping lymphoma [14]. The authors in this paper provide a nice outline of which cytologic procedures are necessary for the various subtypes. For example, cell block preparations are generally adequate for Hodgkin's and high-grade non-Hodgkin's subtypes, whereas low-grade lymphomas and benign hyperplasia are often distinguished by the addition of flow cytometry to cytologic specimens [14].

ROSE can be useful in the diagnosis of benign conditions as well. In particular, sarcoid and infections are often identified on TBNA specimens. EBUS-guided TBNA has shown superiority to conventional TBNA in the diagnosis of sarcoid, with a diagnostic yield of 83.3% compared to 53.8% in the non-EBUS-guided group [15]. ROSE can be helpful in this

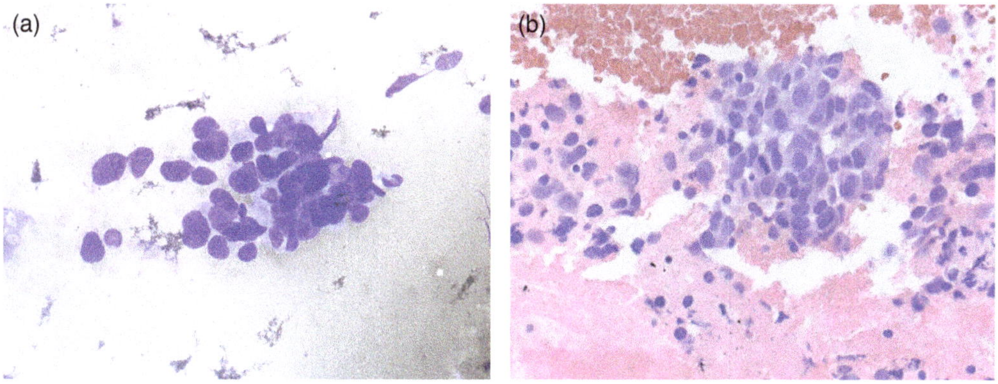

Figure 15.4 (a) Cytology slide using Diff-Quik stain at 400× magnification in a patient with small cell carcinoma. (b) Cell block material prepared from the same patient at 400× magnification. *Source:* Images courtesy of Sharon Sams, MD, and Lisa Litzenberger, Department of Pathology, University of Colorado Denver School of Medicine, USA.

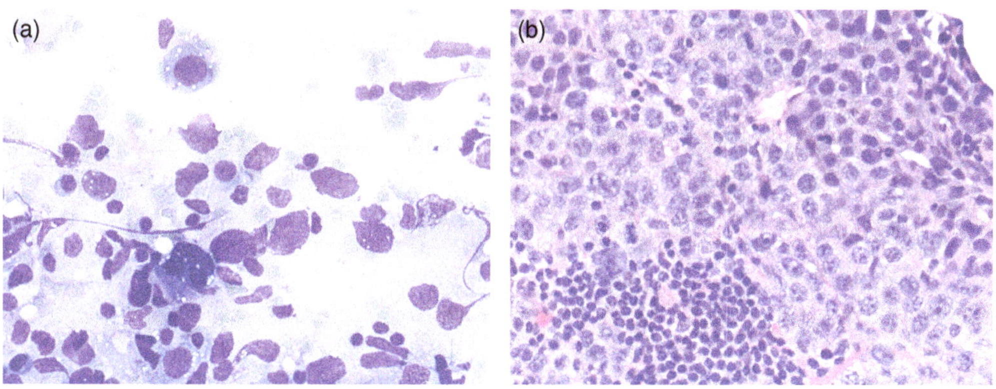

Figure 15.5 (a) Cytology slide using Diff-Quik stain at 400× magnification showing atypical lymphocytes with minimal cytoplasm in a patient with lymphoma. (b) Cell block material prepared from the same patient at 400× magnification. *Source:* Images courtesy of Sharon Sams, MD, and Lisa Litzenberger, Department of Pathology, University of Colorado Denver School of Medicine, USA.

regard, in that identification of the characteristic non-caseating granulomas on TBNA specimens is often diagnostic and can significantly narrow the differential diagnosis in the patient with adenopathy (see Figure 15.6). It remains standard practice to perform additional maneuvers such as bronchoalveolar lavage to rule out infectious causes of granulomatous inflammation in such patients. Aside from sarcoid, EBUS-TBNA is now accepted as a diagnostic tool for diagnosis of tuberculosis as well. A recent large study concluded that EBUS-TBNA, combined with cytologic and microbiologic examination, had a sensitivity of 87.5% for the diagnosis of mediastinal tuberculous lymphadenitis [16]. ROSE should again look for granulomatous inflammation in these patients, although unlike in sarcoid these granulomas often contain necrosis. In addition, adding the Xpert MTB/RIF assay to EBUS-TBNA specimens has been described and may aid in more rapid diagnosis in patients with suspected tuberculosis [17].

Given that ROSE appears to reduce the number of biopsies performed intraoperatively, cost reduction is an additional potential benefit. A recent economic study performed in Canada sought to evaluate the cost-effectiveness of ROSE

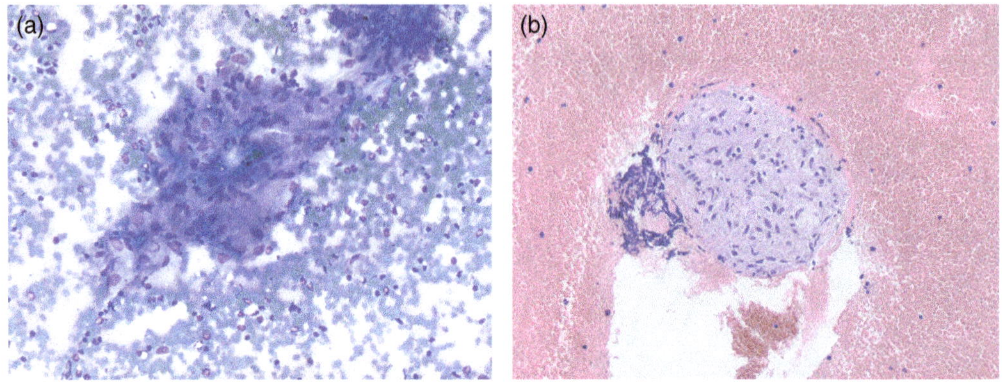

Figure 15.6 (a) Cytology slide using Diff-Quik stain at 400× magnification in a patient with sarcoidosis showing the characteristic non-caseating granulomas. (b) Cell block material prepared from the same patient at 400× magnification. *Source:* Images courtesy of Sharon Sams, MD, and Lisa Litzenberger, Department of Pathology, University of Colorado Denver School of Medicine, USA.

combined with EBUS-TBNA [18]. Based on a simulated model, the authors concluded ROSE to be cost-saving in both cancer as well as sarcoidosis, an increasingly common application of this technology. The projected cost savings were modest, but this finding is noteworthy given that one potential criticism of the use of ROSE is the need for additional trained personnel at the time of the procedure.

Based on the favorable risk to benefit profile, ROSE is now routinely performed during EBUS at most large high-volume centers. The main limitation for the utilization of ROSE is usually local resources, thus for those looking to establish EBUS programs at new centers it is important to develop collaborative relationships with cytopathologists in order to facilitate this process. Currently, multiple expert panels recommend on-site evaluation during EBUS whenever possible. The Pulmonary Pathology Society recently published its recommendations regarding the use of ROSE to aid in EBUS procedures [2]. Likewise, the World Association for Bronchology and Interventional Pulmonology has published similar recommendations [19]. Therefore, those looking to build a successful endobronchial ultrasound program should consider ROSE as an integral feature.

Recent Advances in ROSE during EBUS-TBNA

Recent advances in EBUS-TBNA have mirrored those in thoracic oncology, with current interest in obtaining adequate specimens for testing beyond simple cytopathologic or histopathologic analysis. A recent study sought to develop an algorithmic approach to assessing sample adequacy in real time, using the following criteria: core size ≥2 cm, presence of malignant cells, presence of microscopic anthracotic pigment (MAP), and lymphocyte density (LD) of ≥40 cells/field at 40× magnification [20]. In this study of 300 lymph nodes sampled, when all four criteria were met the sensitivity and accuracy rates of ROSE increased from 64.4% and 64.7% to 98.6% and 97.3%, respectively, when compared to samples that did not meet the criteria [20].

In the age of modern oncology, testing for molecular markers is a particular area of interest given the advances in targeted therapeutics. Thus, an important aim of EBUS-TBNA sampling is not only to provide a diagnosis, but also to obtain adequate tissue to allow for additional testing on specimens. This generally requires that more lymph node or tumor tissue be obtained, although this field is continuing to evolve, and as time progresses we are developing new ways to test different types of cellular specimens, including pleural fluid.

There are several molecular targets of interest, and the role of EBUS-TBNA has rapidly expanded in recent years as more studies have shown that needle aspirate specimens can be used to evaluate for these markers. Studies have shown that molecular analyses such as epidermal growth factor receptor (EGFR), Kirsten rat sarcoma viral oncogene (KRAS), B-raf proto oncogene (BRAF), and phosphoinositide-3-kinase, catalytic, alpha polypeptide (PIK3CA) are feasible on cytologic specimens and provide results which in about 80% of cases are equivalent to those obtained from histologic specimens [21]. Generally adequate tissue for this testing can be obtained by one or two additional passes, on top of the standard three passes performed on each lymph node. TBNA specimens have also shown feasibility for testing for anaplastic lymphoma kinase (ALK) fusion mutations, yet another common molecular target in modern cancer therapeutics [22]. Most importantly, tissue obtained during TBNA can be used to test for multiple mutations, thus limiting the need for larger surgical or histopathologic specimens [23].

Additionally, recent studies have shown that cytology specimens can be used to determine expression of programmed death-ligand 1 (PD-L1) and are comparable to surgical specimens [24]. Use of a 19 gauge core needle to obtain specimens for PD-L1 testing has been reported [25]. However, a recent study comparing diagnostic yield between 19 and 22 G needles showed no difference between the two, and actually suggested that the 19 G needle may be more likely to obtain inadequate, bloody specimens [26]. Therefore, the debate about optimal needle size for obtaining tissue for molecular markers is ongoing, with most clinicians using standard (21 or 22 G) needles during tissue sampling.

One last concept that has been studied is the performance of on-site evaluation by non-cytopathologists. A recent meta-analysis reviewing the literature on this topic showed substantial heterogeneity among the studies, with differences in who performed the evaluations, as well as wide variation in the reported diagnostic accuracy [27]. Based on this, we cannot currently recommend this practice.

References

1 Naylor, B. (2000). The century for cytopathology. *Acta Cytologica* 44 (5): 709–725.

2 Jain, D., Allen, T.C., Aisner, D. et al. (2018). Rapid on-site evaluation of endobronchial ultrasound-guided transbronchial needle aspirations for the diagnosis of lung cancer: a perspective from members of the Pulmonary Pathology Society. *Archives of Pathology & Laboratory Medicine* 142: 253–262.

3 Hahn, P.F., Eisenberg, P.J., Pitman, M.B. et al. (1995). Cytologic touch preparations (imprints) from core needle biopsies: accuracy compared with that of fine-needle aspirates. *American Journal of Roentgenology* 165: 1277–1279.

4 Silverman, J.F. and Frable, W.J. (1990). The use of the Diff-Quik stain in the immediate interpretation of fine-needle aspiration biopsies. *Diagnostic Cytopathology* 6 (5): 366–369.

5 Hirschowitz, S.L., Mandell, D., Nieberg, R.K., and Carson, K. (1994). The alcohol-fixed Diff-Quik stain. A novel rapid stain for the immediate interpretation of fine needle aspiration specimens. *Acta Cytologica* 38 (4): 499–501.

6 Henry, M.J., Burton, L.G., Stanley, M.W., and Horwitz, C.A. (1987). Application of a modified Diff-Quik stain to fine needle aspiration smears: rapid staining with improved cytologic detail. *Acta Cytologica* 31 (6): 954–955.

7 Murgu, S. and Colt, H. (2013). Role of the pulmonologist in ordering post-procedure molecular markers in non-small cell lung cancer: implications for personalized medicine. *Clinical Lung Cancer* 14 (6): 609–626.

8 Oki, M., Saka, H., Kitagawa, C. et al. (2013). Rapid on-site evaluation during endobronchial ultrasound-guided transbronchial needle aspiration for diagnosing lung cancer: a randomized study. *Respiration* 85: 486–492.

9 Sehgal, I.S., Dhooria, S., Aggarwal, A.N., and Agarwal, R. (2018). Impact of rapid on-site cytological evaluation (ROSE) on the diagnostic yield of transbronchial needle aspiration during mediastinal lymph node sampling: systematic review and meta-analysis. *Chest* 153 (4): 929–938.

10 Cardoso, A.V., Neves, I., Magalhaes, A. et al. (2015). The value of rapid on-site evaluation during EBUS-TBNA. *Revista Portuguesa de Pneumologia* 21 (5): 253–258.

11 Joseph, M., Jones, T., Lutterbie, Y. et al. (2013). Rapid on-site pathologic evaluation does not increase the efficacy of endobronchial ultrasonographic biopsy for mediastinal staging. *Annals of Thoracic Surgery* 96: 403–410.

12 Nakajima, T., Yasufuku, K., Saegusa, F. et al. (2013). Rapid on-site cytologic evaluation during endobronchial ultrasound-guided transbronchial needle aspiration for nodal staging in patients with lung cancer. *Annals of Thoracic Surgery* 95: 1695–1699.

13 Schmidt, R.L., Witt, B.L., Lopez-Calderon, L.E., and Layfield, L.J. (2013). The influence of rapid onsite evaluation on the adequacy rate of fine-needle aspiration cytology. *American Journal of Clinical Pathology* 139: 300–308.

14 Moonim, M.T., Breen, R., Fields, P.A., and Santis, G. (2013). Diagnosis and subtyping of de novo and relapsed mediastinal lymphomas by endobronchial ultrasound needle aspiration. *American Journal of Respiratory Critical Care Medicine* 188 (10): 1216–1223.

15 Tremblay, A., Stather, D.R., MacEachem, P. et al. (2009). A randomized controlled trial of standard vs endobronchial ultrasonography-guided transbronchial needle aspiration in patients with suspected sarcoidosis. *Chest* 136 (2): 340–346.

16 Erer, O.F., Erol, S., Anar, C. et al. (2017). The diagnostic accuracy of endobronchial ultrasound-guided transbronchial needle aspiration (EBUS-TBNA) in mediastinal tuberculous lymphadenitis. *Turkish Journal of Medical Sciences* 47 (6): 1874–1879.

17 Lee, J., Choi, S.M., Lee, C.H. et al. (2017). The additional role of Xpert MTB/RIF in the diagnosis of intrathoracic tuberculous lymphadenitis. *Journal of Infection and Chemotherapy* 23 (6): 381–384.

18 Kalluri, M., Puttagunta, L., Ohinmaa, A. et al. (2015). Cost analysis of intra-procedural rapid on-site evaluation of cytopathology with endobronchial ultrasound. *International Journal of Technology Assessment in Health Care* 31 (5): 273–280.

19 Van der Heijden, E.H.F.M., Casal, R.F., Trisolini, R. et al. (2014). Guideline for the acquisition and preparation of conventional and endobronchial ultrasound-guided transbronchial needle aspiration specimens for the diagnosis and molecular testing of patients with known or suspected lung cancer. *Respiration* 88: 500–517.

20 Choi, S.M., Lee, A.R., Choe, J.Y. et al. (2016). Adequacy criteria of rapid on-site evaluation for endobronchial ultrasound-guided transbronchial needle aspiration: a simple algorithm to assess the adequacy of ROSE. *Annals of Thoracic Surgery* 101: 444–450.

21 Pusztaszeri, M., Soccal, P.M., Mach, N. et al. (2011). Cytopathological diagnosis of non small cell lung cancer: recent advances including rapid on-site evaluation, novel endoscopic techniques and molecular test. *Journal of Pulmonary and Respiratory Medicine* S5: 002.

22 Sakairi, Y., Nakajima, T., Yasufuku, K. et al. (2010). EML4-ALK fusion gene assessment using metastatic lymph node samples

obtained by endobronchial ultrasound-guided transbronchial needle aspiration. *Clinical Cancer Research* 16 (20): 4938–4945.

23 Nakajima, T., Yasufuku, K., Nakagawara, A. et al. (2011). Multigene mutation analysis of metastatic lymph nodes in non-small cell lung cancer diagnosed by endobronchial ultrasound-guided transbronchial needle aspiration. *Chest* 140 (5): 1319–1324.

24 Heymann, J.J., Bulman, W.A., Swinarski, D. et al. (2017). PD-L1 expression in non-small cell lung carcinoma: comparison among cytology, small biopsy, and surgical resection specimens. *Cancer Cytopathology* 125: 896–907.

25 Herath, S. and Cooper, W.A. (2017). The novel 19G endobronchial USS (EBUS) needle samples processed as tissue "core biopsies" facilitate PD-L1 and other biomarker testing in lung cancer specimens: case and the view point from the respiratory physician and the pathologist. *Respirology Case Reports* 5 (6): e00271.

26 Chadda, U., Ronaghi, R., Elatre, W. et al. (2018). Comparison of sample adequacy and diagnostic yield of 19- and 22-G EBUS-TBNA needles. *Journal of Bronchology & Interventional Pulmonology* 25 (4): 264–268.

27 Pearson, L., Factor, R.E., White, S.K. et al. (2018). Rapid on-site evaluation of fine-needle aspiration by non-cytopathologists: a systematic review and meta-analysis of diagnostic accuracy studies for adequacy assessment. *Acta Cytologica* 62 (4): 244–252.

16

Future Directions for Endobronchial Ultrasonography

David I.K. Fielding

Royal Brisbane and Women's Hospital, Herston, Queensland, Australia

Peripheral Pulmonary Lesions and EBUS

Izumo et al. have reported [1] on rapid on-site cytologic evaluation (ROSE) during endobronchial ultrasound (EBUS) with a guide sheath (GS). This could become important to reduce procedure time, but also facilitate triaging of specimens for molecular purposes. Modified Giemsa (Diff-Quik) staining was used for ROSE and conventional air-dried slides were also taken. Additional cytology smears were prepared for Papanicolaou staining. Results of 718 cases of ROSE were compared to the final cytology results. The sensitivity, specificity, positive predictive value (PPV), negative predictive value (NPV), and diagnostic accuracy of ROSE during EBUS GS for peripheral pulmonary lesions were 88.6%, 65.9%, 81.2%, 77.7%, and 80.1%, respectively. Regarding triaging in addition to saving specimens for molecular tests, the authors commented that if, for example, ROSE shows that there are several neutrophils or macrophages, bacterial culture would be recommended. It is likely that ROSE use will continue to grow in the era of molecular individualized medicine. Regarding ground-glass opacities, in 167 cases there were slight differences in the diagnostic parameters of ROSE: the sensitivity, specificity, PPV, and NPV were 88%, 54%, 72%, and 80%, respectively.

Steinfort et al. also reported on the benefits of ROSE in 128 cases [2]: where ROSE was positive the procedure time was reduced by 12 minutes on average (19 vs. 31 minutes, $p < 0.0001$). They commented on the benefits of using ROSE (negative) to prompt a move of the sheath to a different subsegment. For malignancy there were PPV and NPV of ROSE of 97% and 68%, respectively.

Maekura et al. [3] have similarly reported from 50 cases with lesions <30 mm PPV and NPV of ROSE for malignancy of 97% and 80%, respectively. They commented on the way ROSE could prompt a change in technique: the use of larger forceps without a GS meant larger samples could be taken. Similarly, negative ROSE could prompt the use of a curette. Others have reposted the use of ROSE to be effective in very large tumors (>70 mm) which have necrotic centers, hence the ability to find viable parts of the tumor by shifting site on the basis of ROSE findings [4].

Genetics of small samples in the lung periphery is another key topic which will undoubtedly be the subject of much study. EBUS GS will be part of this field, especially as it is easier to repeat such samples than with computed tomography fine-needle aspiration (CT-FNA).

Endobronchial Ultrasonography, Second Edition. Noriaki Kurimoto, David I.K. Fielding, Ali I. Musani, Christopher Kniese, and Katsuhiko Morita.

Companion website: www.wiley.com/go/kurimoto2e

Izumo et al. [5] studied rebiopsy for resistant non-small cell lung cancer (NSCLC) after treatment with epidermal growth factor receptor–tyrosine kinase inhibitors (EGFR-TKIs). The goal was to determine how well EBUS GS biopsies could provide tissue for molecular re-evaluation. From 44 patients with peripheral masses, 33 specimens were adequate for reanalysis for mutations (75%). This compared to 100% of 9 cases with repeat samples using EBUS-TBNA (transbronchial needle aspiration). Where positive, either the original mutation was seen (Del 19 or L858R, or L816Q), or an additional T790M. The main limitation to obtaining good tissue was a more peripherally placed tumor. Nonetheless, this form of biopsy is very likely to become commonplace.

Guisier et al. performed a similar study but on newly diagnosed cancers [6]. They assessed the predictive factors of molecular analysis feasibility from samples of peripheral non-squamous NSCLC obtained by EBUS GS and 1.5 mm microbiopsy forceps. Mutations assessed were EGFR, Kirsten rat sarcoma viral oncogene homolog (KRAS), anaplastic lymphoma kinase (ALK), HER2, PI3K, BRAF, c-MET, and ROS1. After cytologic and histologic analysis, unstained slides or paraffin blocks were used for molecular analysis. The feasibility of molecular analysis was assessed by the pathologist on the basis of the remaining material after standard staining and immunostaining. The percentage of tumor cells on hematoxylin and eosin (H&E) slides was quantified, but was not considered a limiting factor for molecular analysis. From 113 procedures (mean nodule diameter 28 ± 15 mm), 41 mutations were identified (23 KRAS,10 EGFR, 2 BRAF, 1 HER2, and 5 ALK rearrangements). Four c-MET overexpressions were noted. Overall multigene molecular analysis could be performed in nearly 80% of paraffin-embedded biopsies or smear specimens sampled. Feasibility of molecular analysis rose from 67% for the first 57 procedures to 89% for the last 56 procedures ($p = 0.02$), likely due to a higher number of biopsies performed (2 ± 1 vs. 3 ± 2, $p = 0.005$). Percentage of tumor cells, size of lesion, and distance to the pleura did not correlate with molecular feasibility.

Factors correlated with the ability to do molecular analysis were biopsy samples (odds ratio [OR] 4.49, 95% confidence interval [CI]: 1.79–11.30, $p = 0.001$) rather than brushing; at least three biopsies performed (OR 4.29, 95% CI: 1.69–10.90, $p = 0.002$); and insufficient material for two or more immunostainings (OR 0.27, 95% CI: 0.11–0.67, $p = 0.005$). The authors commented that these samples provided similar genetic material to that reported in a previous study that used frozen brushing specimens for EGFR and KRAS testing [7] and they are close to the reported molecular analysis from CT-guided transthoracic sampling (transthoracic needle biopsy, TTNB) [8] and to ultrathin bronchoscopy sampling with direct vision of the lesion. The increase in mutant-allele fraction (MAF) was probably due to the higher number of biopsies performed per lesion in the later part of the study, suggesting a clinical learning curve.

Other Technical Innovations Combined with EBUS GS

Optical processing of images for their inherent diagnostic potential is a subject of ongoing study. Other tumor types have been subjected to these types of study, including ultrasound of tumors of breast prostate and endometrial ultrasound images. Nguyen et al. [9] reported grayscale texture computerized analysis of images of EBUS GS localized lesions. Particular regions of interest within the lesion were localized and results compared between malignant and benign lesions. A training set was created by analyzing numerous ultrasound characteristics in 85 lesions (including maximum and minimum pixel values and ultrasound entropy) and tested with a validation set of 82 lesions. Scoring by two different reviewers in the validation set showed sensitivity for malignancy of

75% and 76% for each, and NPV for malignancy of 82% and 100%, respectively. Interestingly, malignant lesions had more homogeneous characteristics than benign lesions. The latter tend to have more open airways (white points scattered through lesions), whereas they are compressed or obliterated in many malignant lesions.

A similar study was reported by Morikawa et al. [10] testing the use of a histogram display of brightness of regions of the ultrasound image. From 60 EBUS GS images, a specified size of region of interest (ROI) was studied, typically 3 to 5 mm radially from the probe histogram height, and width, height/width ratio, standard deviation, kurtosis, and skewness were studied. The best results were obtained for histogram standard deviation; a cutoff value for standard deviation of 10.5 was associated with a diagnostic accuracy for lung cancer of 81.7%.

Both of these studies show promise; however, they were limited to some extent by the necessity for the proceduralist to identify an ROI; ongoing studies are underway to analyze the whole of the EBUS image to counter problems of ROI selection. The method obviously is also operator dependent (as are all ultrasound methods) in terms of generating good-quality concentric EBUS miniprobe images.

A fascinating combination of technologies in the periphery of the lung has been reported [11] to examine the malignant nature of peripheral nodules: EBUS GS, Doppler optimal coherence tomography (OCT), and autofluorescence imaging (AFI). AFI offers sensitive surface identification of suspicious airway sites, while co-registered OCT provides detailed structural information on the airway morphology and deeper vessels [12]. A small 0.9 mm diameter catheter was used in 31 patients. They demonstrated how Doppler OCT and AFI offer complementary information. The method utilizes the well-known difference of tumor vascularity to benign lesion vessels (more tortuous and chaotic). AFI vascular imaging offers visualization of in vivo vascular networks, which had fewer breathing and cardiac motion artifacts compared to Doppler OCT. Conversely, Doppler OCT shows the vessels' blood flow rate/direction and depth resolution (Figure 16.1). Figure 16.2 shows how Doppler OCT can show small nodules to be blood vessels (not realized by radial probe EBUS), hence limiting the chance of bleeding from the biopsy of such a site.

Therapies

Interstitial photodynamic therapy (PDT) is a method whereby a light diffuser is placed within (as opposed to on the surface of) tumors and is necessary for larger tumors than those typically treated with endobronchial PDT. A new 0.5 mm optical fiber for PDT has been used through a 21 gauge EBUS-TBNA needle [13], theoretically demonstrating its potential utility in the management of locally advanced lung cancer. The cylindrical diffuser end was used to deliver the therapeutic light through the 21 G EBUS needle. Safe and effective fiber placements and tumor illumination were accomplished. In addition, computer simulation of light propagation suggests that locally advanced lung cancer tumor can be illuminated. This study demonstrates the potential feasibility of this new therapeutic modality, justifying further investigation in the treatment of locally advanced lung cancers. Applying this through more peripherally placed "fine-needle" PDT has been previously demonstrated in animal models [14, 15] and the way this interstitial PDT could be combined with EBUS GS methods in peripheral tumors is obvious. Further work is needed to maximize the chances of PDT efficacy by optimizing drug and light combinations to enable larger treatment sizes.

The potential for interstitial therapies via the guide sheath does of course exist for brachytherapy and other thermal therapies, including radiofrequency ablation.

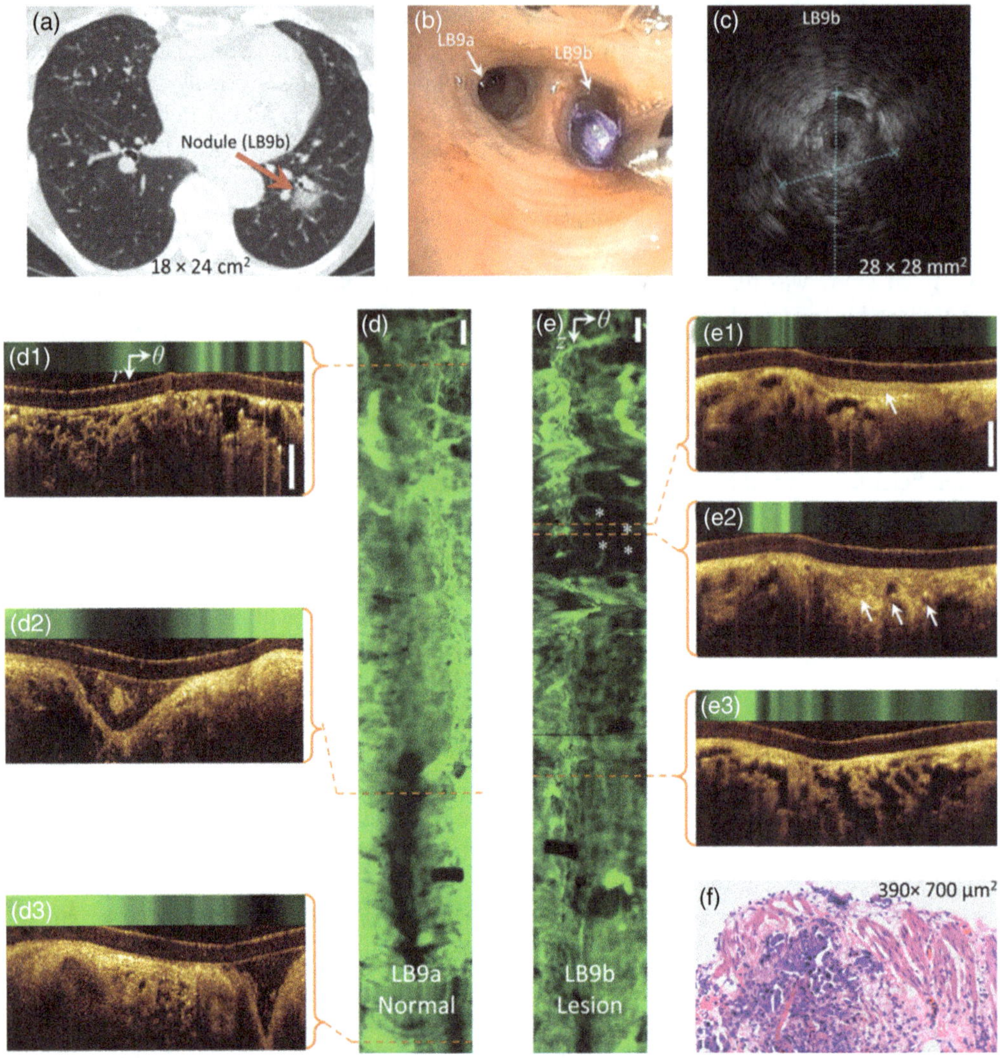

Figure 16.1 Tumor detection by Doppler optimal coherence tomography–autofluorescence imaging (OCT-AFI): (a) A nodule accessible through LB9b detected in computed tomography (CT) scan. (b) White-light image of LB9a and LB9b being imaged by OCT-AFI. (c) Radial endobronchial ultrasound (R-EBUS) image of the nodule. (d, e) Autofluorescence (AF) 2-θ maps of the normal (LB9a) and target (LB9b) airways, respectively; the airway images are oriented distally to proximally top to bottom (d1–d3, e1–e3); cross-sectional OCT-AFI images polar coordinated (r, θ) corresponding to the red dashed lines along the scans of the normal and target airways, respectively. (f) Hematoxylin and eosin (H&E) image of the biopsy sample collected from LB9b. * Indicates suspicious area in the AF images (e) and arrows indicate epithelial thickening and invasive tumor in (e1) and (e2), respectively. Scale bars are 1 mm. *Source:* Pahlevaninezhad et al. [11]. Reprinted with permission from OSA Publishing.

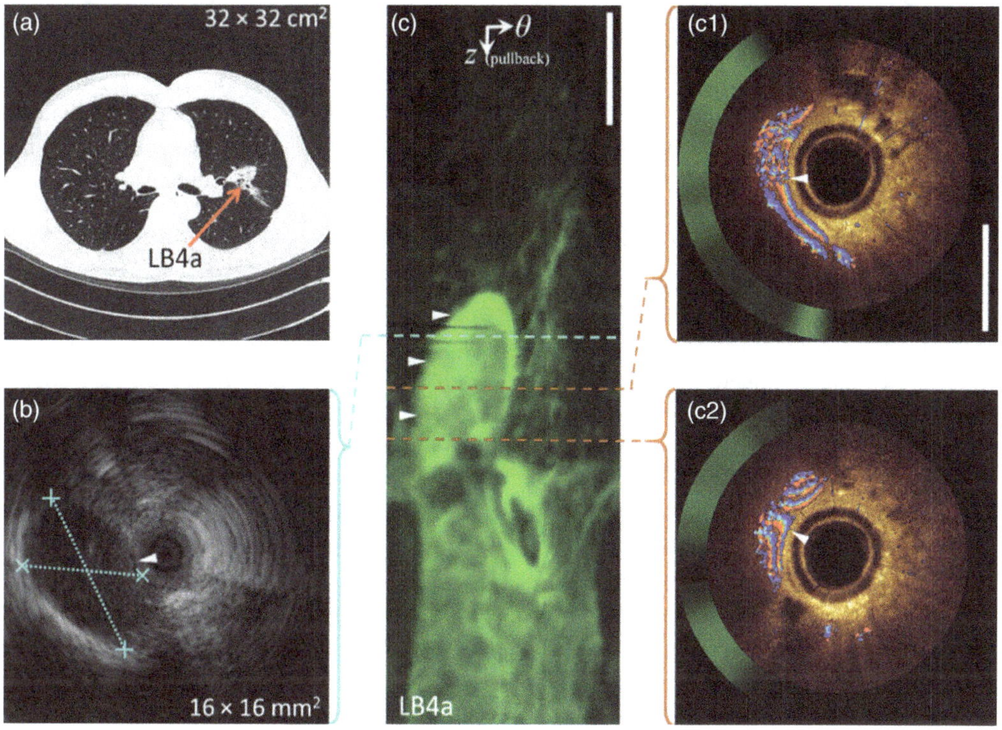

Figure 16.2 Differentiation of large blood vessels from nodules by Doppler optimal coherence tomography–autofluorescence imaging (OCT-AFI). (a) Computed tomography (CT) scan showing a nodule in LB4a. (b) Radial endobronchial ultrasound (R-EBUS) image of the nodule. (c) AF 2-θ map of a pullback from the same airway site (c1–c2), cross-sectional Doppler OCT-AFI in Cartesian coordinates corresponding to the red dashed lines along the pullback. R-EBUS and Doppler OCT-AFI are referenced with respect to the end of the guide sheath. ► indicates vessel location. Scale bars are 1 mm. *Source:* Pahlevaninezhad et al. [11]. Reprinted with permission from OSA Publishing.

References

1 Izumo, T., Matsumoto, Y., Sasada, S. et al. (2017). Utility of rapid on-site cytologic evaluation during endobronchial ultrasound with a guide sheath for peripheral pulmonary lesions. *Japanese Journal of Clinical Oncology* 47 (3): 221–225.

2 Steinfort, D.P., Leong, T.L., Laska, I.F. et al. (2015). Diagnostic utility and accuracy of rapid on-site evaluation of bronchoscopic brushings. *European Respiratory Journal* 45 (6): 1653–1660.

3 Maekura, T., Sugimoto, C., Tamiya, A. et al. (2017). Combination of virtual bronchoscopic navigation, endobronchial ultrasound, and rapid on-site evaluation for diagnosing small peripheral pulmonary lesions: a prospective phase II study. *Journal of Thoracic Disease* 9 (7): 1930–1936.

4 Chen, C.H., Cheng, W.C., Wu, B.R. et al. (2015). Improved diagnostic yield of bronchoscopy in peripheral pulmonary lesions: combination of radial probe endobronchial ultrasound and rapid on-site evaluation. *Journal of Thoracic Disease* 7 (Suppl 4): S418–S425.

5 Izumo, T., Matsumoto, Y., Chavez, C., and Tsuchida, T. (2016). Re-biopsy by endobronchial ultrasound procedures for

mutation analysis of non-small cell lung cancer after EGFR tyrosine kinase inhibitor treatment. *BMC Pulmonary Medicine* 16 (1): 106.

6 Guisier, F., Salaün, M., Lachkar, S. et al. (2016). Molecular analysis of peripheral non-squamous non-small cell lung cancer sampled by radial EBUS. *Respirology (Carlton, Vic.)* 21 (4): 718–726.

7 Ferretti, G.R., Busser, B., de Fraipont, F. et al. (2013). Adequacy of CT-guided biopsies with histomolecular subtyping of pulmonary adenocarcinomas: influence of ATS/ERS/IASLC guidelines. *Lung Cancer (Amsterdam, Netherlands)* 82 (1): 69–75.

8 Shiau, C.J., Babwah, J.P., da Cunha Santos, G. et al. (2014). Sample features associated with success rates in population-based EGFR mutation testing. *Journal of Thoracic Oncology* 9 (7): 947–956.

9 Nguyen, P., Bashirzadeh, F., Hundloe, J. et al. (2015). Grey scale texture analysis of endobronchial ultrasound mini probe images for prediction of benign or malignant aetiology. *Respirology (Carlton, Vic.).* 20 (6): 960–966.

10 Morikawa, K., Kurimoto, N., Inoue, T. et al. (2015). Histogram-based quantitative evaluation of endobronchial ultrasonography images of peripheral pulmonary lesion. *Respiration; International Review of Thoracic Diseases* 89 (2): 148–154.

11 Pahlevaninezhad, H., Lee, A.M.D., Ritchie, A. et al. (2015). Endoscopic Doppler optical coherence tomography and autofluorescence imaging of peripheral pulmonary nodules and vasculature. *Biomedical Optics Express* 6 (10): 4191–4199.

12 Lam, S., Standish, B., Baldwin, C. et al. (2008). In vivo optical coherence tomography imaging of preinvasive bronchial lesions. *Clinical Cancer Research* 14 (7): 2006–2011.

13 Harris, K., Oakley, E., Bellnier, D., and Shafirstein, G. (2017). Endobronchial ultrasound-guidance for interstitial photodynamic therapy of locally advanced lung cancer—a new interventional concept. *Journal of Thoracic Disease* 9 (8): 2613–2618.

14 Fielding, D.I., Buonaccorsi, G., Cowley, G. et al. (2001). Interstitial laser photocoagulation and interstitial photodynamic therapy of normal lung parenchyma in the pig. *Lasers in Medical Science* 16 (1): 26–33.

15 Fielding, D.I., Buonaccorsi, G.A., MacRobert, A.J. et al. (1999). Fine-needle interstitial photodynamic therapy of the lung parenchyma: photosensitizer distribution and morphologic effects of treatment. *Chest* 115 (2): 502–510.

Appendix: Videos

Case A1

A 64-year-old man was under radiological surveillance for a number of pulmonary nodules. He had multiple rounded calcified nodules; however, an index lesion among these nodules had slowly grown. Over the previous six months it had gone from 15 x 10 mm to 22 x 16 mm. A previous bronchoscopy washing in the right upper lobe was negative. There was a background of a 40 pack-year history of smoking, with ongoing smoking and moderate to severe chronic obstructive pulmonary disorder (COPD) with forced expiratory volume (FEV1) of 47% predicted and gas transfer 32% predicted. A virtual planning bronchoscopy revealed the position of the nodule adjacent to the RB3A1 bronchus. It was clearly not suitable for a guide sheath transbronchial lung biopsy given its position adjacent to the bronchus. Using the virtual bronchoscopy plan a miniprobe confirmed the position of the nodule next to the airway. The guide sheath was then removed and a 22 gauge transbronchial needle aspiration (Wang) needle was used to puncture the wall directly at this site. On one pass the rose was positive for non-small cell carcinoma. See **Video Clip 1**. The procedure was uneventful. He was subsequently referred for curative external beam radiotherapy and this was completed successfully, with no growth of the lesion over 18 months.

Video Clip 1

This shows first of all the virtual bronchoscopy pathway to the lesion in the right upper lobe (RUL). Then the endobronchial ultrasonography guide sheath (EBUS GS) image, then the directed transbronchial needle aspiration (TBNA) into the lesion.

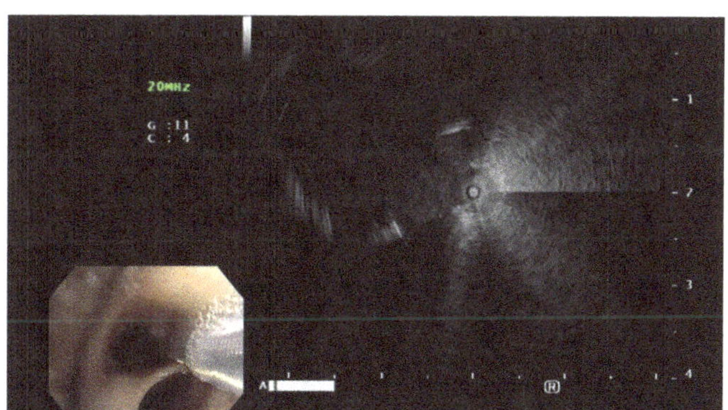

Case A1.1 EBUS guide sheath.

Endobronchial Ultrasonography, Second Edition. Noriaki Kurimoto, David I.K. Fielding, Ali I. Musani, Christopher Kniese, and Katsuhiko Morita.

Companion website: www.wiley.com/go/kurimoto2e

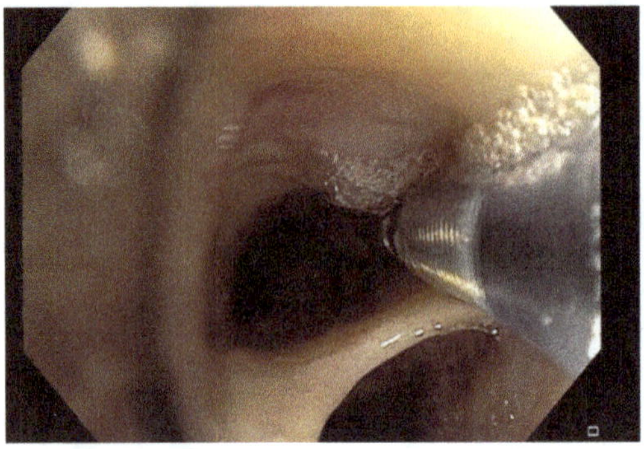 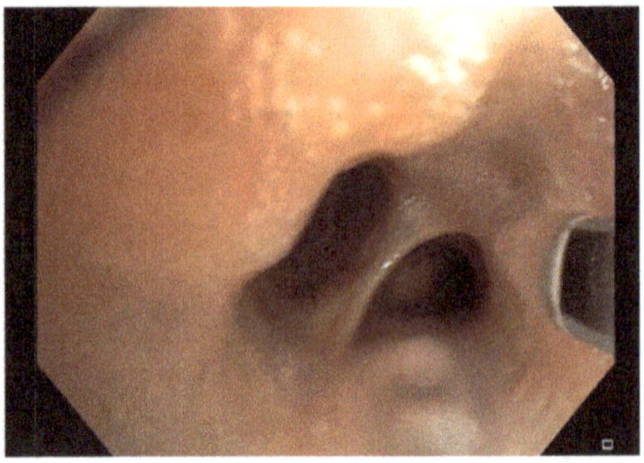

Case A1.2 Wang needle procedure.

Case A2

A 25-year-old woman was referred with a persistent and slowly increasing subtle pulmonary nodularity on computed tomography (CT) scan in the right upper zone, along with small but persistent bilateral hilar and mediastinal lymphadenopathy. There was non-specific chest pain and some exertional breathlessness. Previously colleagues at an external hospital had performed transbronchial needle aspiration (TBNA) on the lymph nodes, which showed only non-specific lymphocyte material and no granulomas. In addition, a conventional transbronchial lung biopsy was performed, which also was negative for granulomas.

An endobronchial ultrasonography guide sheath (EBUS GS) procedure was initially performed, which was able to localize some nodularity on the EBUS images in the upper part of the anterior segment of the right upper lobe. Standard transbronchial biopsies were initially performed through the guide sheath. Keeping the same position for the bronchoscope, a tamponade balloon was initially deployed in the right upper lobe bronchus by the sleeve on a Bronchoflex® endotracheal tube. Then two cryobiopsies were performed from the exact position where the guide sheath mini probe had localized the best nodularity. There was only 5 ml of blood loss with the use of the tamponade balloon. See **Video Clip 2**. The cryobiopsies showed multiple non-caseating granulomas consistent with the diagnosis of sarcoidosis. In addition, deep mucosal biopsies from the right upper lobe bronchus also showed granulomas. Of note is that the conventional transbronchial lung biopsies once again did not have any endobronchial granulomas. The patient responded well to oral corticosteroids.

Video Clip 2

This shows first of all EBUS GS with some parenchymal nodularity seen on ultrasound images. Then balloon deployment and subsequent cryobiopsies.

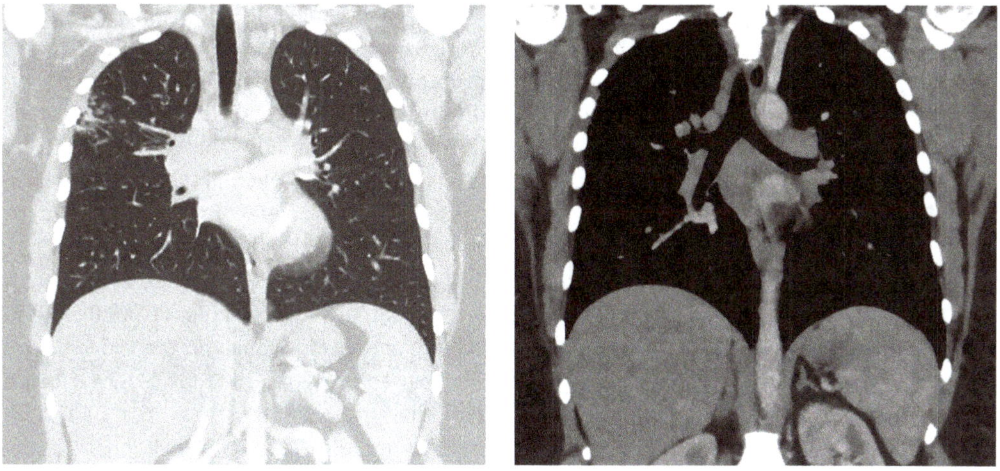

Case A2.1 CT chest.

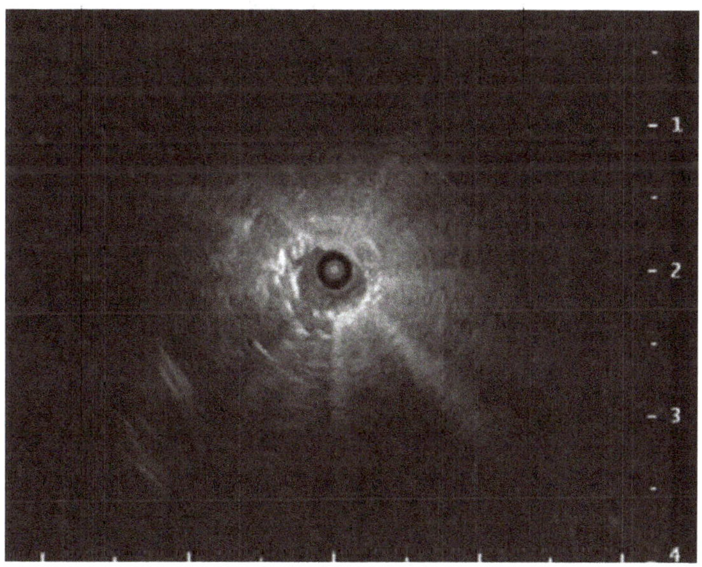

Case A2.2 EBUS guide sheath.

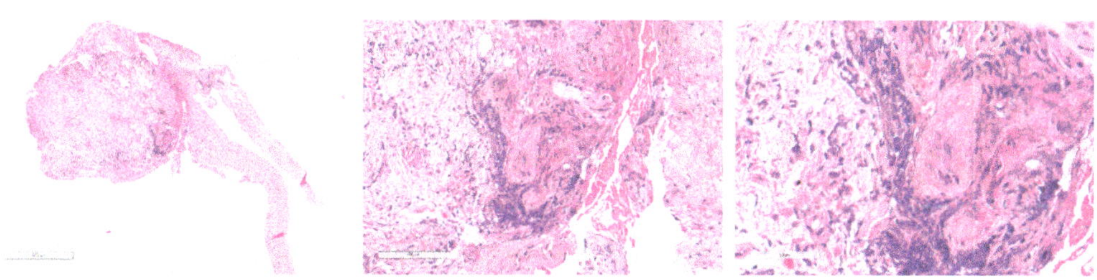

Case A2.3 Histopathology low power high power.

Case A3

A 73-year-old man under the care of the head and neck cancer group was referred with an incidentally detected right middle lobe nodule. He previously had undergone parotidectomy and neck dissection for scalp and parotid squamous cell carcinoma. There was a background of 25 pack-years of smoking, ceasing some 30 years previously. A number of calcified lymph nodes had been seen symmetrically on computed tomography (CT) scan and these had not progressed over a number of years; however, there was now a new nodule in the right middle lobe measuring 30 mm. A positron-emission tomography (PET) scan showed that the nodule had significant PET avidity. There was symmetrical lymph node uptake in the hilar and mediastinal nodes, which was similar to five years previously and was regarded as being consistent with his work in a foundry with coal dust exposure.

Lung function tests were normal.

At bronchoscopy, no endobronchial lesions were seen. The mass was noted prior to the procedure to be adjacent to the right pericardium and in a watershed area between the lower lobe and middle lobe. A endobronchial ultrasound transbronchial needle aspiration (EBUS TBNA) convex probe bronchoscope was used to directly advance into the bronchus 5B2, and samples from this were consistent with squamous cell carcinoma on Rose and subsequent cell block analysis. See **Video Clip 3**. The patient was referred for external beam radiotherapy. Note that the man had large enough middle lobe bronchi to permit the entrance of the convex probe bronchoscope, as he was over 185 cm tall.

Video Clip 3

This shows localization of the EBUS TBNA bronchoscope into a distal airway to allow direct EBUS TBNA sampling of the primary lung mass.

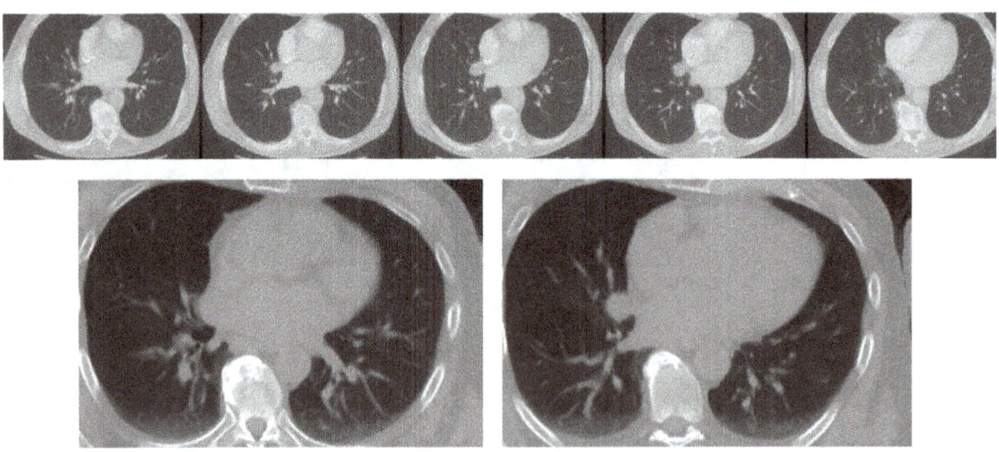

Case A3.1 CT.

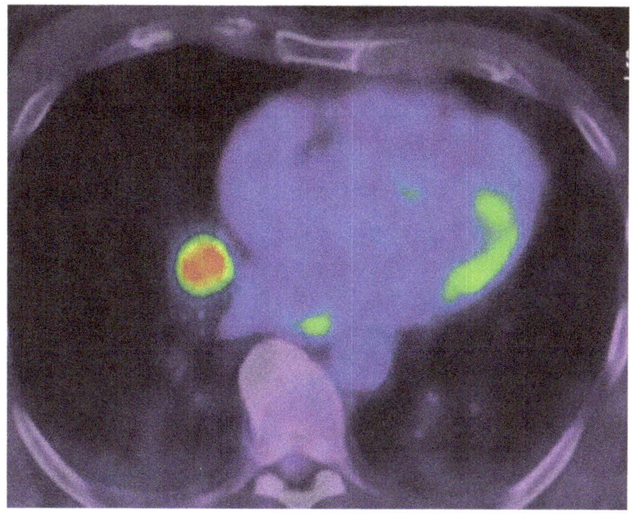

Case A3.2 PET CT.

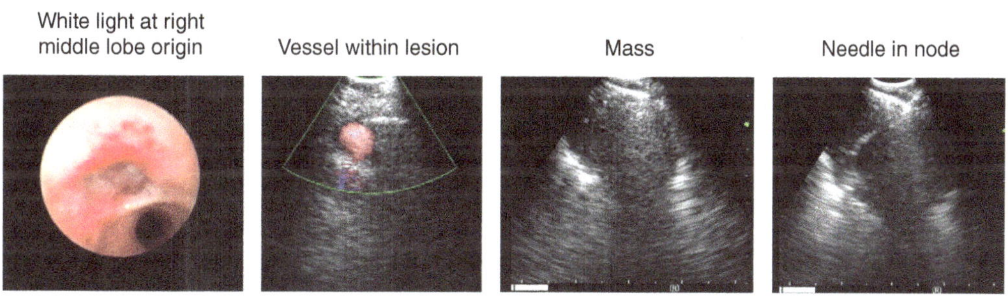

Case A3.3 White light and EBUS TBNA images.

Case A4

A 75-year-old woman with a heavy smoking history presented with chest infection symptoms. These were treated with antibiotics. A chest X-ray and computed tomography (CT) chest scan at the time, however, showed a coincident mass in right segment 6b. A positron-emission tomography (PET) CT showed that the mass was moderately PET avid. In addition, there was faint uptake in a station 7 lymph node. At bronchoscopy, first of all endobronchial ultrasound transbronchial needle aspiration (EBUS TBNA) was performed. A very small 4L node was seen (4 mm) and not sampled. The station 7 node was oval shaped and had large intranodal vessels (see **Video Clip 4**). Three samples from this node were negative for malignant cells. Then with a bronchoscope change, samples were taken using the EBUS guide sheath (GS) method. A concentric EBUS GS image was obtained from RB6B and Rose from bronchial brushings confirmed non-small cell carcinoma. See **Video Clip 4**. Final histopathology on cell block on the node revealed copious normal lymphocytes and no malignant cells. Brushings and biopsy of the peripheral nodule confirmed squamous cell carcinoma. The patient was considered medically unsuited for surgery and was referred for curative radiotherapy.

Video Clip A4

This shows initial EBUS TBNA sampling of small mediastinal lymph node followed by EBUS GS of peripheral lesion with concentric EBUS GS images.

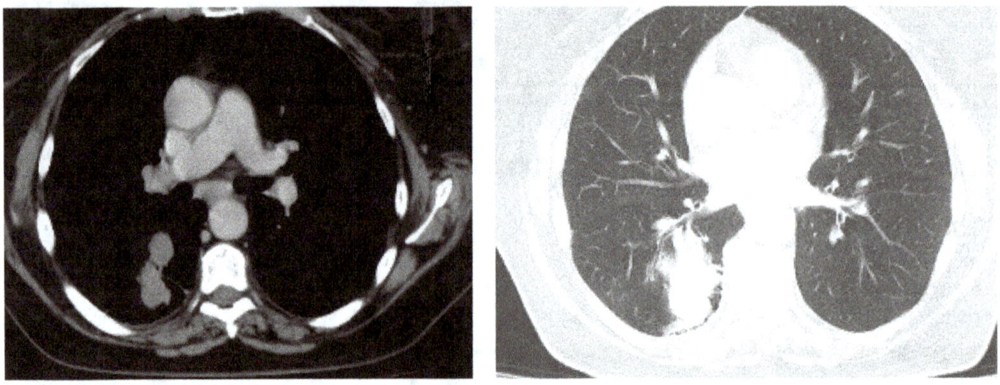

Case A4.1 Chest X-ray and CT scan.

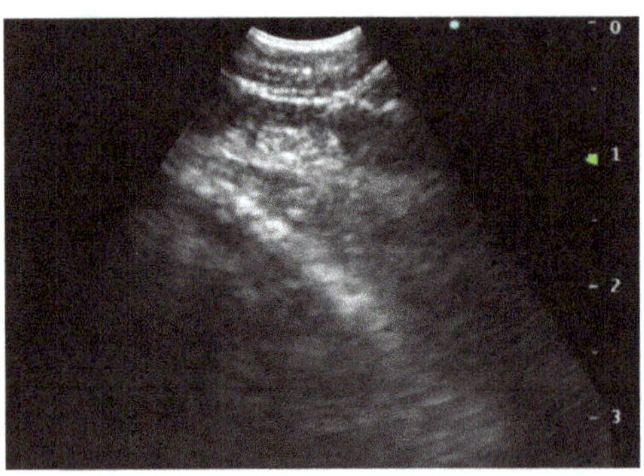

Case A4.2 EBUS TBNA.

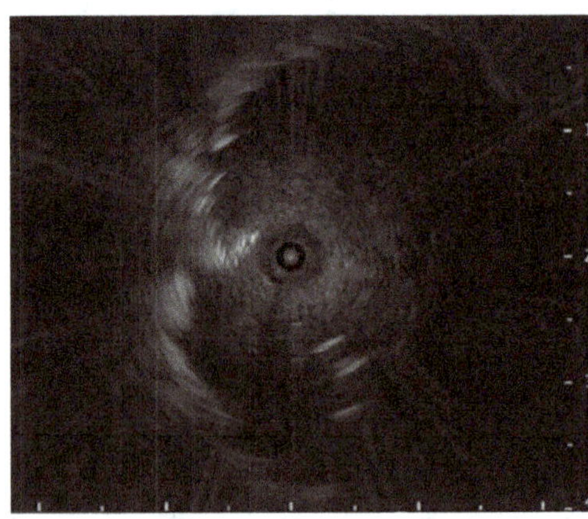

Case A4.3 EBUS guide sheath.

Case A5

A 75-year-old woman with severe chronic obstructive pulmonary disorder (COPD) was referred with a productive cough and a 12 mm oval-shaped lesion in the left upper lobe. Positron-emission tomography/computed tomography (PET/CT) showed only low-grade uptake in the lesion. A virtual bronchoscopy was performed; however, there was limited airway visualization due to airway mucus plugging at the time of the CT chest.

Using the Kurimoto method (rotating the CT to have the left upper lobe openings at the lower part of the side on CT images), a paper plan was made of the pathway to the lesion (see matching CT images and corresponding drawings on the paper plan). It was anticipated the lesion would be in LB1&2 B, subsegment b, with the most likely site at the medial side of that bronchus (**), with a less likely site at the lateral side of that bronchus (*). Indeed, the lesion was located, albeit with eccentric images, in LB1&2 Bii beta (see **Video Clip 5**). Samples from this showed chronic inflammation and fibrosis; antibiotics were prescribed and follow-up CT over 12 months showed a slight reduction in the size of the lesion.

Video Clip 5

Endobronchial ultrasound guide sheath (EBUS GS) sampling.

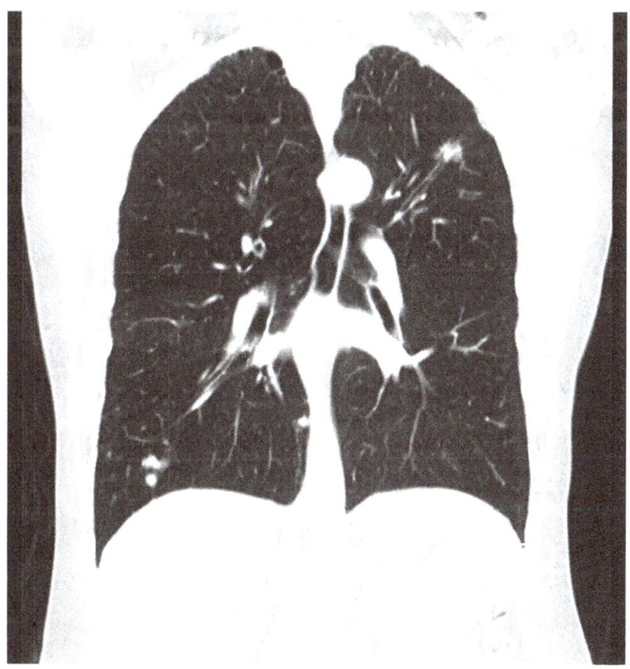

Case A5.1 PET/CT.

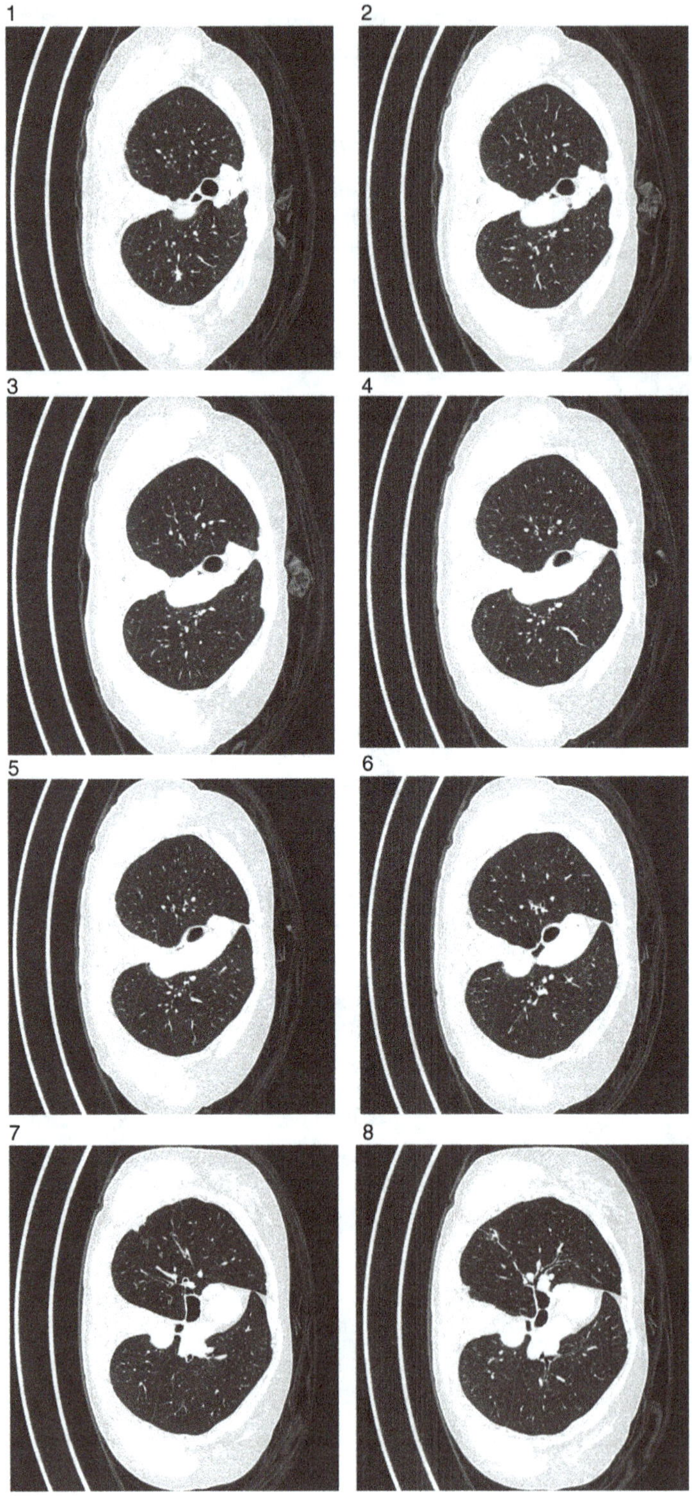

Case A5.2 Scrolling CT images.

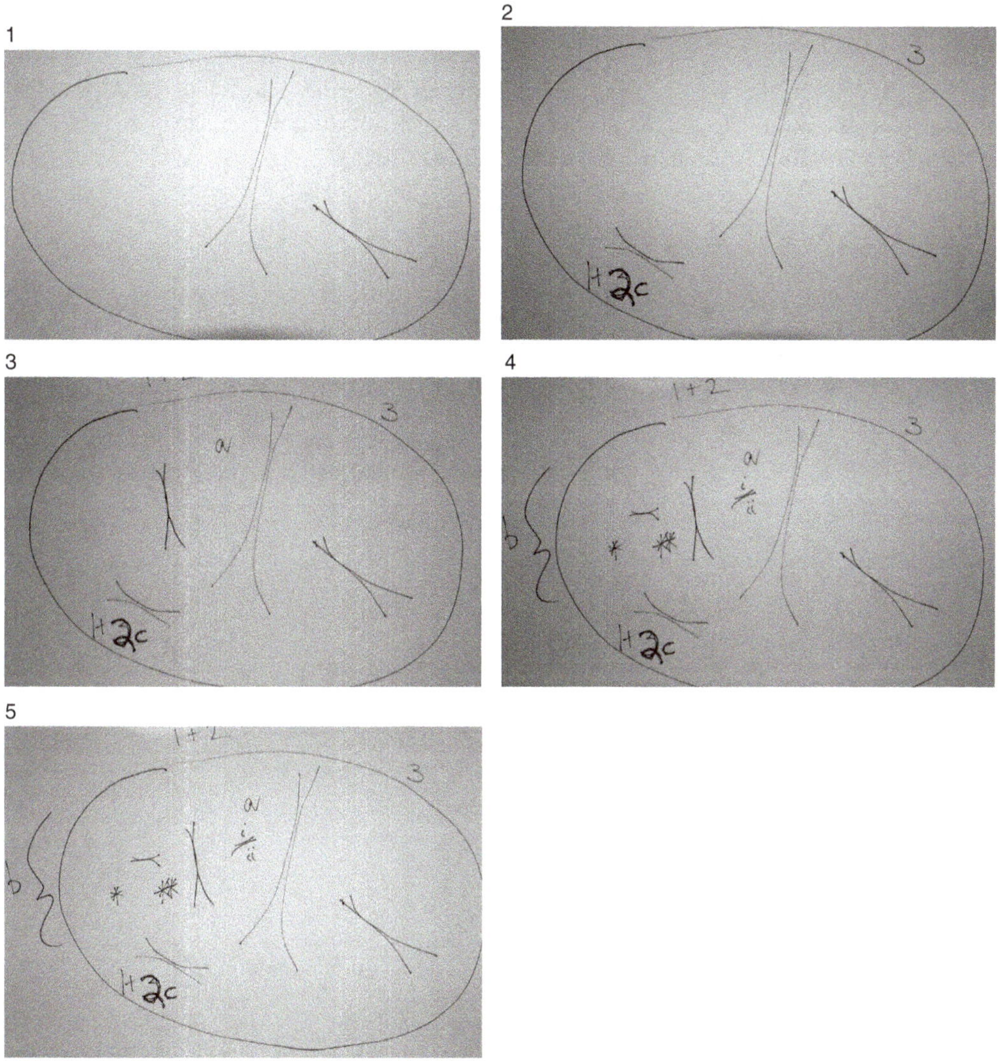

Case A5.3 Making the paper plan by the Kurimoto method.

Case A6 Right B^2biiαx leads to the lesion

The part-solid lesion was detected in the S^2b of the right lung. Reading CT anatomy showed that B^2biiαx entered the lesion. The tip of the thin-bronchoscope advanced into B^2bii. The probe/GS inserted into B^2biiα. EBUS revealed hyperechoic points without an open vessel (see **Video Clip 6**).

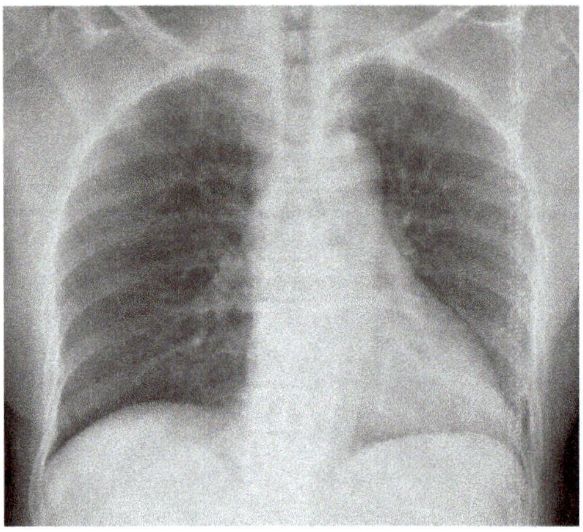

Chest XP (posteroanterior or PA view). No abnormal shadow is detected.

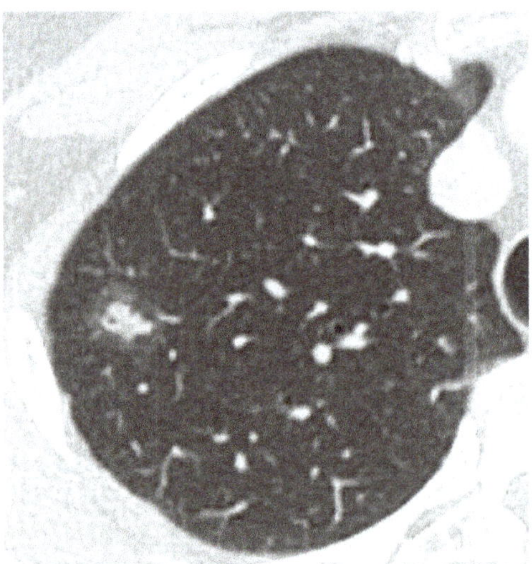

Chest computed tomography (CT, lung window).

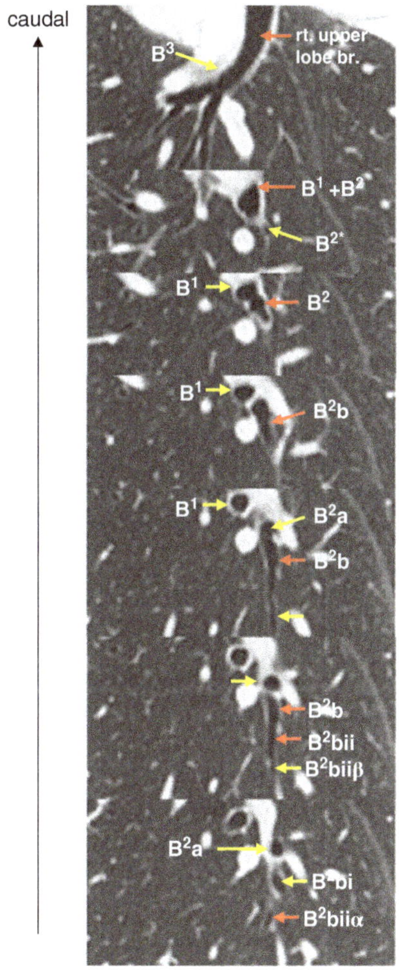

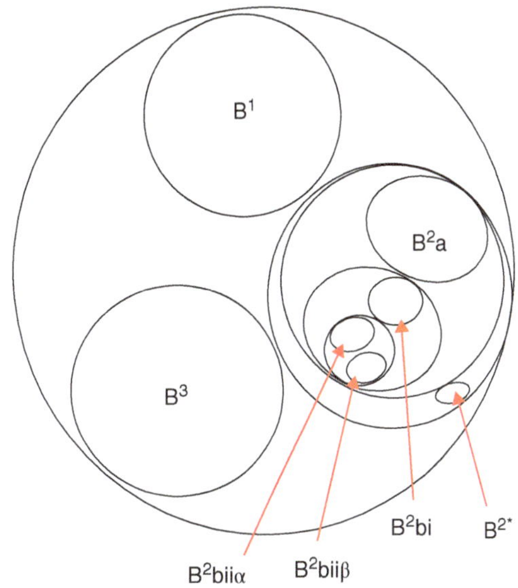

The axial CT images are rotated 90° counterclockwise. The right upper lobe bronchus branches into B^1, B^2, and B^3. B^2 branches into B^2a (cranial and dorsal) and B^2b (caudal and ventral).
B^2b branches into B^2bi (cranial and dorsal) and B^2bii (caudal and ventral). B^2bii branches into $B^2bii\alpha$ (cranial and ventral) and $B^2bii\beta$ (caudal and dorsal).

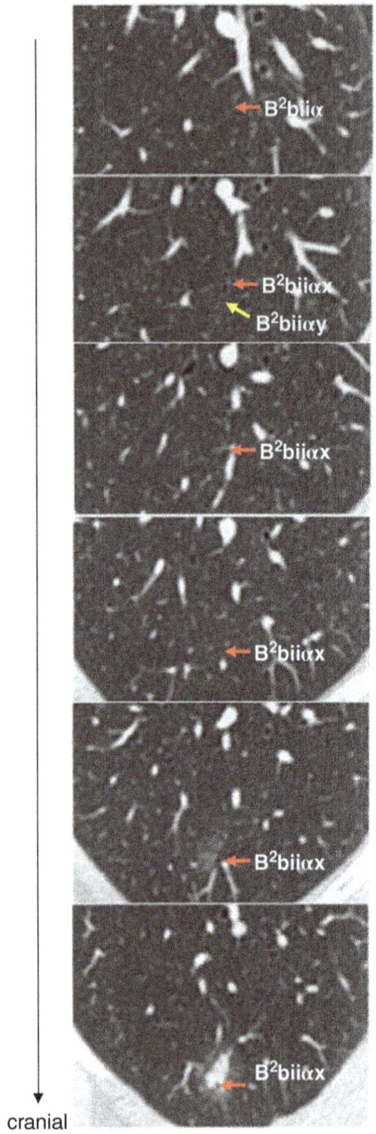

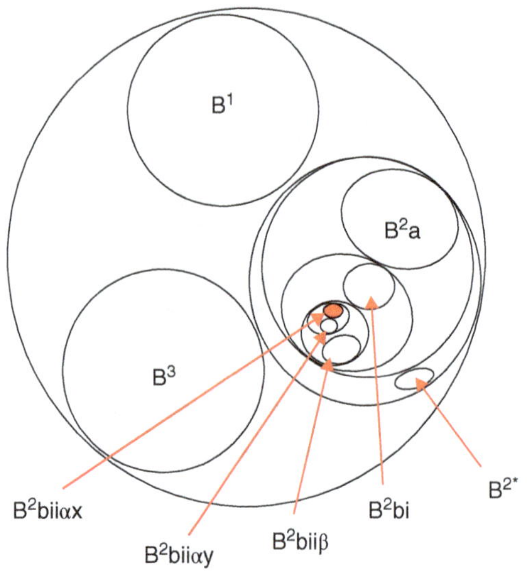

B^{2}biiα branches into B^{2}biiαx (cranial) and B^{2}biiαy (caudal).
B^{2}biiαx enters the lesion.

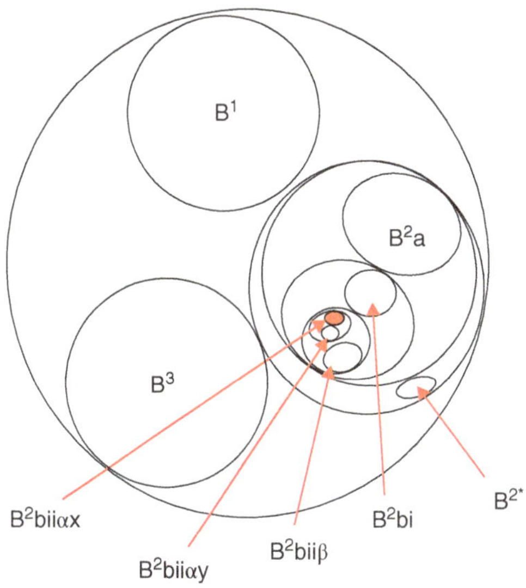

The tip of the bronchoscope advanced into B^2bii.

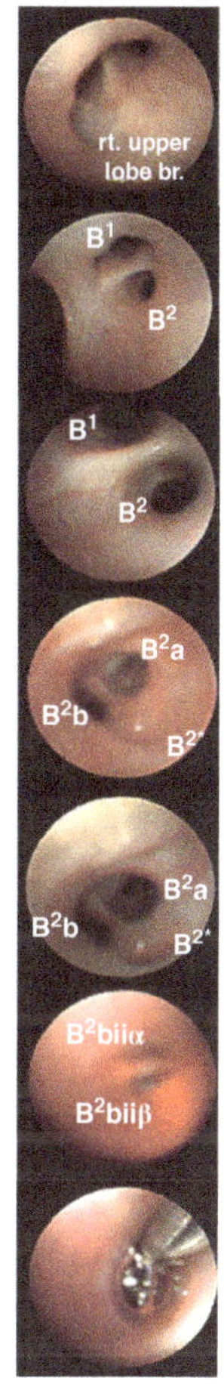

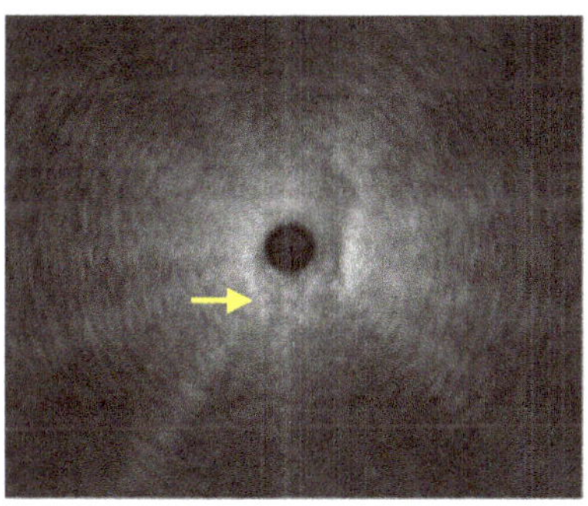

Endobronchial ultrasound (EBUS).

The tip of the bronchoscope is advanced into B^2bii and the probe/guide sheath (GS) inserted into B^2biiα. EBUS reveals hyperechoic points (→) without an open vessel. This lesion is classified as Type IIa.

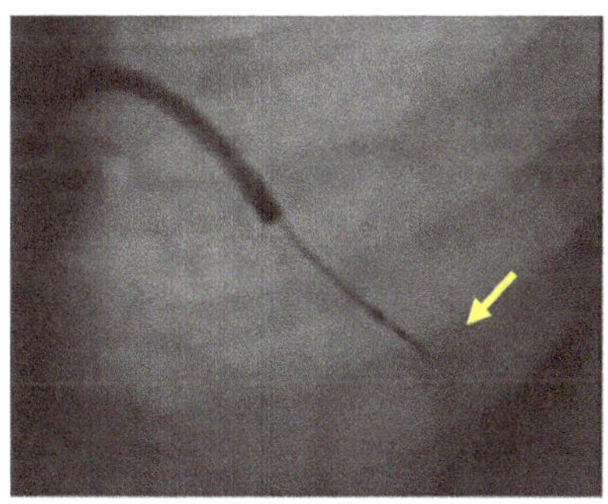

Fluoroscopy.

The probe/GS is advanced into the lesion (→).

Case A7 Right B^3aiiαyxx leads to the lesion

The part-solid lesion was detected in the S^3a of the right lung. Reading CT anatomy showed that B^3aiiαyxx entered the lesion. The tip of the thin-bronchoscope advanced into B^3aii. The probe/GS inserted into B^3aiiα. EBUS revealed hyperechoic points and an open vessel (see **Video Clip 7**).

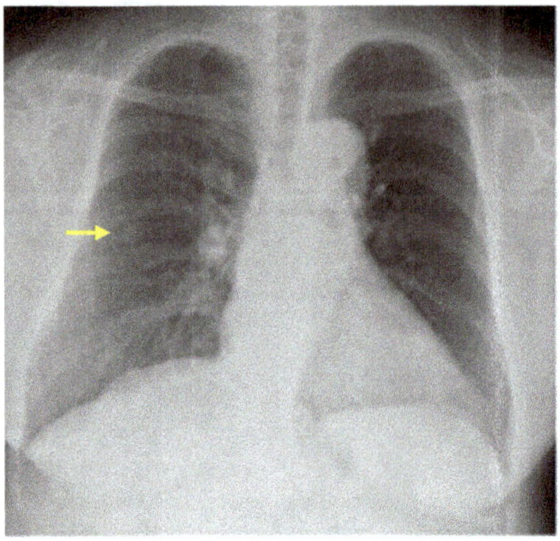

Chest XP (posteroanterior or PA view).
An abnormal shadow (→) is detected in the middle lung field of the right lung.

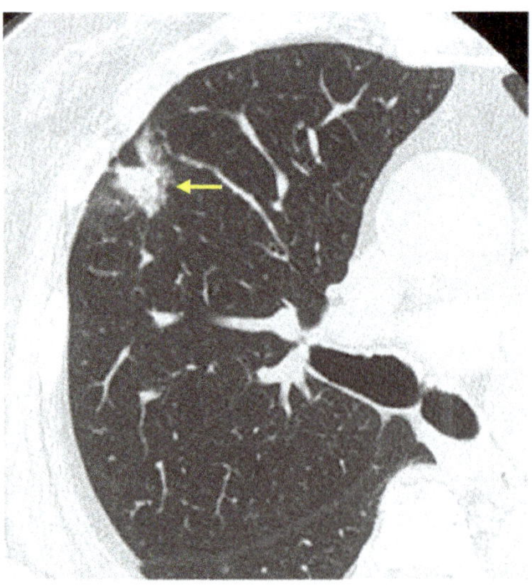

Chest computed tomography (CT, lung window).
An abnormal shadow (→) is detected in the S^3a of the right lung.

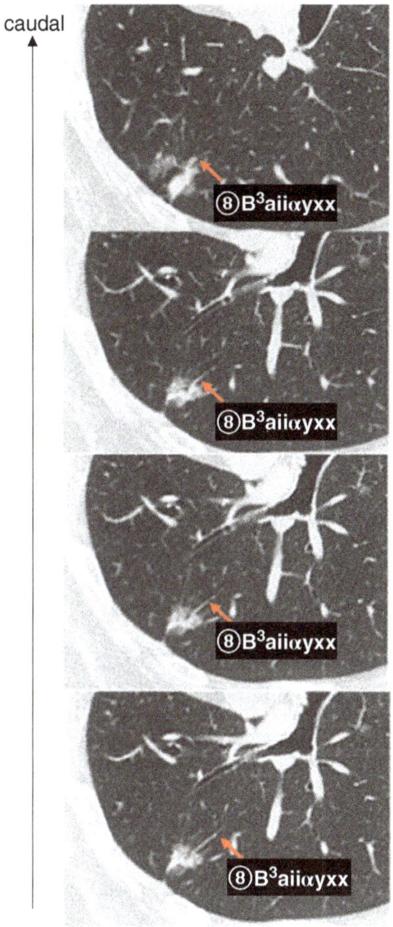

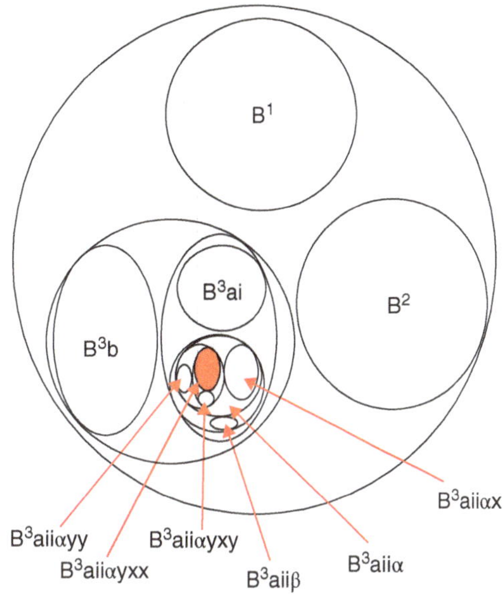

The axial CT images are rotated 90° counterclockwise. The right upper lobe bronchus branches into B^1, B^2, and B^3.

On the next page, first check the CT images.

B^3aiiαyxx enters the lesion.

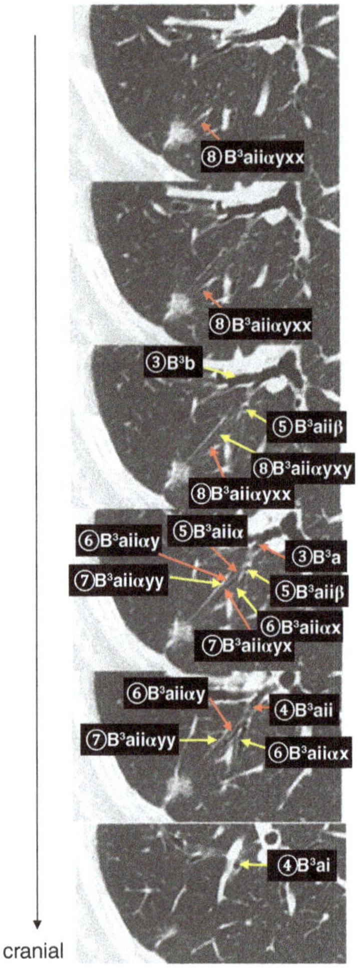

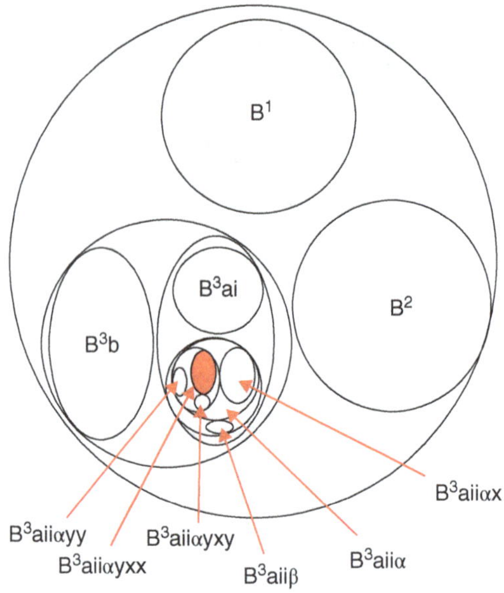

B^3 branches into B^3a (dorsal) and B^3b (ventral).
B^3a branches into B^3ai (cranial) and B^3aii (caudal).
B^3aii branches into B^3aiiα (cranial) and B^3aiiβ (caudal).
B^3aiiα branches into B^3aiiαx (dorsal) and B^3aiiαy (ventral).
B^3aiiαy branches into B^3aiiαyx (dorsal) and B^3aiiαyy (ventral).
B^3aiiαyx branches into B^3aiiαyxx (cranial) and B^3aiiαyxy (caudal).

The numbers in front of the bronchus name refer to the generation of the bronchus. In Japan, the lobar bronchus is considered to be the first generation.

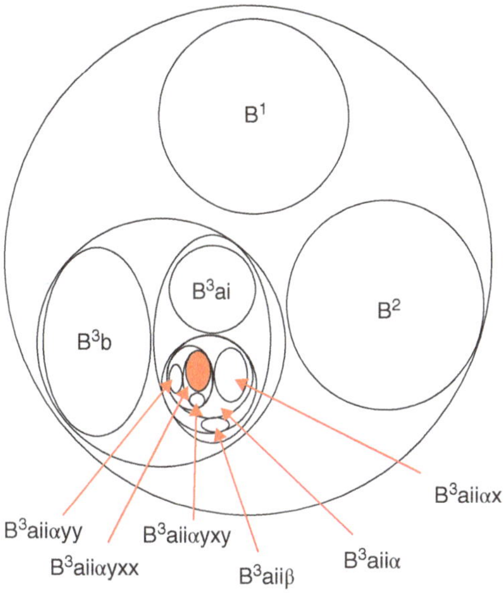

The tip of the bronchoscope is advanced into B^3aii.

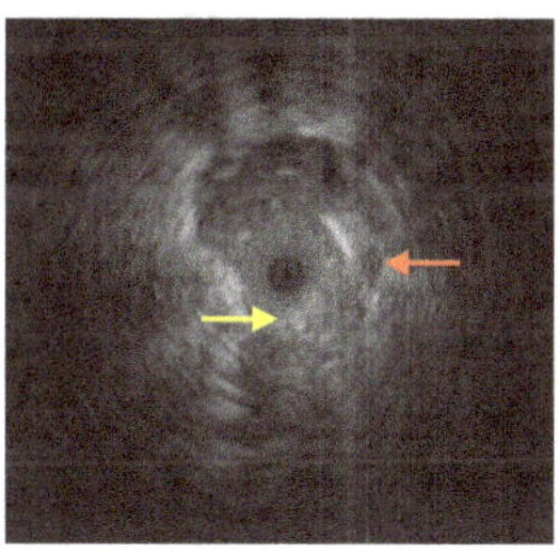

Endobronchial ultrasound (EBUS).
The tip of the bronchoscope is advanced into B^3aii and the probe/guide sheath (GS) inserted into $B^3aii\alpha$. EBUS reveals hyperechoic points (yellow arrow) and an open vessel (red arrow). This lesion is classified as Type IIb.

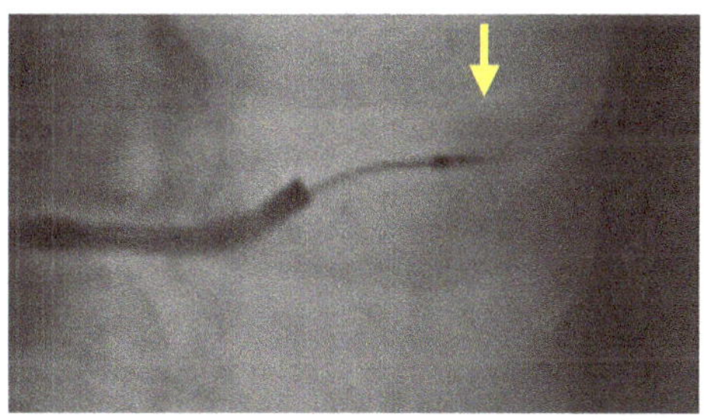

Fluoroscopy.
The probe/GS is advanced into the lesion (→).

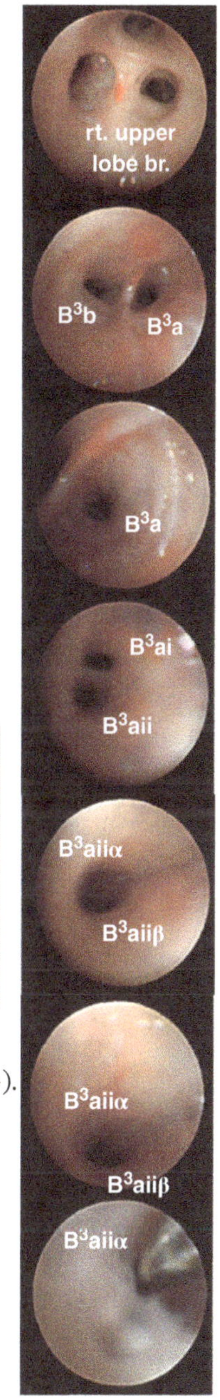

Case A8 Right B^3aiβxyx leads to the lesion

The cavitary lesion was detected in the S^3a of the right lung. Reading CT anatomy showed that B^3aiβxyx entered the lesion. The tip of the thin-bronchoscope advanced into B^3aiβx. The probe/GS inserted into B^3aiβx. EBUS revealed hyperechoic points without an open vessel (see **Video Clip 8**).

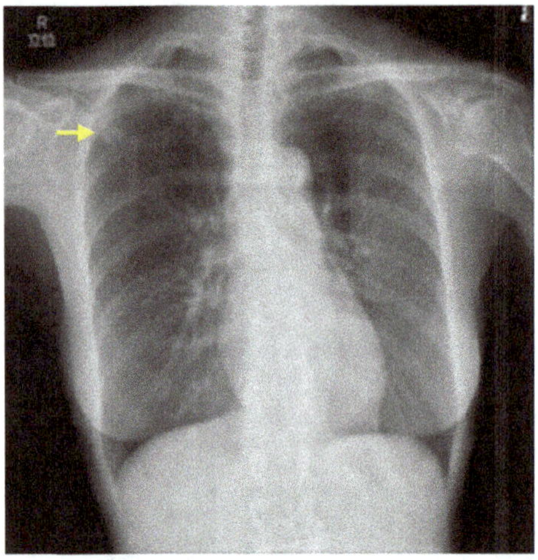

Chest XP (posteroanterior or PA view).
An abnormal shadow (→) is detected in the upper lung field of the right lung.

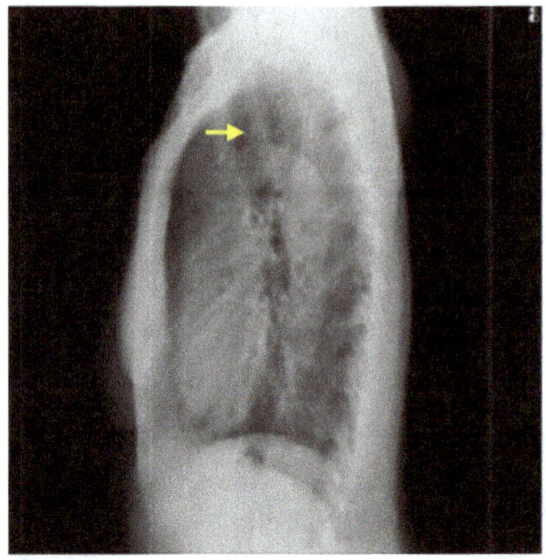

Chest XP (lateral view).
An abnormal shadow is detected (→).

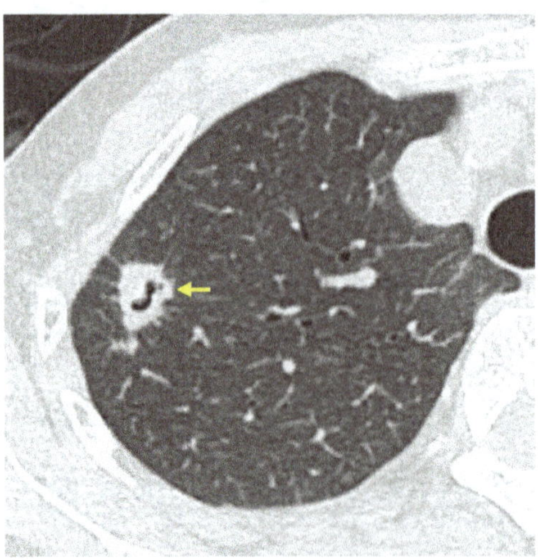

Chest computed tomography (CT, lung window).
An abnormal shadow (→) is detected in the S^3a of the right lung.

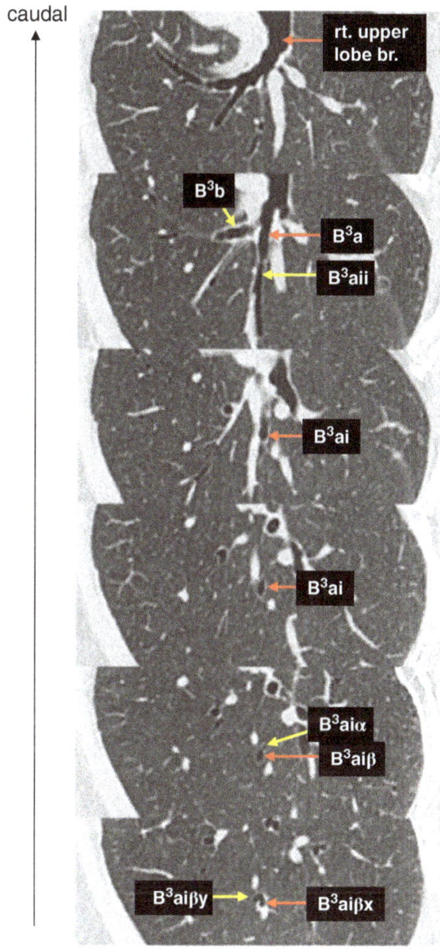

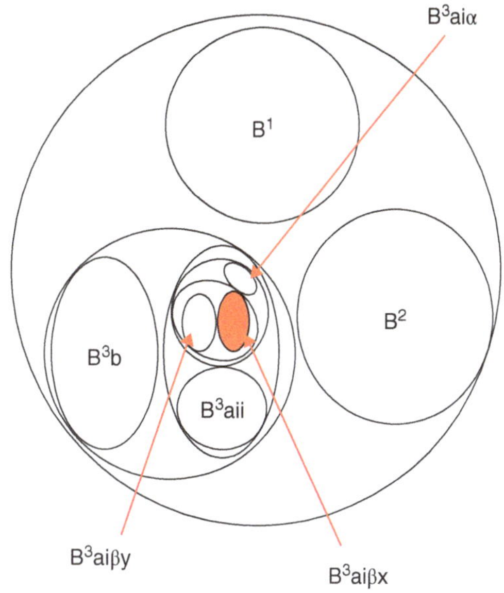

The axial CT images are rotated 90° counterclockwise.
The right upper lobe bronchus branches into B^1, B^2, and B^3.
B^3 branches into B^3a (dorsal) and B^3b (ventral).
B^3a branches into B^3ai (cranial) and B^3aii (caudal).
B^3ai branches into B^3aiα (cranial and dorsal) and B^3aiβ (caudal and ventral).
B^3aiβ branches into B^3aiβx (dorsal) and B^3aiβy (ventral).

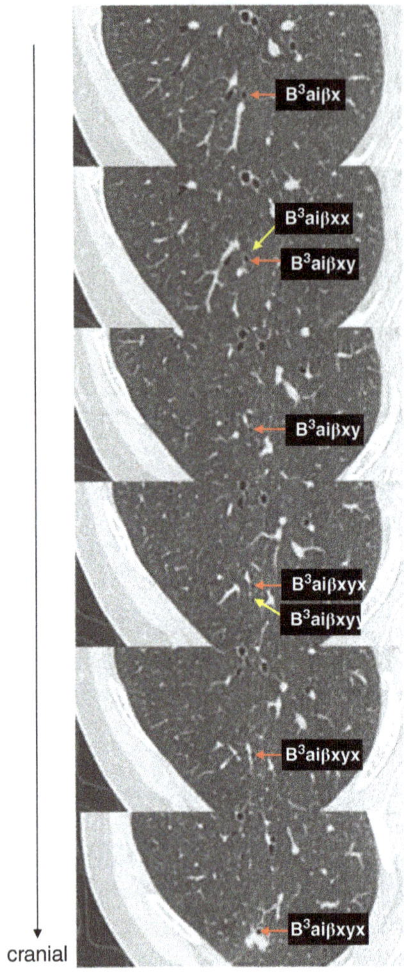

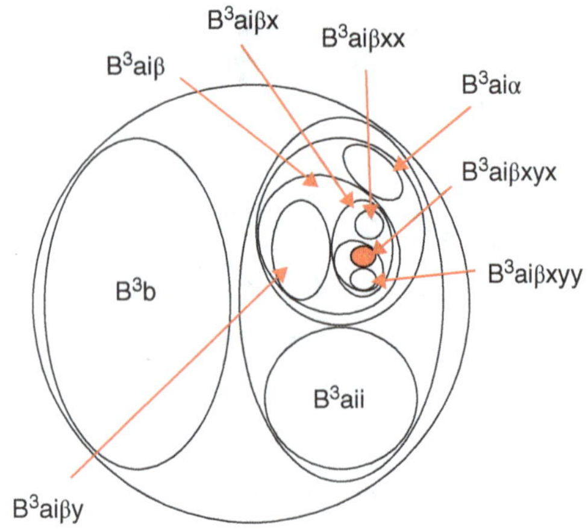

B^{3}aiβx branches into B^{3}aiβxx (cranial and dorsal) and B^{3}aiβxy (caudal and ventral).
B^{3}aiβxy branches into B^{3}aiβxyx (cranial) and B^{3}aiβxyy (caudal).

B^{3}aiβxyx enters the lesion.

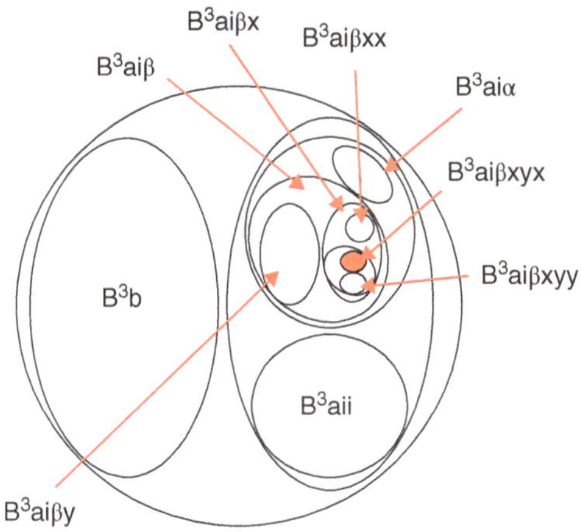

The tip of the bronchoscope is advanced into $B^3ai\beta$.

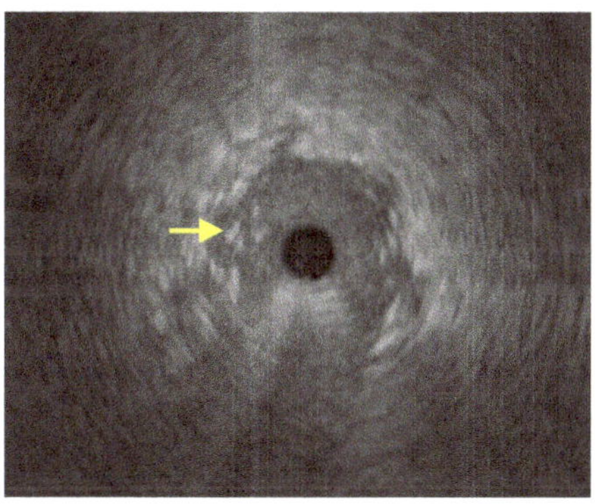

Endobronchial ultrasound (EBUS). The tip of the bronchoscope is advanced into $B^3ai\beta$ and the probe/guide sheath (GS) inserted into $B^3ai\beta x$. EBUS reveals hyperechoic points (→) without an open vessel. This lesion is classified as Type IIa.

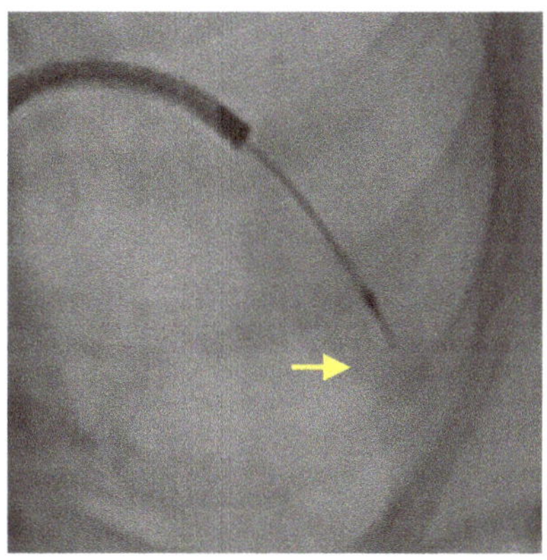

Fluoroscopy.
The probe/GS is advanced into the lesion (→).

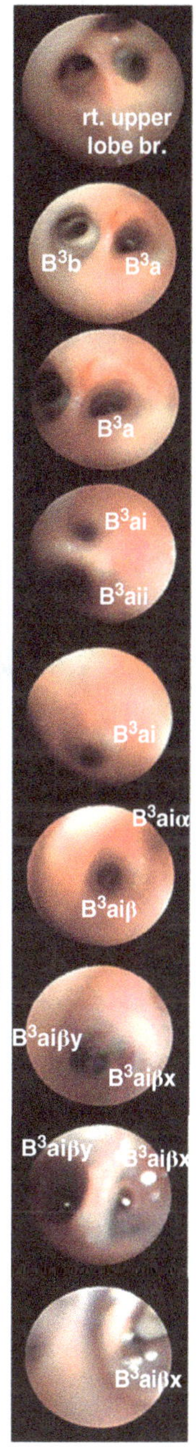

Case A9 Left $B^{1+2}ci\alpha$ leads to the lesion

The solid lesion was detected in the $S^{1+2}c$ of the left lung. Reading CT anatomy showed that $B^{1+2}ci\alpha$ entered the lesion. The thin-bronchoscope was rotated 180° clockwise at the left main bronchus. The thin-bronchoscope was advanced into the left upper lobe bronchus, left superior segment bronchus, B^{1+2}, $B^{1+2}c$, and $B^{1+2}ci$. The probe/GS inserted into $B^{1+2}ci\alpha$. EBUS revealed hyperechoic points and an open vessel (see **Video Clip 9**).

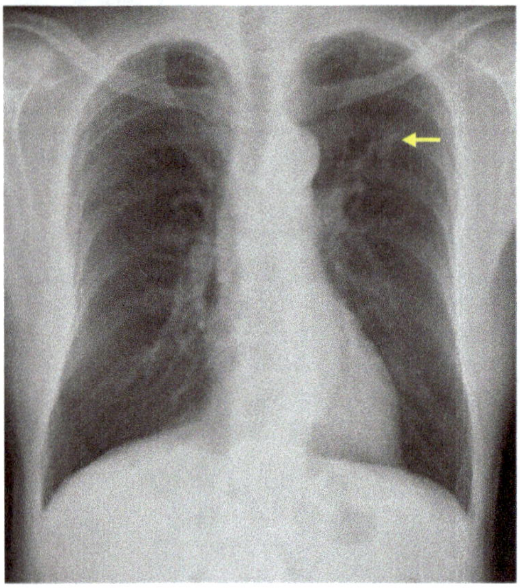

Chest XP (posteroanterior or PA view). An abnormal shadow (→) is detected in the upper lung field of the left lung.

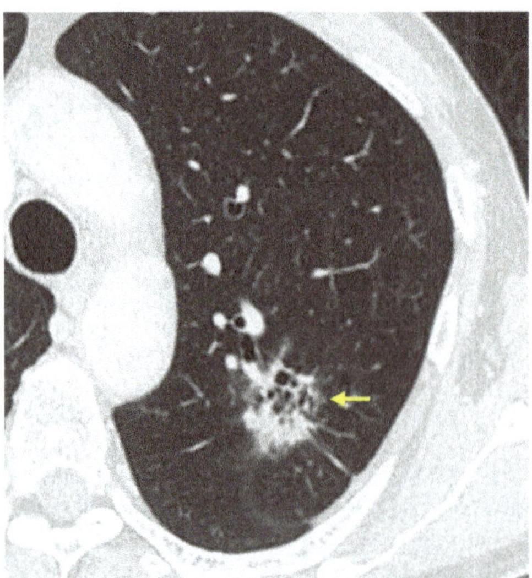

Chest computed tomography (CT, lung window). An abnormal shadow (→) is detected in the $S^{1+2}c$ of the left lung.

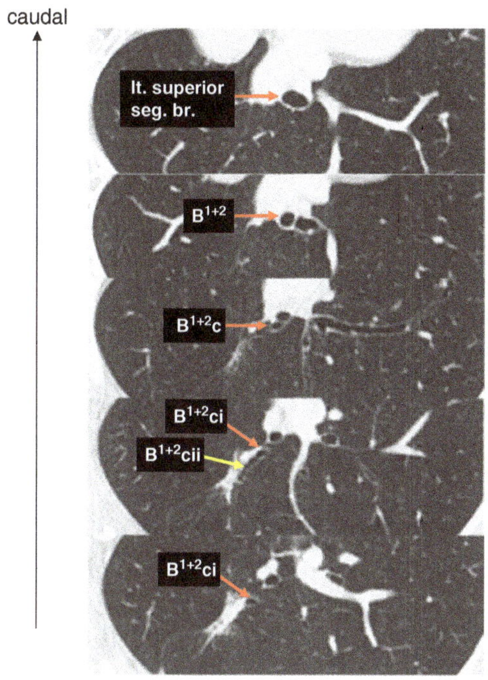

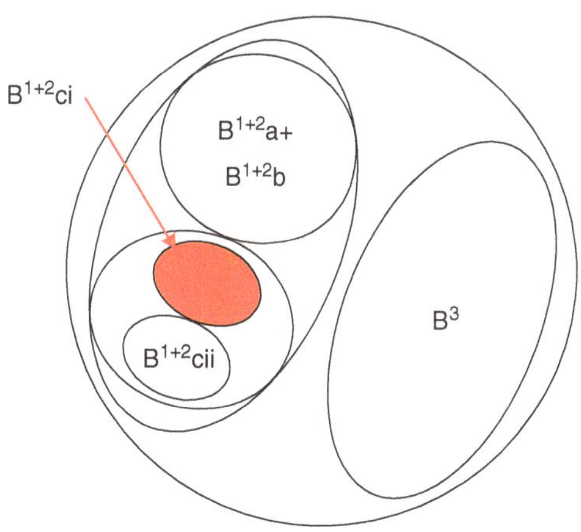

The axial CT images are rotated 90° clockwise. The left superior segment bronchus branches into B^{1+2} and B^3.
B^{1+2} branches into $B^{1+2}a+B^{1+2}b$ (cranial) and $B^{1+2}c$ (caudal, dorsal, and lateral).
$B^{1+2}c$ branches into $B^{1+2}ci$ (cranial) and $B^{1+2}cii$ (caudal).

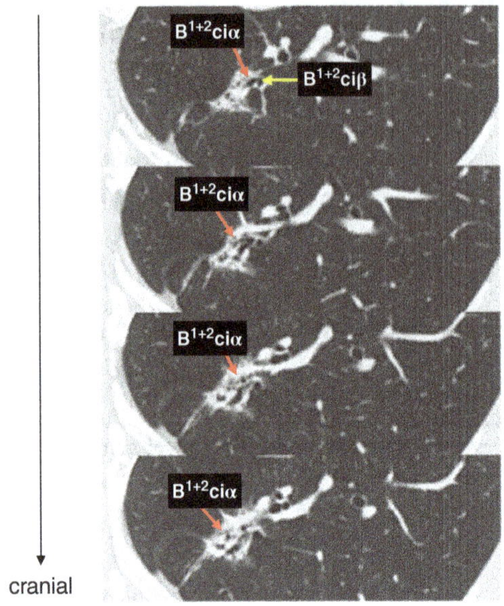

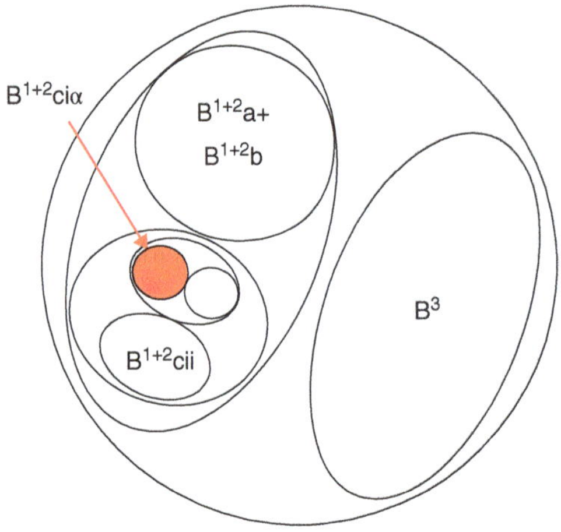

B^{1+2}ci branches into B^{1+2}ciα (dorsal) and B^{1+2}ciβ (ventral).
B^{1+2}ciα enters the lesion.

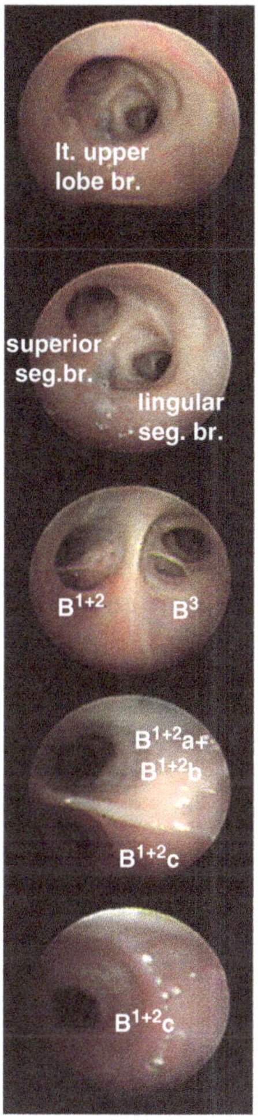

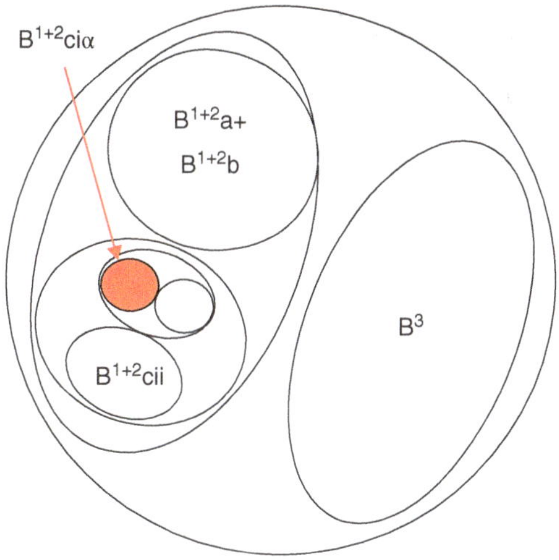

The tip of the bronchoscope is advanced into $B^{1+2}ci$

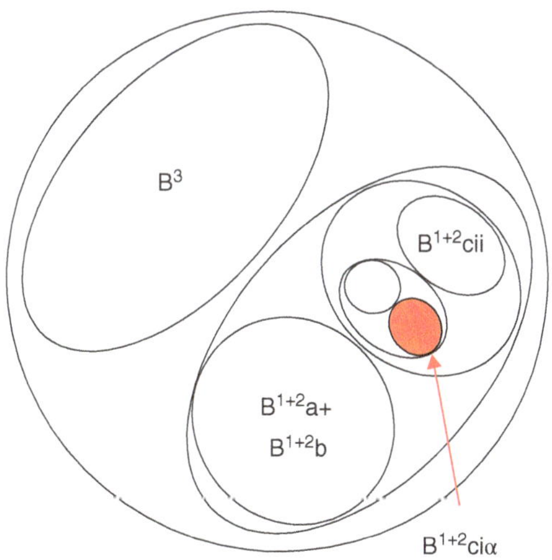

The branchoscope is rotated 180° clockwise at the left main bronchus. The tip of the bronchoscope is advanced into the left upper lobe bronchus and then via the superior segment bronchus, B^{1+2}, and $B^{1+2}c$ into $B^{1+2}ci$.

The bronchoscope is rotated 180° clockwise

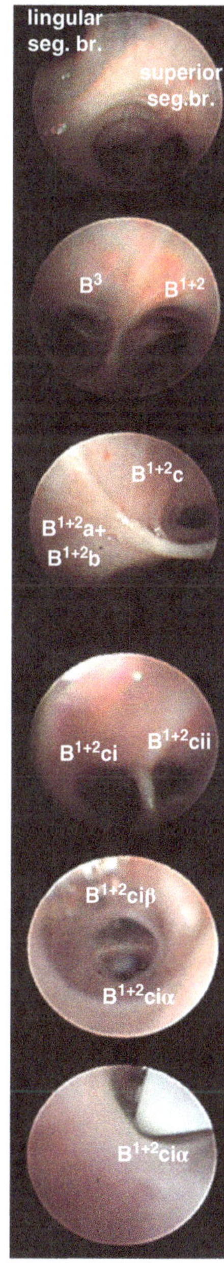

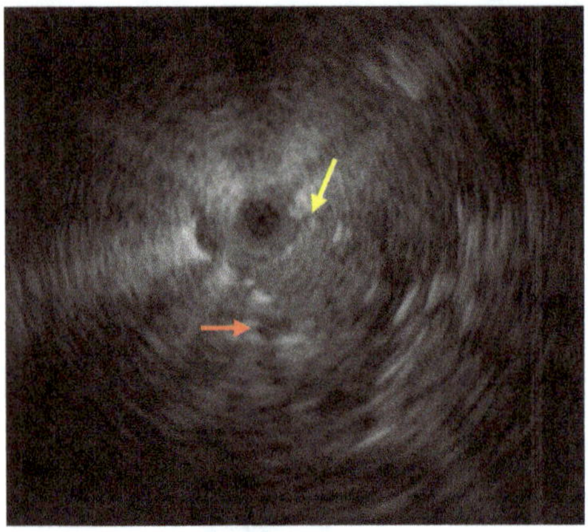

Endobronchial ultrasound (EBUS).
The tip of the bronchoscope is advanced into B^{1+2}ci and the probe/guide sheath (GS) inserted into B^{1+2}ciα. EBUS reveals hyperechoic points (yellow arrow) and an open vessel (red arrow). This lesion is classified as Type IIb.

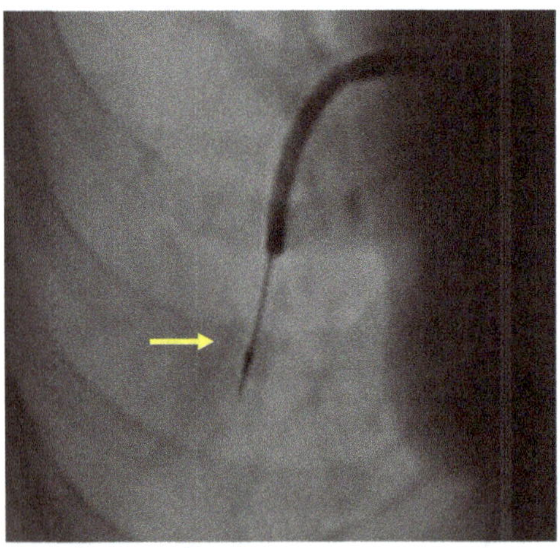

Fluoroscopy.
The probe/GS is advanced into the lesion (→).

Index

The following abbreviations are used in the index: EBUS: endobronchial ultrasonography; EUS-FNA: endoscopic ultrasound-guided fine needle aspiration; GS: guide sheath; PPLs: peripheral pulmonary lesions; TBNA: transbronchial needle aspiration.

Endobronchial Ultrasonography, Second Edition. Noriaki Kurimoto, David I.K. Fielding, Ali I. Musani, Christopher Kniese, and Katsuhiko Morita.

Companion website: www.wiley.com/go/kurimoto2e

C

m

n

o

p

www.ingramcontent.com/pod-product-compliance
Lightning Source LLC
Chambersburg PA
CBHW080455260726
48474CB00005B/193